W0050749

Recent Advances in
Biological Psychiatry

Officers of

SOCIETY OF BIOLOGICAL PSYCHIATRY

for 1961–62

Lauretta Bender, M.D., *President*
Paul I. Yakovlev, M.D., *First Vice-President*
Amedeo S. Marrazzi, M.D., *Second Vice-President*
George N. Thompson, M.D., *Secretary-Treasurer*

Councilors

William H. Gantt, M.D.
Paul H. Hoch, M.D.
Joseph Wortis, M.D.
Jules Masserman, M.D.
Margaret A. Kennard, M.D.

Committee on Public Relations

George A. Ulett, M.D., *Chairman*
Benjamin Pasamanick, M.D.
Henry W. Brosin, M.D.

Committee on Program

John I. Nurnberger, M.D., *Chairman*
Williamina Himwich, Ph.D.
Jackson A. Smith, M.D.
Herman C. B. Denber, M.D.

Committee on Publications

Joseph Wortis, M.D., *Chairman*
Margaret A. Kennard, M.D.
Howard D. Fabing, M.D.

Committee on Membership

Leo Alexander, M.D., *Chairman*
Hudson Hoagland, Ph.D.
Frank J. Ayd, Jr., M.D.

Committee on Research Awards

Harold E. Himwich, M.D., *Chairman*
Warren McCulloch, M.D.
George N. Thompson, M.D.
Seymour Kety, M.D.

VOLUME IV

Recent Advances in Biological Psychiatry

THE PROCEEDINGS OF THE SIXTEENTH ANNUAL CONVEN-
TION AND SCIENTIFIC PROGRAM OF THE SOCIETY OF BIO-
LOGICAL PSYCHIATRY, ATLANTIC CITY, N. J., JUNE 9-11, 1961

Edited by

Joseph Wortis, M.D.

*Associate Clinical Professor of Psychiatry,
State University of New York, Downstate
Medical College, Brooklyn, New York*

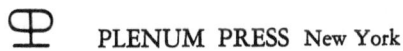 PLENUM PRESS New York

ISBN 978-1-4684-8308-6   ISBN 978-1-4684-8306-2 (eBook)
DOI 10.1007/978-1-4684-8306-2

Library of Congress Catalog Card Number 58-14190
Copyright 1962 Plenum Press Inc.
Softcover reprint of the hardcover 1st edition *1962*
227 West 17th St., New York 11, New York
All rights reserved

*No part of this publication may be reproduced
in any form without written permission
from the publisher*

Contents

Part IV: CLINICAL STUDIES

Presidents of the Society of Biological Psychiatry

1947—J. M. Nielsen

1948—Percival Bailey

1949—S. Bernard Wortis

1950—Harry C. Solomon

1951—Roland P. Mackay

1952—Abram E. Bennett

1953—Ladislas J. Meduna

1954—Harold E. Himwich

1955—Howard D. Fabing

1956—Margaret A. Kennard

1957—Jules H. Masserman

1958—Joseph Wortis

1959—Paul H. Hoch

1960—W. Horsley Gantt

1961—Lauretta Bender

Contributors

AARONS, LOUIS, PH.D.—Instructor in Neurology and Psychiatry, Northwestern University Medical School, Chicago, Ill.

ALEXANDER, LEO, M.D.—Director, Neurological Unit and Research Clinic, Division of Psychiatric Research, Boston State Hospital, Boston, Mass.

APRISON, M. H., PH.D.—Principal Research Investigator in Biochemistry, The Institute of Psychiatric Research; Associate Professor of Biochemistry, Departments of Biochemistry and Psychiatry, Indiana University Medical Center, Indianapolis, Ind.

ASTRUP, CHRISTIAN, M.D.—U.S.P.H. Research Fellow, Pavlovian Laboratory, Johns Hopkins University School of Medicine, Baltimore, Md.

AX, ALBERT F., PH.D.—Head, Psychophysiology Laboratory, Lafayette Clinic, Detroit, Mich.

BECKETT, PETER G. S., M.D.—Assistant Director, Administration, Lafayette Clinic, Detroit, Mich.; Wayne State University, College of Medicine, Detroit, Mich.

BENDER, LAURETTA, M.D.—Departmental Consultant, Children's Unit, Creedmoor State Hospital, Queens Village, N. Y.

BERGEN, JOHN R., PH.D.—Senior Scientist, The Worcester Foundation for Experimental Biology, Shrewsbury, Mass.

BLOCK, JAMES D., PH.D.—Assistant Professor of Psychology, Albert Einstein College of Medicine, New York, N. Y.

BRIDGER, WAGNER, M.D.—Assistant Professor, Department of Psychiatry, Albert Einstein College of Medicine, New York, N. Y.

BROWN, CLINTON C., PH.D.—Director, Psychophysiologic Research Laboratories, VA Hospital, Perry Point, Md.

COCHRAN, BURT JR., M.D.—Assistant Professor, Department of Internal Medicine, College of Medical Evangelists School of Medicine and Medical Consultant, Los Angeles County Hospital Psychiatric Unit, Los Angeles, Cal.

COHEN, BERTRAM D., PH.D.—Head, Division of Psychology, and Professor of Psychology, Lafayette Clinic and Wayne State University, Detroit, Mich.

DELAY, JEAN, M.D.—Professor of Psychiatry and Director of the University Psychiatric Clinic, University of Paris, Paris, France.

DENBER, HERMAN C. B., M.D.—Director of Psychiatric Research, Manhattan State Hospital; Associate Clinical Professor of Psychiatry, New York Medical College, New York, N. Y.

ELLINGSON, R. J., PH.D.—Chief Electroencephalographer, Nebraska Psychiatric Institute, Omaha, Neb.

FINK, MAX, M.D.—Director, Department of Experimental Psychiatry, Hillside Hospital, Glen Oaks, Long Island, N. Y.

FREEDMAN, ALFRED, M.D.—Professor and Chairman, Department of Psychiatry, New York Medical College, Flower and Fifth Avenue Hospital, New York, N. Y.

FREEMAN, HARRY, M.D.—Director of Research, Medfield State Hospital, Harding, Mass.

FROHMAN, CHARLES E., PH.D.—Director Biochemistry, Lafayette Clinic, Detroit, Mich.

GANTT, W. HORSLEY, M.D.—Director, Pavlovian Laboratory, Johns Hopkins School of Medicine; Principal Scientist, Perry Point Veterans Administration Hospital, Perry Point, Md.

GLUCKMAN, MELVYN I., PH.D.—Pharmacologist, Wyeth Research Laboratories, Philadelphia, Pa.

GOLD, ELEANOR, B.A.—Research Assistant, Children's Unit, Creedmoor State Hospital, Queens Village, N. Y.

GOLDMAN, DOUGLAS, M.D.—Clinical Director, Longview State Hospital; Assistant Clinical Professor of Psychiatry, University of Cincinnati, Cincinnati, Ohio.

GOLDSCHMIDT, LOTHAR, M.D.—Neurology and Psychiatry, Staff Member, Creedmoor State Hospital, Queens Village, N. Y.; Goldwater Memorial Hospital, Kew Gardens General Hospital, N. Y.

GOTTLIEB, JACQUES S., M.D.—Director, Lafayette Clinic; Professor of Psychiatry, Wayne State University, College of Medicine, Detroit, Mich.

GROSS, MARTIN, M.D.—Research Director, Springfield State Hospital, Sykesville, Md.

HART, E. ROSS, PH.D.—Chief, Division of Neurophysiology and Neuropharmacology, Veterans Administration Research Laboratories in Neuropsychiatry, Pittsburgh, Pa.

HIMWICH, HAROLD E., M.D.—Research Director, Thudichum Psychiatric Research Laboratory, Galesburg State Research Hospital, Galesburg, Ill.

HIMWICH, WILLIAMINA A., PH.D.—Medical Research Associate IV, Galesburg Research Hospital, Galesburg, Ill.

HOAGLAND, HUDSON, M.D., PH.D., SC.D.—Executive Director, The Worcester Foundation for Experimental Biology, Shrewsbury, Mass.

HOROVITZ, ZOLA P., PH.D.—Research Investigator, University of Pittsburgh School of Pharmacy, Department of Pharmacology, Pittsburgh, Pa.; Veterans Administration Research Laboratories in Neuropsychiatry, Pittsburgh, Pa.

JOHNSON, J. E., M.D.—Assistant Professor of Medicine, University of Texas, Medical Branch, Galveston, Texas.

JOHNSON, MARGARET, B.S., R.N.—Research Assistant, Washington University School of Medicine, Neuropsychiatric Research Department, St. Louis, Mo.

KAUFFMAN, DOROTHY, R.N.—Head Nurse, Research Division, Manhattan State Hospital, New York, N. Y.

KOELLA, WERNER, M.D.—Senior Scientist, The Worcester Foundation for Experimental Biology, Shrewsbury, Mass.

KRIS, ELSE B., M.D.—Director of Psychiatric Research (Social Psychiatry), Research Unit, Manhattan After-care Clinic, New York, N. Y.

LEHRMAN, DANIEL, PH.D.—Professor of Psychology, Rutgers University, Newark, New Jersey.

MACKAY, ROLAND, M.D.—Professor of Neurology, Northwestern University Medical School, Chicago, Ill.

MARBACH, EDWARD P., PH.D.—Biochemist, College of Medical Evangelists Metabolic Research Laboratory, Los Angeles County Hospital, Los Angeles, Cal.

MARRAZZI, AMEDEO S., M.D.—Director, Veterans Administration Research Laboratories in Neuropsychiatry; Professor of Physiology and Pharmacology, University of Pittsburgh School of Medicine, Pittsburgh, Pa.

MASSERMAN, JULES H., M.D.—Professor of Psychiatry and Neurology, Northwestern University Medical School, Chicago, Ill.; Director of Education, Illinois State Psychiatric Institute, Chicago, Ill.

MERLIS, SIDNEY, M.D., F.A.C.P.—Director of Psychiatric Research, Research Division, Central Islip State Hospital, Central Islip, N. Y.

MOLTZ, HOWARD, PH.D.—Assistant Professor, Department of Psychology, Brooklyn College, Brooklyn, N. Y.

MOORE, A. ULRIC, PH.D.—Assistant Director, Behavior Farm Laboratory, Cornell University, Ithaca, N. Y.

MOWRER, MARIE O., M.D.—Director, Outpatient Department, Malcolm Bliss Mental Health Center; Instructor, Department of Psychiatry and Neurology, Washington University School of Medicine, St. Louis, Mo.

NURNBERGER, JOHN I., M.D.—Professor and Chairman, Department of Psychiatry, Indiana University Medical Center, Indianapolis, Indiana.

PENNELL, ROBERT B., PH.D.—Director, Protein Foundation, Boston, Mass.

PETERS, HENRY A., M.D.—Associate Professor of Psychiatry and Neurology, University of Wisconsin Medical School, Madison, Wis.

PFEIFFER, CARL, M.D.—Head, Section on Pharmacology, Bureau of Research in Neurology and Psychiatry, New Jersey Neuro-Psychiatric Institute, Princeton, New Jersey.

POLLACK, MAX, PH.D.—Senior Research Associate, Department of Experimental Psychiatry, Hillside Hospital, Long Island, N. Y.

RAJOTTE, PAUL, M.D.—Associate Research Scientist (Psychiatry), Manhattan State Hospital, New York, N. Y.

RODRIGUEZ, JOSÉ M., M.D.—Research Neurologist, Veterans Administration Research Laboratories in Neuropsychiatry, Pittsburgh, Pa.

SANKAR, D. BARBARA, B.A.—Research Assistant, Biochemical Research Laboratory, Children's Unit, Creedmoor State Hospital, Queens Village, N. Y.

SANKAR, SIVA D. V., PH.D.—Senior Research Scientist, Biochemical Research Laboratory, Children's Unit, Creedmoor State Hospital, Queens Village, N. Y.

SARAVIS, CALVIN A., PH.D.—Staff Member, Protein Foundation, Boston, Mass.

SCHEIBEL, ARNOLD B., M.D.—Associate Professor, Departments of Psychiatry and Anatomy, UCLA Medical Center, Los Angeles, Cal.; Consultant to Brentwood and Sepulveda V A. Hospitals, and California State Mental Hospitals.

SCHEIBEL, MADGE E.—Departments of Psychiatry and Anatomy, UCLA Medical Center, Los Angeles, Cal.

SCHULMAN, JEROME L., M.D.—Assistant Professor of Psychiatry, Northwestern University Medical School, Chicago, Ill.; Director, Child Guidance Clinic, Children's Memorial Hospital, Chicago, Ill.

SILA, BASRI ARAS, M.D.—Resident Psychiatrist, Barnes Hospital; Washington University, Department of Psychiatry and Neurology, St. Louis, Mo.

SMITH, R. B., B.A.—Student Fellow in Psychiatry, University of Texas, Medical Branch, Galveston, Texas.

STEIN, LARRY, PH.D.—Department of Psychopharmacology, Basic Sciences Research Division, Wyeth Laboratories Inc., Philadelphia, Pa.

SUTHERLAND, GEORGE F., M.D.—Director of Psychiatric Education and Training, Rosewood State Training School, Owings Mills, Md.

THOMPSON, GEORGE N., M.D.—Research Associate and Neurophysiologist, St. Joseph Hospital; Associate Clinical Professor of Neurology and Psychiatry, University of Southern California, Burbank, Cal.

TOURNEY, GARFIELD, M.D.—Assistant Director in Charge of Education, Lafayette Clinic, Detroit, Mich.; Associate Professor of Psychiatry, Wayne State University, College of Medicine, Detroit, Mich.

ULETT, GEORGE A., M.D.—Professor of Psychiatry, Malcolm Bliss Mental Health Center and the Department of Psychiatry and Neurology, Washington University School of Medicine, St. Louis, Mo.

WHITMAN, JAMES, PH.D.—Chief, Clinical Applications, Psychophysiologic Research Laboratories, Veterans Administration Hospital, Perry Point, Md.

WILSON, W. P., M.D.—Associate Professor of Psychiatry, Duke University Medical Center, Durham, North Carolina.

WORTIS, JOSEPH, M.D.—Associate Clinical Professor of Psychiatry, State University of New York, Downstate Medical Center, Brooklyn, N. Y.; Director, Division of Pediatric Psychiatry, Jewish Hospital of Brooklyn, Brooklyn, N. Y.

YAKOVLEV, PAUL I., M.D.—Director, Research Laboratory, Perinatal Neuropathology; Clinical Professor of Neuropathology, Emeritus; Consultant in Neuropathology, Massachusetts General Hospital, Boston, Mass.

ZIMMAR, GEORGE P., M.A.—Research Assistant in Neurology and Psychiatry, Northwestern University Medical School, Chicago, Ill.

ZISKIND, EUGENE, M.D.—Clinical Professor of Psychiatry, University of Southern California School of Medicine, Burbank, Cal.

I JOINT MEETING OF THE PAVLOVIAN SOCIETY AND THE SOCIETY OF BIOLOGICAL PSYCHIATRY

Preface

The present volume of proceedings of the most recent meeting of the Society of Biological Psychiatry again attempts to do two things: to present a picture of advances in the broad field of experimental psychiatry as they are reflected in the papers presented at our meeting, and to conduct symposia of timely interest. Traditionally the Society's president not only gives expression to his views and interests in the Presidential Address, but also influences the composition of the annual program. In this instance our president, W. Horsley Gantt, pupil and translator of Pavlov, organized a joint meeting with the Pavlovian Society, and the symposium was the result. Some ten years ago Dr. Gantt helped found the American Pavlovian Society, a small group of active research workers in this field that meets from time to time in different settings. Though the Pavlovian approach has long been integrated into the field of experimental psychology, its influence in psychiatry has been much too small, and the Pavlovian Society has served a useful function in cultivating this work.

Ethology is, strictly speaking, the systematic observation of animal behavior in its natural state but has become associated with the special views of Lorenz and of Tinbergen on instincts, imprinting, etc. These theories have aroused considerable interest among psychiatrists in recent years so that it seemed appropriate to organize a small symposium on the theme. It is not surprising that two of the three participants are psychologists, for in this field it is the psychiatrists who must learn from them.

JOSEPH WORTIS, M.D.

CHAPTER 1

Ivan Petrovich Pavlov
PRESIDENTIAL ADDRESS

By W. HORSLEY GANTT, M.D.

My justification for speaking on the work of Pavlov and its later development rests upon the fact that only about six or seven pupils of Pavlov are still alive and actively working—it has been a quarter of a century since his death. Of these, three are still working in Russia—Kupalov, Asratyan, and Anokhin—and three, to my knowledge, outside Russia—Konorski in Poland and Harold Wolff* and myself in this country. Liddell (Cornell) visited Pavlov's laboratory in 1926 while I was there. Paul Yakovlev (Harvard) and Peter Karpovich (Springfield, Massachusetts) were pupils of Pavlov in Petrograd. Also in Russia are Ivanov-Smolensky, Krasnogorsky, and Speransky, but all of these men are, as I hear, too feeble to work. During the past two years three eminent pupils of Pavlov—Bykov, Orbeli, and Vollorth— have died.

EARLY WORK: TECHNIQUES

After graduating from the University of St. Petersburg, Pavlov spent two years in Germany, in the laboratory of Heidenhain in Breslau and of Ludwig in Leipzig. In Heidenhain's laboratory he devised the Pavlov pouch, which preserves the vagal fibers to the stomach. While with Ludwig he studied vasomotor functions. Pavlov discovered independently but at the same time as Gaskell the trophic nerves to the heart. These nerves Pavlov considered increase the force of the heart beat without changing its rate.

From his work on the heart Pavlov extended his idea of a trophic function of nerves having to do with the nutrition of tissues. Although the experiences of clinicians, especially of surgeons, for a long time

---

*Harold Wolff, who was my first collaborator in the Pavlovian Laboratory, Johns Hopkins School of Medicine, died February 21, 1962.

have tended toward a belief in trophic nerves, physiology has been unable to demonstrate their existence. The surgeon often sees evidence of trophic disturbances, but physiology has lagged behind in the explanation of these phenomena. Pavlov later further extended his concept. As he explained [1]:

> In my laboratory, though not experimentally, but clinically, I leaned toward the views of the clinicians about the existence of special trophic nerves. In the course of many years, while operating on the digestive tracts of animals, I often unexpectedly observed strange symptoms in the animals that lived. I noted trophic disturbances—tetany, paresis, ascending paresis, and shock—which had two issues, either death or temporary lethargy.
>
> These observations confirmed my opinion that these symptoms could be explained as the reflexes from abnormally stimulated centripetal nerves of the alimentary tract to inhibitory nerves to different tissues. It was assumed that the metabolism of every tissue was regulated by special centrifugal nerves by two opposing principles. One set of nerves augments, the other diminishes its vitality, and if extremely irritated destroys altogether the resistance of the tissue.

During his work with cardiac function, before 1890, Pavlov's skill and capabilities with the chronic experiment enabled him to measure the blood pressure in an unanesthetized dog. With the dogs standing quietly on the table in the laboratory, Pavlov trained them so that they would submit to a cannula being inserted into the artery. With such animals Pavlov was able to measure the influence of both emotional stimuli and pharmacological agents. It is noteworthy that by using this procedure Pavlov achieved a difficult task which even at present is rarely duplicated; I do not know of a laboratory where this is being routinely done.*

Pavlov's later work on the conditional reflex derived from his method of the chronic fistula, which he evolved with Heidenhain during his sojourn in Germany. The miniature stomach (Pavlov pouch) that he devised had the advantage over the Heidenhain pouch in that, unlike the Heidenhain pouch, it did not require severance of the vagal nerves. Pavlov preserved these nerves by constructing a bridge between the main and small stomachs. In this way the se-

---

*There are, of course, laboratories where cardiovascular functions are successfully being studied in the unanesthetized dog, such as in Rushmer's laboratory at the University of Washington in Seattle, and Irvine Page's Cleveland Clinic.

cretion of the small stomach is a true reflection of gastric digestion in the main stomach. Besides the gastric pouch, Pavlov used other fistulas in the study of gastrointestinal secretions — salivary, gall-bladder, pancreatic, and Thiry-Vella fistulas. This externalization of secretions enabled him to study these functions in a normal healthy animal over its lifespan.

The substitution of the chronic for the acute experiment was responsible for Pavlov's contribution to the physiology of secretion as well as for the development of the conditional reflex theory. The method made it possible for him to observe the adventitious fluctuations of secretion characteristic of the normal instead of the pathological specimen. These fluctuations are in essence products of conditional reflexes, in contrast to the unconditional reflex characteristic of the acute experiment. In the latter it was, of course, impossible to obtain any conditional reflexes.

A second advance in Pavlov's methodology consisted in the isolation of the stimuli acting upon the animal. This necessitated the confinement of the dog in a sound-proof room, the so-called "camera." But, in the beginning, before the construction of the new laboratory, about 1911, the dog was not separated from the experimenter. However, as the research progressed, Pavlov realized that in order to attain precise laws it would be necessary to eliminate all stimuli, especially the presence of the experimenter, except those intentionally introduced.

A third feature of his methodology concerned the quantitative measurement of the relevant responses of the animal. This included both specific functions, e.g., salivation, and the more general ones, such as respiration and movement. Salivation was recorded electrically when I first saw his laboratory in 1922.

It is important to emphasize these three characteristics of Pavlov's early experimentation: (1) the chronic experiment, (2) the isolation of the animal and the measured stimulus, and (3) the quantitative and graphic recording of response. It is astonishing and regrettable that those investigating behavior in the latter half of the twentieth century do not often observe these precautions, especially the isolation of the animal from the experimenter.

Another innovation of Pavlov's at that time was the introduction of asepsis in the physiological operation. As far back as 1890 Pavlov constructed a surgical laboratory consisting of a series of four rooms devised so that one could not get to the final one containing the operating table except by passing through the other three. These were successively: (1) washroom for bathing and scrubbing (by tub

bath) the animal, (2) preparation room for the animal, (3) preparation room for the surgeon, and (4) operating room [2]. I have not
seen a duplicate of such a well-devised operating room in a modern
physiological laboratory, although the use of antibiotics diminishes,
but does not obviate, the necessity for aseptic technique.

LATER WORK: CONCEPTS

Pavlov's choice of the salivary gland as the quantitative measure
of the conditional reflex, although necessary at that period, was
perhaps unfortunate for medicine. The very reasons why salivation
is advantageous for recording the conditional reflex make it un-
interesting for clinical medicine because the salivary function is
of little importance except for its ancillary function in digestion.
The fact that the salivary glands have few connections with any
function other than the ingestion of food means that there are few
interferences from outside stimuli Pavlov undoubtedly was aware
of the role of the cardiovascular and respiratory systems in relation
to the conditional reflex, but he did not use these systems as indicators because of their multifarious connections with other functions.
Had Pavlov chosen the cardiovascular system, e.g., the heart rate,
as the index of the conditional reflex, his teachings would probably
long ago have been incorporated into clinical medicine. Through the
use of the salivary gland, however, he could during the incipiency
of his studies better see the laws governing the conditional reflex.

As Dr. Wortis has devoted the bulk of his paper to a discussion
of Pavlovian concepts,* I shall review these only briefly. Concerning
the anatomy of the conditional reflex, Pavlov formulated an idea of
the analyzer, by which he meant to include the sensory pathways
and all the central connections. He considered that the conditional
reflex function is concentrated in certain brain areas, e.g., the
visual, in the area striata, but that it has widespread cortical repre-
sentations. Therefore, in order to abolish completely the visual
conditional reflexes, the whole cortex has to be removed. His law
of induction, positive and negative, taken from the current neurology
of the period, finds its parallel in Sherrington's work. But induction
as part of the conditional reflex operates not only over short periods
of time—seconds and minutes—but for much longer intervals—days
and weeks.

Besides the laws of generalization and differentiation, phenomena
well known as part of the learning process, Pavlov discovered the

*Page 13.

more controversial laws of irradiation and concentration. In these laws, he postulated the movement of either an excitatory or inhibitory process spreading over the cortex and then contracting to its original point, an action requiring seconds or minutes. The theory was based upon experiments in which tactile stimuli were applied as conditional stimuli along the leg of a dog. Neurophysiologists have objected to the length of time required for the spread of Pavlov's inhibitions. Recently, however, electrophysiological studies have found similar slowly spreading processes.

Much has been written about inhibition. I shall pause only long enough to say a word concerning the essential Pavlovian inhibition. The father of Russian physiology, Sechenov, described central inhibition, the inhibition evoked by stimulating the optic thalamus in a frog with sodium chloride. When there is a rival stimulation irrelevant to the function in action, such as the opening of a door while a dog is listening to the signal for food, and the new stimulus stops the conditional reflex, Pavlov termed this "external inhibition" because the focus in the nervous system is outside the focus of the original activity. When the excitatory conditional reflex develops into an inhibitory one, such as during non-re-enforcement of the conditional stimulus, this is "internal inhibition" because the inhibition develops within the same function. Sleep, according to Pavlov, is due to a spread of internal inhibition over the cortex; the inhibition is no longer localized but is generalized.

Pavlov considered that the psychical function, or what he called the "higher nervous activity," depends upon two opposite processes, excitation and inhibition, at the basis of which are chemical substances liberated in the brain. It is worth noting that Pavlov's concept of excitatory and inhibitory substances was formulated a decade or more before the discovery of such a substance as acetylcholine.

Seeing behavior disturbances in his dogs as a result of a difficult differentiation between excitatory and inhibitory stimuli (1921), Pavlov thought that the "experimental neurosis" resulted from a "collision" between cortical excitation and inhibition. He found that there are phases detectable in the conditional reflexes leading up to the full-fledged experimental neurosis. These phases (paradoxical, ultraparadoxical) become apparent in the changes in the relationships between strong and weak, or excitatory and inhibitory, reflexes with the strong ones becoming weak and vice versa, or the inhibitory ones becoming excitatory and vice versa. When the conditional stimulation becomes excessively intense, inhibition results. Pavlov considered this reaction a protection against overstimulation and damaging fatigue.

Since all dogs do not give parallel reactions to corresponding stimuli, Pavlov saw the need for classifying his animals according to their reactivity. For this purpose he used the Hippocratic temperaments as bases, the extreme ones (choleric and melancholic) representing pathological types and the two well-balanced, central categories (sanguine and phlegmatic) representing normal types. The recognition of a functional basis for classification was an extremely important step forward in getting away from the rigidity of statistical classifications, etc., which do not include the individual. Unfortunately there is no entirely satisfactory criterion for the classification of individuals into types. The recent work of Krasutsky in Bykov's laboratory, using drugs such as caffeine and considering hereditary types, seems promising.

At about the age of 80 Pavlov began to study intensively patients in psychiatric clinics. He attempted to explain their psychoses through analogies with the laws he had found valid in dogs. The results of this preoccupation are described in Pavlov's "Conditioned Reflexes and Psychiatry." As an example of this is Pavlov's explanation of paranoia as an inertness or stereotypy of the conditional reflexes. Once formed in castrated dogs, it becomes difficult to modify conditional reflexes. Pavlov related this to a clinical observation that paranoiac individuals are deficient in sexual function.

Although Pavlov cautioned against making premature analogies between the laboratory and the clinic, he perhaps fell into the error that he exhorted others to avoid. Another one of his errors was accepting too literally the various formulations and theories of psychiatric disorders given by psychiatrists. Nevertheless, his formulations provide interesting theories for future work, especially since his theories were constructed on the basis of the facts he collected.

Perhaps Pavlov's greatest contribution in explaining human behavior was his enunciation of the "second signalling system," viz., the function of language. Pavlov recognized that this human development represents a function not present in the lower animals, that language represents a generalization, an elaboration new in the animal kingdom, a novel cerebral function peculiar to the human brain. The great possibilities of connections based on language, explicit or implicit, are responsible for the marvellous achievements of the human as well as for his tragedies.

EXTENSION OF PAVLOV'S WORK

Among those in Russia who have been most active in extending Pavlovian work to the human being have been Krasnogorski and Ivanov-Smolensky. In 1907 Krasnogorski started working with the salivary conditional reflex chiefly in children. Recently he has devoted considerable attention to the development of speech—the second signalling system—in infants. Ivanov-Smolensky, a pupil of Bekhterev as well as of Pavlov, has investigated the conditional reflexes of both children and adults. He is the author of a number of books on this subject and a pioneer in the application of conditional reflex knowledge to education.

The pupil of Pavlov's who has done the most to extend the work in the fields interesting for medicine has been Bykov, who was made an honorary member of the American Psychiatric Association in 1958 and who died after a prostatectomy in 1959. As early as 1925 Bykov demonstrated to me the formation of urinary conditional reflexes by the use of externalized ureters in the dog. Since then, he has shown that many visceral functions, as well as hormonal secretions and metabolic changes, can become conditional reflexes. Bykov and his collaborators have included the kidney, suprarenals, spleen, and cardiovascular system as well as diurnal temperature regulations and ovarian function in their studies of the conditional reflex. In 1957 Bykov's Physiological Institute of the Academy of Sciences in Leningrad and Koltushi had a staff of 700, including 200 professional investigators. One of his active pupils has been Airapetiantz. The Institute is now under the direction of Chernigovsky. Bykov's work is described in his book "The Cerebral Cortex and the Internal Organs" [3].

The orienting reflex is now receiving considerable attention in both Russia and the United States. Liddell has based his attractive theory of vigilance upon this function. In 1943 Robinson and I began the study of the cardiac component of the orienting reflex. During Pavlov's lifetime there had been only a few papers from his laboratory on the orienting reflex. Since the war Luria and Sokolov in Moscow and many other Russians have published articles and books on the orienting reflex, and it has been studied in this country by Bridger, Winokur, Newton, Dykman, and others. It may lie at the basis of learning, and its exaggeration or abolition may be characteristic of certain psychiatric disorders.

My own work and that of my collaborators, begun in this country in 1929 when the Pavlovian Laboratory at The Johns Hopkins School of Medicine was initiated, have differed somewhat from that being carried on in Russia. While the Russians have attempted to extend and generalize Pavlovian concepts to include all the functions of the organism, I have been chiefly concerned with discovering the principles governing conditioning, the delimitation of reactions that can become conditional reflexes, and the role of the central versus the peripheral structures. My especial attention has been given to the inclusion of the cardiovascular system in the study of the conditional reflex. This I have carried out from two points of view: first, because of the importance of the cardiovascular system in medicine, especially in view of the great mortality from cardiovascular diseases; and second, because a study of the cardiovascular component of the conditional reflex reveals mechanisms at the basis of the development of psychopathological disturbances.

From the inclusion of the cardiovascular function we are able to see the precise role of the "person" in both normal and abnormal behavior. Also, certain principles are found to govern cardiovascular and other autonomic functions which are not apparent in the more specific and observable components of the conditional reflex, such as movement and salivation. "Schizokinesis" is the term used for the split between the general autonomic function and the specific conditional reflex. Paradoxically, the cardiovascular conditional reflexes form more quickly but are much longer lasting, thus showing a certain rigidity. In fact, cardiovascular conditional reflexes may persist in certain dogs after all attempts have been made to eradicate these reflexes by the ordinary methods of conditional reflex extinction. Schizokinesis is in opposition to the principle of Claude Bernard and elaborated by Cannon under the term "homeostasis." Schizokinesis throws new light on Pavlovian inhibition; what formerly appeared to be complete inhibition can now be seen as only a state of partial inhibition in which the motor and specific secretory components may be in abeyance but with the cardiovascular and respiratory conditional reflexes still active. If homeostasis were universally true, death would not occur.

In the experimental neurosis I have studied the development of symptoms during the lifespan of several dogs ("Nick" and "V3," each fourteen years). From such a prolonged study new principles appear. For instance, aberrant sexual phenomena are seen simply as a spreading from the original focus of disturbance to include many physiological systems. The sexual function is especially liable to perversion from neurotic disturbances in other systems [4].

"Autokinesis," seen in the development of new symptoms over a period of months or years, indicates that new relationships may occur, viz., new arrangements between foci of excitation in the brain. We have seen functional evidence of this. The recent work of Eccles and Jerzy Rose may provide a neurological basis for the theory of autokinesis. There may be positive as well as negative autokinesis. As an example of positive autokinesis is a continuing and progressive improvement observable in patients after one or two experiences or psychiatric conferences. The exact laws at the basis of autokinesis, especially the intraneural relationships, constitute an enormous field for future exploration [5].

PAVLOV THE MAN

In concluding this address to the Society of Biological Psychiatry and to the Pavlovian Society, I shall say a few words about Pavlov's character as an investigator and as a person. He was par excellence a masterful experimenter, a genius in devising methods appropriate to the function he was studying. He had extraordinary powers of observation as well as imagination. Many of his concepts are still being proven a half century later. A perusal of his works even today furnishes a wealth of material for investigation. Although his writings are replete with theories, he felt that a theory was useful to test the facts but that it should not outlive nonconforming facts. Facts were to him what the earth was to Atlas. Over the portals of his new laboratory in Koltushi he had engraved the words "Observation and Observation."

Precise and aggressive in his enunciation of theories, he was nevertheless unrelenting in his dependence upon objectivity and clarity of thinking. Although intolerant of slipshod or inaccurate experimentation, he exercised a softness toward his co-workers; it is said that he never discharged anyone from the laboratory over his long life.

Pavlov had a nineteenth century, adolescent, idealistic attitude toward science. He believed it would wrest the human from his despicable condition [6]:

Let the mind rise from victory to victory over surrounding nature, let it conquer for human life and activity

not only the surface of the earth but all that lies between the depth of the seas and the outer limits of the atmosphere, let it command for its service prodigious energy to flow from one part of the universe to the other, let it annihilate space for the transference of its thoughts—yet the same human creature, led by dark powers to wars and revolutions and their horrors, produces for itself incalculable material losses and inexpressible pain, and reverts to bestial conditions. Only science, exact science about human nature itself, and the most sincere approach to it by the aid of the omnipotent scientific method, will deliver man from his present gloom, and will purge him from his contemporary shame in the sphere of interhuman relations.

Pavlov remained a scientist to the end. Within one-half hour of his death, he was making observations on his own pathological condition.

As a pupil of Pavlov's, I cannot refrain from a word about his character. Besides his idealism, expressed in the preceding quotation, his courage was perhaps unparalleled in the entire history of science. He consistently stood for the truth, irrespective of monarchy or proletariat dictatorship; he defied both Czar and Commissar and even challenged Stalin's manipulation of science for political purposes. There has never been a scientist more truthful, or a human being more courageous and uncompromising in defending his beliefs. The enigma is that, although Pavlov lived under the most ruthless dictatorship, he died a natural death at the age of eighty-six.

REFERENCES

1. Gantt, W. H.: Medical Review of Soviet Russia, London, Brit. Med. Assoc., 1928, p. 112.

2. Pavlov, I. P.: Work of the Digestive Glands, London, 1910, p. 21.

3. Bykov, K.: The Cerebral Cortex and the Internal Organs, New York, Chemical Publ., 1957.

4. Gantt, W. H.: Experimental Basis for Neurotic Behavior, New York, Hoeber, 1944.

5. Gantt, W. H.: Principles of Nervous Breakdown—Schizokinesis and Autokinesis, New York Acad. Sci. 56 : 143, 1953.

6. Pavlov, I. P.: Lectures on Conditioned Reflexes (translated and edited by W. H. Gantt) New York, International Publ., 1928.

Pavlovianism and Clinical Psychiatry

By JOSEPH WORTIS, M.D.

As a clinical psychiatrist with some research interests I cannot speak to you about Pavlovian physiology from the interior position of a physiologist but rather as an outsider whose clinical understanding and approaches are much indebted to the work of Pavlov and his school.

If we define Pavlovianism as the system of basic views of Pavlov and his school, it is timely to describe these views and to relate them to clinical psychiatry. Although Pavlov had a strong influence and a large following outside his country, especially in the United States, the persistent application of his teachings to psychiatric problems has been largely a Russian development. Now that scientific intercommunication is being re-established between the United States and Russia, it is a stimulating experience to enter this Russian storehouse of science—like entering a vault long buried underground—to share and enjoy its valuable possessions.

For the sake of simplicity I have reduced Pavlov's theories to seven main principles, and I have related each of them to some current lines of research and to some pertinent clinical problems. These principles are [1]:

1. The conditioned reflex or theory of temporary connections [2, 3].
2. Excitation and inhibition.
3. The theory of types.
4. The experimental neurosis.
5. The nature of psychoses.
6. Protective inhibition.
7. The secondary signal system.

Supported by a grant from the National Institute of Mental Health (MY-2679) for the translation and interpretation of Russian psychiatric literature.

THE CONDITIONED REFLEX

The lid blink to a flash of light, the pupillary response, the swallowing reflex, the salivary response to stimulation of the tongue, and a host of other reflexes are inborn. The association of a new sensory stimulus with any one of these reflexes builds up a conditioned response to the new stimulus; this response is maintained but usually needs reinforcement from time to time, although a powerful experience can sometimes maintain the conditioned reflex indefinitely. The site of the coupling reaction is the cortex, although there has been some recent experimental evidence that under certain conditions subcortical conditioning can occur. Although pure and simple conditioned reflexes are rare in animals and even rarer in man, whose nervous processes are complex, highly integrated, and varied, nevertheless there are important applications of the simple conditioned reflex concept even for the human subject. Nail biting, bed wetting, phobias, and fetishisms can often be best understood as manifestations of conditioning and treated by conditioning concepts, reinforcing the habit by positive conditioning and discouraging it by negative conditioning. To cite another example: a human subject's urge to urinate can be altered so that it does not correspond to his actual physiological state by training him to observe the increased readings of a manometric bladder pressure indicator as his own urge to urinate develops and by then altering the indicator without his knowledge. When the indicator shows a low pressure, he inhibits his urge to urinate even though the bladder is full; conversely, when the indicator reading is high, the urge to urinate develops even though the bladder is far from full [4].

Conditioned reactions may not only modify an unconditioned reaction but may actually oppose it. Bykov [5] indicated that a conditioned sleep response to the striking of a sheet of metal with a hammer can be induced. Alcoholic reactions may be prevented after the ingestion of alcohol by the hypnotic suggestion that it is water [6].

Much work has been done in defining and refining the laws of operation of conditioned reactions. For example, it has been found that within certain limits a response will increase with the strength of a stimulus but that beyond a certain point (ultramaximal) a stimulus will provoke inhibition ("frozen by fear," "paralyzed by fright," etc.). But consideration of other details of the conditioning phenomenon would lead us too far afield.

There are myriad instances of relatively simple conditioned responses. As an example, may I remind you of the gun-shy dog. Not infrequently we see children who have been badly frightened by sudden and unexpected noises, such as the child who develops a fear of toileting because of the strange and frightening flushing noise. I recall a woman patient with an enormous fear of everything pertaining to glass ever since she had been terribly frightened by the sudden crashing of an object through her skylight while she was sleeping. There have been patients who became highly sensitized to the sound of planes or to the unsteadiness of ferry decks after frightening war experiences. Many cases of sexual perversion are related to early conditioning experiences. The placebo effect, so often misunderstood in clinical research, can often explain the effectiveness of an inert substance after prior conditioning by an active agent.

Conditioning responses of one type can be transferred to another. Kasatkin [7] and others have shown by simple though fascinating examples that an infant trained to develop sucking movements to a nursing bottle presented in a blue case but none to an empty bottle in a red case could at the age of five months immediately selectively grasp the proper bottle; infants without this training needed many trials. The capacity to transfer a learned response from one motor path to another has its sensory analogies; John [8] and others have shown that a learned response to a rhythmic flicker greatly facilitates a learned response to a rhythmic buzz of the same frequency.

THEORY OF EXCITATION AND INHIBITION

The conditioning process is complicated and varied, as we can see when we actually analyze what happens when conditioning occurs. If, for example, a dog is trained to salivate whenever pressure is applied to the lower portion of his foreleg, the dog at first will also respond to pressure to the upper portion; but as reinforcement follows only the application of pressure to the lower portion of the limb, the dog begins to discriminate. There is clear evidence from many experiments that what happens is this: during the first trials the conditioned stimulus radiates from the corresponding cortical area to the surrounding area. The cortical area of stimulation, however, is surrounded by a circle of inhibition lying concentrically around the stimulated area, like a circle of wetness around a fire, to contain the stimulation. As discrimination proceeds in successive trials, the circle of inhibition moves inward to confine the stimulus to a small point. This inhibition is an active physiological process and not the mere absence of excitation. If the upper portion of the leg is stimulated, a spread of actual inhibition that also radiates is induced; but at the same time a circle of excitation, which contains the area of inhibition like a circle of heat containing an area of wetness, is also induced.

The phenomenon of inhibition is of great interest and importance to psychiatrists. Under certain conditions a response will become inhibited and the inhibition will deepen and spread, as for example when there is a long delay between two stimuli. To illustrate: If the arrival of food is delayed after a bell has rung, a dog will grow sleepy or even fall asleep. Sleep, said Pavlov, is a state of general inhibition, but inhibition can differ in intensity, cortical locus, or depth of penetration into subcortical structures. As inhibition spreads and deepens, it undergoes phases during which the brain as a whole acts peculiarly: a stage of equalization in which all stimuli tend to produce equal reactions, then a paradoxical phase in which only weak stimuli are effective, a further phase in which only inhibitory stimuli are effective, and a final phase of complete inhibition. Hypnosis, said Pavlov, is some such state of partial sleepiness or inhibition. In hypnosis much of the conscious cortical control is lost, the still small voice of the hypnotist carries the force of a command, and inhibited catatonic or cataleptic postures are easily suggested. Hysterical blindness or paralysis results from focal inhibitions. Most important of all, schizophrenia is a state of partial inhibition.

THEORY OF TYPES

Pavlov in his work with dogs observed different constitutional types which he categorized as follows: (1) an unbalanced weak melancholic type characterized by constant recurrence of weak but readily irradiating inhibitory tendencies, (2) an unbalanced strong choleric type with both strong excitatory and inhibitory tendencies but with the excitatory tendency predominant so that these animals tend to be excited and unrestrained, (3) a normal but calm, imperturbable phlegmatic type with relative rigidity of the nervous functions, and (4) a normal but active, mobile sanguine type with relative lability of the nervous functions. Contemporary Pavlovians in the Soviet Union do not believe that this classification of types is directly applicable to human subjects, although it does suggest a basis for classification.

Pavlov made an important distinction between two types of human subjects, the distinction depending on the relative dominance of concrete sensory stimulation (primary signal system) or the dominance of verbal stimulation and preoccupation (secondary signal system). It was one of Pavlov's brilliant insights that he was able to describe the personality characteristics of human beings in whom the first or the second signal systems seemed to dominate. When the first system dominates, individuals are vivid, easily reactive, intense, and responsive and in extreme cases can develop hysterical symptoms. Pavlov characterized such people as artistic types. Those in whom the secondary signal system predominates are the quiet, sedentary, ruminative, inward people—the thinking types—who in extreme cases develop psychasthenic symptoms. In the social scene those in whom the primary system dominates often emerge to prominence and leadership, while those dominated by the secondary system, although also sometimes influential, tend to retire to background roles.

Despite this distinction, human personality, according to Pavlov, can never merely reflect constitutional type; it must also reflect the organism's life experience, its health or condition, and the situation in which it lives. In his report on a recent important symposium on human typology held in the Soviet Union, Zimkina [9] concludes that the problem is far from solved and adds significantly that so far no effective way of isolating the reactive pattern of an individual from his past experience or from the pervasive influence of the secondary signal system has been found.

THE EXPERIMENTAL NEUROSIS

The three classical methods of inducing the breakdown and disorganization of higher nervous function that Pavlov characterized as the experimental neurosis are: (1) the presentation of difficult or insoluble problems of differentiation and discrimination, (2) the exposure of the organism to overwhelming stimulation, and (3) the exhaustion of the organism by repetitious stimulation.

Miasishchev [10] says it is questionable whether a neurosis constitutes a specific clinical entity, although he thinks it at least represents a group of functional and usually psychogenic disorders. Physical predisposing factors are sometimes important, and physiological or medical disorders not infrequently develop from them. It is just as wrong, says Miasishchev, to investigate the psychic history of an individual and neglect the physiological state as it is to examine the physiological state and neglect the psychological one. "The development of Pavlov's teachings requires not the elimination of the psychic but the integration of the psychological and physiological." Only a detailed understanding of the history and psychological make-up of the individual, he goes on to say, can explain why a particular experience may be innocuous to one individual and constitute overwhelming stress to another. Weakness and vulnerability of the organism need not involve the entire nervous system but merely certain functional areas, such as the motor or the visceral system.

Of particular medical importance is the relation of neurotic states to medical disease, for at one point a reversible physiological imbalance may become an irreversible pathological state. We must recognize that not only diencephalic but also cortical systems can affect autonomic functions. Moreover, afferent interoceptors, as well as exteroceptors, can induce neuroses, as Bykov and his school have shown. Neurotic symptoms may involve not only motor acts but trophic (according to Bykov related to the metabolism of nerve cells at rest) and visceral disturbances as well. Children are especially prone to develop somatic symptoms from neuroses [11]. Even immunological reactivity has been found to be altered in neurasthenic states. Since the early stages of physical disease can also predispose to neurotic developments, careful clinical judgment is required to analyze each clinical problem anew.

In the course of the life history of an individual, according to Pavlov, special areas of sensitivity develop, so-called "sore points" (Pavlov's term; recent writers prefer to use "pathodynamic structure" to avoid the implication of a specific anatomical focus) which become the foci of obsessive thoughts, phobias, or irritable feelings from which disturbances flow. To rest these sore points and to develop competing foci of excitation, new interests or excitements can be very helpful.

The treatment of neuroses thus involves several simultaneous approaches: the discovery and elimination of sore points by means of discussion, suggestion, or changes in environment or experience; the resting of the tired brain; the elimination of excessive excitation; the creation of competing points of excitation; and the general strengthening of the organism. Similarly, the prevention of neuroses involves the ordering of the individual's experience to minimize stress while at the same time the individual must be trained early in life to assimilate life's inevitable strains and stresses. The individual should be armed with understanding while his health and good condition are maintained.

THE NATURE OF PSYCHOSES

Manic states can be readily understood as states of excessive excitation and weakened inhibition with perhaps a chemical basis involving excessive neural transmission substances, such as acetylcholine and catecholamines, or deficient cholinesterase or monoaminoxidase. Depressive states may involve an inhibition of deeper subcortical formations, and schizophrenia (or "délire chronique" of the French) may be associated with the dream-like state of partial inhibition pictured by Pavlov.

In manic states, according to Pavlov, the entire brain is in a state of excitation with a marked increase in associative activity leading to chaotic activity of the large hemispheres and with a marked dominance of subcortical excitation. In depression there is a corresponding decrease in brain activity with marked subcortical exhaustion and a suppression of instinctive patterns.

Soviet workers [12] picture a variety of psychiatric symptoms in Pavlovian terms. Delusions involve either a disruption of the efficiency of the cortical analyzers of sensation or a disruption of the relations between the verbal analyzers and other cortical functions. Hypochondriacal delusions involve a similar disruption of interoceptive and proprioceptive analyzers. Incoherence is pictured as an inhibition specifically of the secondary signal system [13] or as an excessive and chaotic radiation of excitatory processes freed from the constraining and selective force of inhibition, etc. [14]. These concepts are not merely semantic; they direct attention to a specific locus of derangement and suggest the specific physiological malfunctioning involved.

In many instances experimental data can confirm the validity of these concepts. The late Popov [15], for example, regarded hallucinations as a phase of partial inhibition when weak stimuli, in this case trace or adventitious stimuli, acquire the force of primary stimuli and induce a subjective sensation of reality. Popov adduced experimental evidence for this hypothesis by direct cortical stimulation of hallucinating patients. Similar phenomena are encountered in hypnogogic hallucinations, in the reactivation of hallucinations just before insulin coma supervenes, or in the nocturnal delusions of the aged when inhibitory tendencies grow dominant at night [16]. Bridger and Gantt [17] nicely demonstrated these phenomena in their experimental work on mescaline intoxication. Similarly, the presence of negative tendencies—refusal of food, violence to a loved object, immoral impulses, and the like—probably relate to the paradoxical phase of partial inhibition in which reactions tend to become negative or contrary.

The general concept that hallucinations are due to states of partial inhibition also gains support from certain pharmacological experiments showing that cortical stimulants like caffeine temporarily diminish or abolish hallucinations and cortical depressants like bromides reinforce them [12]. The extent to which hallucinatory phenomena are due to inert foci of stimulation or to inhibitory states needs to be further elaborated through experimental work. Probably both factors operate in different cases.

Pavlov felt that the state of partial inhibition which generally characterized schizophrenia was caused by a weakness of the nervous system. Since partial inhibition also implicates vegetative centers, many if not most of the vascular, visceral, endocrine, or immunological abnormalities of reaction that are encountered may be secondary to changes in nervous control. Although gross brain damage is rare in schizophrenia, minimal brain damage of infectious origin is not. Kameneva [18] reports 55 such cases following lues, sepsis, grippe, rheumatism, malaria, pneumonia, and paranatal infections. The actual encephalitis may be mild or unnoticed, and delayed development of symptoms is possible, especially when later infection, head trauma, exhaustion, or psychogenic stress is superimposed.

PROTECTIVE INHIBITION

The concept of weakness or exhaustion of the nerve cells is commonly employed to denote a general diminution of reactivity, a state sometimes occurring after prolonged or intensive activity or after exposure to stress. Chistovich [14] regards confusion, or amentia, as an extreme instance of such weakness, the weakness appearing at all levels of brain activity. In such cases the cortical points of excitation are too weak to induce negative inhibition so that the discrete selectivity of spread of excitation goes awry and chaotic cortical activity with incoherence in thought and speech results. There is a disruption of the relations between the primary and secondary signal systems with the secondary system most affected; even unconditioned reflex activity (orienting, defense, and feeding reflexes) is disturbed, and all vegetative activity is disrupted.

These considerations are the basis for the wide use of sleep treatment in the Soviet Union, where sleep is employed as the therapeutic form of protective inhibition to rest and revive exhausted brain cells. These considerations also throw some light on the rationale of patient care in Soviet psychiatric hospitals with their great emphasis on quiet, sleep, gentle management, and maximum freedom from stress.

Interesting work is being done to determine the correlations of brain chemical states with levels of activity. Kreps [19] declares that the general phosphorus turnover is markedly diminished during all inhibitory states, and Sytinsky [20] also reports decreased organic phosphorus levels as well as increased ATP levels in sleep. A number of investigators, Vladimirova [21] among them, have demonstrated a rapid increase in the ammonia content of the brain under states of excitation, with a decline in inhibitory states.

THE SECONDARY SIGNAL SYSTEM

Although Pavlov laid the basis for the study of the secondary signal system, "the signals of signals," he had little opportunity to develop investigations on the symbolic word system peculiar to man, being mainly preoccupied with animals and with the relatively gross disturbances encountered in human psychoses. However, Russian psychologists, especially Vygotsky [22] and his pupil Luria [23], and the psychiatrist Platonov [6] have done a great deal to demonstrate the importance and power of language in man and its intimate relation to thought.

The work on the secondary signal system has opened the way to a rational scientific approach to psychotherapy and provides an important bridge connecting the physiological interests of Russian psychiatry with the psychological and psychotherapeutic preoccupations of western, especially American, psychiatry of recent years. An appreciation of the importance of the secondary signal system will help bring Pavlovianism closer to the special and distinctive problems of human mental disorder.

CONCLUSION

Contrary to some current notions, most Pavlovian workers are very cautious in applying to man the data of animal experiments and recognize the vast difference between the higher nervous activity of man and that of all other living organisms. This difference derives not only from the far greater complexity of man but also from his peculiar dependence on social life. Pavlov wrote [1]:

There is no doubt that we must use the greatest care in relating our animal work to man... and we have the obligation to check these data again when we deal with human organisms. The early exact but elementary knowledge we have gained in animal work requires extreme caution when applied to man. It is precisely his higher nervous activity which raises man so high above the whole animal series. It would be truly naive to regard these first steps in the study of the physiology of the hemispheres, which initiated our studies but did not complete them, as in any sense a fulfillment of the difficult task of investigating human nature. Any premature attempt to bring some settled order into these current investigations can only reflect a certain narrow concept of the problem.

I cannot vouch for the validity of all of the experimental data and conclusions presented in this paper; some of them must certainly be wrong since they contradict each other. However, regardless of the validity of particular conclusions, Pavlovian work represents a method, a frame of reference, an approach that cannot fail to answer many questions and to stimulate our work. Its great virtue is that it comprehends, as no other point of view can, all the complexities of mental processes and makes it possible to incorporate psychological, physiological, anatomical, and chemical data, not as competing elements, but as essential and complementary features of the complex phenomena of mind.

REFERENCES

1. Pavlov, I. P.: Sämtliche Werke, Akademie-Verlag, Berlin (D.D.R.), 1954, 6 vols. (Ger.)

2. Pavlov, I. P.: Lectures on Conditioned Reflexes, vol. I, 1928, 414 pp; Conditioned Reflexes and Psychiatry, vol. II, 1941, 199 pp.; International Publishers, New York. (Gantt, W. H., Trans.)

3. Pavlov, I. P.: Conditioned Reflexes, Oxford Press, New York, 1927, 445 pp. (Anrep, G. V., Trans.)

4. Airapetiantz, E. S. H.: [Recherches sur le mécanisme des analyseurs internes de l'activité nerveuse supérieure], La Raison 7:63, 1953. (Fr.)

5. Bykov, K.: The Cerebral Cortex and the Internal Organs, Foreign Languages Publishing House, Moscow, 1959, 459 pp. (Hodes, R., Trans.)

6. Platonov, K. I.: The Word as a Physiological and Therapeutic Factor, Foreign Languages Publishing House, Moscow, 1959, 452 pp.

7. Kasatkin, N. I.: [Early ontogenesis of reflex activity in children], Zh. Vyssh. Nerv. Deyat. Pavlov 7:805, 1957. (Rus.)

8. John, E. R.: Higher nervous functions. in Brain Functions and Learning, Ann. Rev. Physiol., 1961.

9. Zimkina, A. M.: [On the typological characteristics of higher nervous activity in humans], Probl. Psikhol. 3:179, 1957. (Rus.)

10. Miasishchev, V. N., Ed.: [Neuroses. in Transactions of the Conference on the Problems of Neuroses, June 1955], Gos. izd-vo Kar., A.S.S.R., Petrozavodsk, 1956, 230 pp. (Rus.)

11. Simson, T. P.: [Neuroses in Children], Medgiz, Moscow, 1958, 215 pp. (Rus.)

12. Kerbikov, O. V., Ozeretskii, N. I., Popov, E. A., and Snezhnevskii, A. V.: [Textbook of Psychiatry], Medgiz, Moscow, 1958, 364 pp. (Rus.)

13. Ivanov-Smolensky, A. G.: Essays on the Patho-Physiology of the Higher Nervous Activity, Foreign Languages Publishing House, Moscow, 1954, 349 pp.

14. Chistovich, A. S.: [The role played by purulent infections in the causation of some psychoses], Zh. Nevropat. Psikhiat. Korsakov, No. 11, p. 843, 1955. (Rus.)

15. Popov, E. A.: [Application of I. P. Pavlov's teaching in the domain of psychiatry], ibid., No. 6, p. 673, 1957. (Rus.)

16. Khokhlov, L. K.: [Pseudo-hallucinations between sleep and wakefulness], ibid., No. 9, p. 704, 1954. (Rus.)

17. Bridger, W., and Gantt, W. H.: The effect of mescaline on differentiated conditional reflexes, Amer. J. Psychiat. 113:352, 1956.

18: Kameneva, E. N.: [The interrelationship between schizophrenia and organic brain damage of infectious origin]. in Giliarovskii, V. A., Ed.: Problems of Psychiatry, Min-vo zdravookhr. S.S.S.R., Moscow, 1956, p. 47. (Rus.)

19. Kreps, Ye. M.: [Biochemical characteristics of activity of the cortex of the larger hemispheres of the brain.] Zh. Vyssh. Nerv. Deyat. Pavlov 7:75, 1957. (Rus.)

20. Sytinsky, I. A.: [Variations of the adenosine triphosphate system in brain tissue in different functional states of the central nervous system], Biokhimiya 21:361, 1956. (Rus.)

21. Vladimirova, G. E.: [Functional biochemistry of the brain], Fiziol. Zh. S.S.S.R. Sechenov, 39:3, 1953. (Rus.)

22. Vygotsky, L. S.: [Problems in the psychological development of children], Izd-vo Akad. ped. nauk R.S.F.S.R., Moscow, 1956, 517 pp. (Rus.)

23. Luria, A. R.: The Role of Speech in the Regulation of Normal and Abnormal Behavior, Pergamon Press, London, 1961, 100 pp.

The Traditional and the New in Pavlov's Theory of "Higher Nervous Activity"

By PAUL I. YAKOVLEV, M.D.

Two phases are recognizable in the elaboration of Pavlov's theory of higher nervous activity, the traditional and the new. The traditional phase is customarily dated to Sechenov, Pavlov's teacher; the new phase has emerged since the Revolution of 1917. The contraposition of the subjective-private reality against the objective-public reality has been traditional in Russian scientific thought and is particularly clear and sharp in Pavlov's work. Of the measurable, public reality one is the measurer; of the immense (not measurable) reality of the private self one is the measure.

In the Russia of Pavlov's upbringing, reverence for the "exact" sciences was high. The bodily self-occupying structured physical space and the environment as a physical space filled with objects and events unfolding in a kaleidoscope of time as a dimension are cardinal parameters of objective reality of the exact sciences. It should be noted that the qualification "exact" does not connote, as frequently imputed, a claim of an ultimate truth or finite precision but specifies the method of inquiry, namely, sciences which derive the information from the act (ex-acto) of measuring the observed (ex-acto mensurandi). The subjective, private reality is neither more nor less "real" than the public reality of exact sciences. However, neither are the parameters of exact sciences commensurate with nor is the method ex-acto mensurandi applicable to the immense realities of this private sort. And so the subjective reality is not "exactly" scientific. Pavlov left it to psychologists. He never argued the private validity of subjective psychological generalizations. He rejected the claims for their public validity and regarded the psychologists critique of his experimental method on introspective grounds as the limit of impertinent irrelevance.

It may be of interest to review briefly the origin and development of Pavlov's theory of higher nervous activity in the context of the development of other systems of thought envisaging man as an action system, particularly those of Hughlings Jackson, Ivan Sechenov, and Sigmund Freud. From such a review broader implications may be drawn for understanding the nature of some of the intellectual conflicts of our time, particularly in psychiatry.*

The evolution of biological action systems is traditionally envisaged in the Spencerian sense as a process of differentiation from simple to complex systems and from highly organized, stable modalities of organization such as a living cell to the least organized, labile modalities such as human society—a cenobiosis of action systems in constant evolution.

Jackson, a contemporary of Spencer and of Darwin, followed this envisagement of evolution in his conception of "levels" of organization of brain functions from the lower level of stable, fixed functions represented in the spinal cord and brain stem and common to all vertebrates, to the middle level of organization represented in the sensory-motor cortex of mammals, to the highest level of organization, the level of transcortical, labile, ever-changing functions represented in the rest of the cerebral hemispheres, mainly in the frontal lobes, and taxonomically particular to man.

Spencer's and Jackson's conceptions were constructed within the framework of the information and ideas of their time, the age of the Industrial Revolution. They reflect the time of the immutable strata of mid-Victorian society, the time of smokestacks of Manchester factories rising in tiers as the symbol of the then new social structure. This framework shaped the thought of a whole generation of eminent neurologists coming after Jackson. In this framework the levels of organization of functions rise in vertical superposition of latitudinal strata from lower to higher, the higher levels "controlling" the lower and the lower levels constantly seeking to "escape" or be "released" whenever the higher levels are "abrogated" in some way.

At the turn of the century Freud, who in his concept of a mental apparatus was one of the first on the Continent to acknowledge Jackson's ideas, came out with the outspokenly anatomical diagram of the structure of the apparatus in which the symbolic id, ego, and superego are also strata. However, these strata are no longer con-

---

*The following is extracted with slight alterations in wording from my James Arthur Lecture, "Body, Brain, and Behavior," at the American Museum of Natural History, New York City, 1961, to be published in full elsewhere.

ceived in the vertical superposition of Jacksonian latitudinal levels but in concentric formation. In Freud's schema the id is an indefinable, inchoate, and unconscionable (subconscious) core and represents the lowest level of organization; the ego is a cortical layer interposed between the id and the superego; and the superego is that self-righteous and censorious force (the conscience) which molds and shapes the ego from the primordial stuff of the id. And so, from this primeval swamp of inchoate and shapeless id, the conscious, i.e., symbolized thought, arose like a sinful orchid—beautiful and guilty. Freud's was a great empirical generalization of our time. But there were other ideas abroad.

It is of interest that in his book, "Reflexes of the Brain," published in 1863 (and therefore without the least possible prejudice to Freud's diagram), Sechenov proposed a concept which offers interesting food for thought on what the id, ego, and superego of Freud's system might be in more readily definable and measurable terms, or, to put it otherwise, how Freud's mental apparatus might be envisaged if the immense notion of psyche as used in his psychodynamic system were sloughed off. Sechenov proposed that spinal reflexes are reflexes with the peripheral ends buried in the body so that the body itself is the special domain and end of their adaptive action. On the other hand, cerebral reflexes are reflexes with the peripheral ends cast out into the external environment so that the special domain of their adaptive action is the world of objects and events (and of other selves) about the body rather than the body as their end. It should be evident that the abrasive radionalism of Sechenov's essentially Cartesian conception of man as an action system of reflexes divests the Cartesian conception of its ambiguous dualism and reduces the immensity of the Aristotelian notion of psyche (entelechy, mind, final cause) in Freud's conception of mental apparatus to measurable terms. In these terms the id becomes a measurable force of the physical agents of universal change and motion; the ego (the private self) becomes the palpable, substantial body; and the superego becomes the measurable, public world about the body (the enviroment).

In a retrospect of the past one hundred years of evolution of physiological thought, it is justifiable to say that Sherrington and his school proved in the conception of proprioceptive reflexes the general validity of Sechenov's generalization with regard to the Jacksonian lower level—the spinal cord and brain stem—and middle level—the sensory-motor cortex. But beyond this middle level, i.e., with regard to Jackson's higher level, Sherrington stopped short and with awed "ignoramus!" threw in the sponge, as it were. However, almost at the same time or slightly later Pavlov, Sechenov's pupil, and a rather ruthless man, took up the challenge. In the framework of Ludwig's "Maschinenlehre des lebendigen Organismus"* (rather than of Freud's psychical conception) Pavlov and his school built an impressive body of measurable facts in support of Sechenov's conception of brain reflexes. In the framework of these widely known experimental facts the responses to unconditional stimuli, i.e., physical agents (e.g., light, mechanical and thermal stimuli, gravity), are universal to all organisms. However, the responses to conditional stimuli-signals of physical agents, or conditional reflexes, are corollaries of the evolution of a central apparatus of integration and emerge with the emergence of the cerebral cortex. For Pavlov the cerebral cortex is a definitive mechanism for the induction of the properties of a stimulus-physical agent or a combination of such unconditional stimuli-agents with another set of stimuli-agents by association in time of action of these different sets of agents at least once. The induction is a measurable cortical process. It endows the random stimuli-physical agents, hitherto meaningless in themselves to the organism except as agents, with the meaning of a signal of the specific stimuli-agents whereby these random stimuli now become as effective in evoking alone the appropriate (i.e., meaningful) response as the specific stimuli-physical agents of that particular response.†

The sphere of responses to unconditional stimuli-physical agents is clearly comparable to the lowest level of the Jackson schema and to the core, or the id, of Freud's diagram. The sphere of responses to conditional stimuli-signals of physical agents, or Pavlov's "first system of signals," is comparable to the middle level of the Jacksonian hierarchy of functions but not to the higher transcortical level, and, in a sense, it is also comparable to the ego of Freud's system but not to the superego. An empirical pragmatist, Pavlov constantly strove to fit his theory built upon facts from the experimental laboratory to the realities of human experience. The Revolution of 1917 and the events of "the great experiment" which unfolded on a planetary scale with humanity (rather than dogs) as the medium and object of observation had a great impact on Pavlov's thinking.

---

*Quoted from frontispiece to one of Pavlov's published lectures.

†I have borrowed the succinct terminology "stimuli-agents," "stimuli-signals," and "stimuli-symbols" from Viaud.

Expanding his theory to include specifically human experience, Pavlov and his school crossed the Rubicon in the concept of the "second system of signals," the system of stimuli-symbols of the conditional signals (essentially language) particular to man. And here Pavlov found himself treading upon the same ground as Freud, although each used a radically different mode of locomotion upon their common empirical ground.

It should not be difficult to see a logical link between the Jacksonian hierarchy of lower, middle, and higher levels; the Freudian hierarchy of the id, ego, and superego; and the Pavlovian hierarchy of the stimuli-physical agents, the signals of these agents, and the symbols of the signals. In all three systems the tripartite logical apparatus is similar in their spatiotemporal structure. The Jacksonian levels conceived in vertical superposition of static horizontal strata, or latitudinal levels, are conceptually structured as proceeding from "below up." Freud's diagram of the mental apparatus and Pavlov's and Sechenov's systems of reflex arcs developing from unconditional reflexes with the ends buried in the body to conditional ones with the ends cast out into the world of objects and events (first system of signals) and of specifically human social experience (second system of signals) are concentric and dynamic in the assumption that man as an individual and human society as a collective action system evolve and develop outwards from within. The radical difference lies in the direction of inquiry for which the Freudian and Pavlovian logical apparatus are used and for which each was constructed. Pavlov's apparatus is directed toward the measurable public reality, Freud's toward the immense reality of the private self. Freud faces the millennial riddle of the sphinx; Pavlov admits of no riddles except as a venerable rubble of the centuries.

In the search for relevant answers, one might follow Freud and dig deeper and deeper into the unfathomable nether world of the private, subjective experience, or one might strike out into the open public world of objects and events about us. We know all too well how man's house is divided on this issue into "idealists" and "realists." And yet, one might try to synthesize the information from both directions, be it for no other reason than to satisfy the human need to think, with a hope that some relevant answers fit to act upon may ultimately come from the synthesis.

Salivary Conditional Reflexes in Man

By GEORGE F. SUTHERLAND, M.D.

With improved instrumentation and technique, it is now possible by means of the parotid secretion to make a direct comparison of the conditional responses described by Pavlov in animals with those in man. In addition to changes in the conditional reactions, the series of fluctuations that characterize the salivary curve in eucrasia are modified in abnormal states. A low flat curve tends to be associated with depression of spirits; a high flat curve tends to be associated with anxiety symptoms.

As Lord Adrian has remarked,* advances in science have often been dependent upon concomitant improvements in techniques and instrumentation. For these reasons, until recent years it has been difficult to repeat in man Pavlov's findings in animals. This is attributed to the ease with which inhibition is elaborated in the human subject and the resultant relatively scanty parotid secretion, the measurement of which requires a sensitive recording device and a procedure that ensures a preponderance of excitation [1, 2].

In bridging this gap between animal studies and those in man, it became apparent that there were two problems to be solved. The first arose by virtue of the fact that no precise available instrument had been devised for recording the salivary flow in man; the second lay in certain aspects of the technique that had not been adapted for use in the human subject. The essential defect in previous instrumentation was a delay introduced by the employment of air and rubber tubing in the conducting system; the principal error in technique was due to faulty design which failed to make allowance for the fact that in man the flow of saliva is easily inhibited.

Supported by grant-in-aid by the Foundation's Fund for Research in Psychiatry and assistance from Friends of Psychiatric Research, Incorporated.
*In an address before the World Congress of Psychiatry, Montreal, June 1961.

MATERIALS AND METHODS

The method of conducting the experiments followed the convention of isolating the observer from the subject in separate rooms during the procedure. The daily test was performed at the same hour on successive days. The positive signals were reinforced by 1 ml of sweetened lemon juice.

In the illustrations (Figs. 1–4) an event marker indicates the moment of application of the signal and the reinforcement. In the body of the record each short vertical line represents one drop of saliva (c. 50/ml); the curved line indicates the rate (in 5-second intervals) at which the drops were secreted.

Figure 2 is a striking example of the usefulness of the method in determining the response to medication. In this instance the drug prescribed had the untoward effect of enhancing the patient's anxiety, as shown in the upper tracing. After the drug had been discontinued, the patient's anxiety diminished, as revealed by the lower tracing.

While we rely upon laboratory findings to assist us in the diagnosis and treatment of strictly physical ailments, no such conviction attends the receipt of similar information calculated to reflect abnormalities in the emotional sphere. Why this strange paradox, if the same meticulous care is exercised in obtaining the data? What inherent defect exists in the customary clinical procedures that, however precisely carried out, reveal only gross changes in function whereas more subtle variations escape detection?

Considering those tests regarded as valid indices of malfunction, it becomes apparent that they are largely based upon measurement of a specific unconditional reflex. The reliability of such a test depends upon how closely the measurement is restricted to the particular reflex involved. Under ordinary circumstances, the probability of attaining this ideal is so remote that only gross changes in function can be determined. Attempts to include the more subtle changes by refining the measurement are frustrated because the results become increasingly inconclusive. The dilemma arises by virtue of the fact that one is hoping (whether or not he realizes it) to include an evaluation of the conditional reflex as well, but trying to accomplish this by an inadequate measure. The only solution is to adopt a technique originated by Pavlov for measuring both of these quantities concomitantly.

More than fifty years ago, when Pavlov was in the process of making his monumental contribution to the scientific understanding

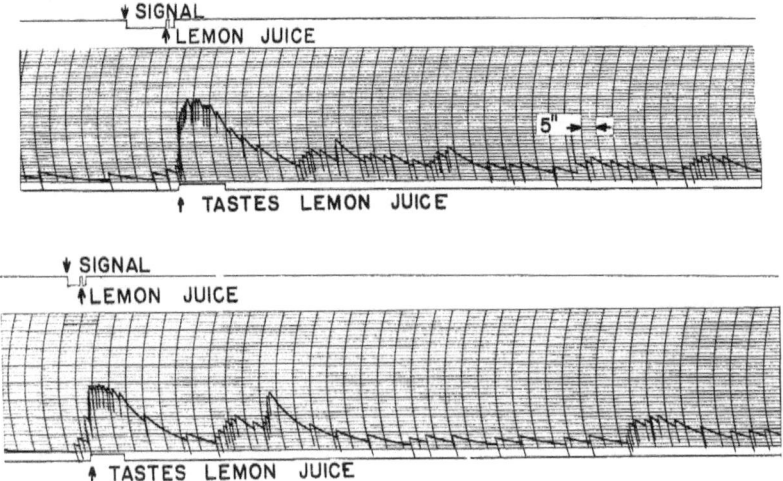

FIG. 1. Graphic depiction of a normal human subject's salivary response to a signal and its reinforcement.

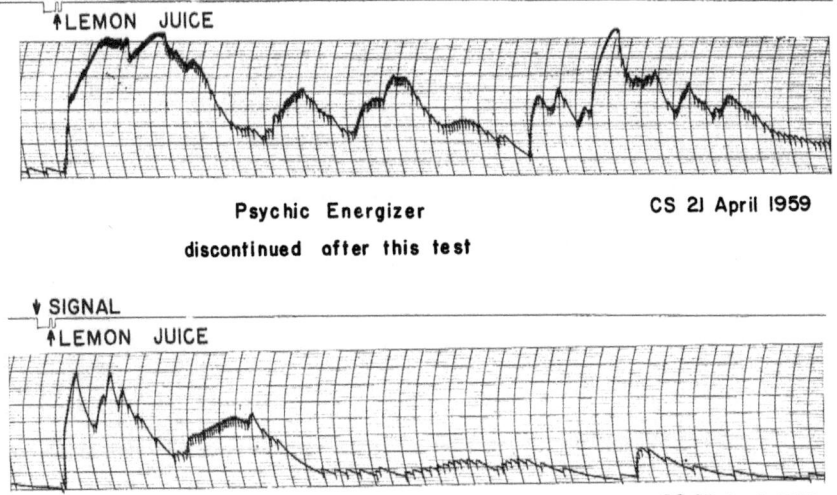

FIG. 2. Graphic depiction of human subject's response to medication as determined by measurement of salivary conditional reflex with lower tracing showing response to test after discontinuance of medication.

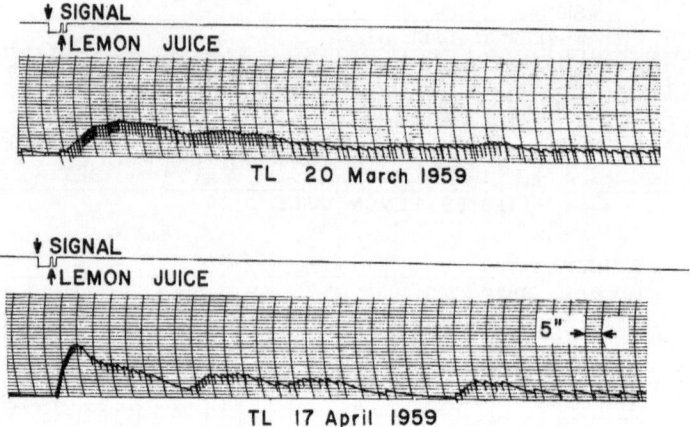

FIG. 3. Graphic depiction of anxiety and depression as revealed by salivary conditional reflex determinations with lower tracing showing improvement after one-month period.

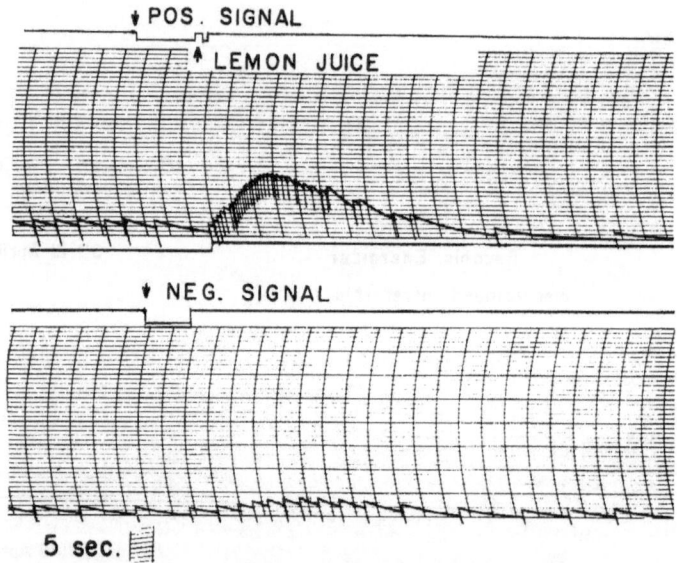

FIG. 4 Graphic depiction of increased internal inhibition as revealed by salivary conditional reflex determinations with upper tracing showing result of a positive signal and lower tracing of a negative one.

of the digestive system, he was struck with the fact that the flow of digestive juices could be elicited in a hungry dog by the mere anticipation of receiving food. At first his interest was directed to these "psychic reflexes," as he called them, because he could no longer ignore their effect during the measurement of the quantity of secretion evoked by specific amounts of different foods. It was only later that his entire attention was devoted to exploring the function of the nervous system by means of the conditional reactions.

Under certain circumstances, the conditional reaction may be of sufficient magnitude to preclude a precise measurement of the unconditional reaction. Thus, one physician found that his readings of the blood pressure in a group of patients suffering from cardiovascular disturbances were erratic, usually too high in comparison with those taken at frequent intervals by the ward nurse. It is obvious that the difference can be attributed to the increased apprehension of the patient when the doctor made the determination. Thus, the readings were c o n d i t i o n a l upon the circumstances under which they were taken.

Failure to take cognizance of the conditional as well as the unconditional factors involved may vitiate, nullify, or confuse the findings. A useful rule in evaluation is to apply the criteria of orientation, namely: time, place, person, and significance as factors that can influence, modify or distort the resultant measurement. The individual trained in the technique of eliciting conditional reactions is frequently shocked to observe the utter disregard of the multitude of extraneous stimuli entering into the clinical experiment or test, as if the organism were expected to exercise some sort of prescience in selecting the proper ones to which to respond. These were the errors that concerned Pavlov and led him to devise a procedure for the precise determination of physiological function. His experiments were chiefly confined to animals, and the salivary conditional reflex was for the most part used as an indicator. This reflex could not be demonstrated satisfactorily in man until recently because the means of measurement and verification were wanting, and as a consequence little attempt has been made to apply Pavlov's precepts to clinical studies.

The continous registration of the rate of salivary flow during the entire test procedure enlarges the scope of the observations. It has become clear that the "interval secretion" (that occurs between successive applications of the signal) serves as a forecast of the nature and extent of the conditional reaction to be elicited.

The interval secretion lasts from 3 to 8 minutes (according to the design of the protocol), allowing for leisurely observation in contrast to the brief reaction that occurs during the conditional signal. In fact, it appears that the observation made during the interval is more likely to reveal consistent information with respect to the state of the internal milieu of the subject than the actual conditional reflex. This method obviates the shortcomings of the method wherein the resultant data depend entirely upon the sucessful demonstration of the conditional salivary reflex in the human subject. It no longer appears to be necessary to regard eliciting the reflex as the essential finding because similar and more information can be obtained by adopting the new procedure. For this reason, to a large extent the conclusions drawn were based upon this part of the record.

The reliability of the findings is enhanced by observing the interval secretion as well as the conditional reactions. Chance extraneous stimuli are easier to detect in a 30-minute period than during four or five 10-second applications of the stimulus. Also, the extraneous stimulus may distort the record just at the moment that the conditional stimulus is applied, negating the response. By modification of the technique to include the entire 30-minute period, the instrument lends itself to clinical use.

RESULTS

It might be supposed that after the application of an adequate stimulus to the normal subject the flow of saliva would rise until it reached a maximum and then decline gradually until it resumed the former level of base-line secretion, but this is not so. Instead, the saliva is secreted in a series of spurts of ever-diminishing amplitude continuing for a considerable period beyond (at least the apparent) application of the stimulus (Fig. 1). The secretion begins with a relatively small response to the positive conditional signal. This is succeeded by a rapid rise that may reach 200 drops per minute immediately following the application of the lemon juice. Then it declines somewhat more slowly until near the end of the second minute it has overshot the base-line. By the third minute a spontaneous secretion appears, similar in contour to the initial reaction to the lemon juice but much diminished in magnitude.

Under ideal circumstances, experimental work has demonstrated that if this pattern is continued, a succession of fluctuations of ever-diminishing amplitude and duration supervene until a point is reached at the end of 8 or 10 minutes when the base-line resumes its initial value. Pavlov postulated that this phenomenon is a manifestation of induction following a stimulus. This means that after the stimulus has ceased, its effects persist, taking the form of alternating phases of positive and negative induction.

Furthermore, he showed that a second stimulus applied during this period becomes modified in accordance with the phase of induction in progress at the particular instant. It follows that a positive phase of induction magnifies the absolute value of the response whereas a negative phase reduces it. This is particularly apparent in the conditional reactions. Consequently, the absolute value of the response to the stimulus can only be determined by making allowance for the effect of the induction. As a rule, this is quite difficult, and so one chooses the resting state—when induction is not operating—to make the determination. With the continous method of recording, this becomes a much easier task.

DISCUSSION

Particular attention should be paid to the inductive effects of extraneous stimuli. Induction arising in this manner affects other modalities. The alternate phases of positive and negative induction are thought to indicate that the base-line (that is, the homeostasis) is re-established by a feedback mechanism of quite precise proportions with respect to amplitude and duration. A departure from this curve indicates a disturbance of homeostasis, whether due to some extraneous stimulus or to part of an internal malfunction of the organism.

As a means of detecting unwanted interference, the conditional reflex technique is far superior to all others because it offers quantitative measurement of the extraneous stimulus, even though it does not identify the modality. Attempts to evaluate unknown factors by the use of controls, the administration of inert substances, or the execution of placebo studies are relatively crude.

In the clinical use of the instrument, disturbances in the emotional sphere may be apparent from the very beginning of the record. If, instead of the base-line secretion approximating 0.03 ml per minute, there is hardly any secretion at all, one suspects that this may be a manifestation of internal inhibition (in the Pavlovian sense). When this is so, the application of the positive signal (e.g., the metronome) elicits no response, with even the reinforcement (1 ml of sweetened lemon juice) producing a relatively meager secretion which subsides in a short period of time to its former low level. A record in which this is consistently demonstrated denotes central inhibition, commonly noted in those phases of an illness associated with depression of spirits.

In contrast to inhibition, irritation manifests itself as an elevated rate of secretion that continues throughout the record. Under these circumstances it is also difficult to demonstrate a positive conditional reflex but for a different reason, namely, the mere addition of a few drops of saliva scarcely alters the record. The high level of basic secretion thus masks the much smaller conditional response. For the same reason, the response to the lemon juice, while clearly detectable, is not as striking as in the normal curve. This type of curve is frequently associated with a state of inner tension.

The upper tracing of Fig. 3 illustrates the record that anxiety and depression produces; in this instance, the depressive features were the more prominent, as shown in the relatively flat low trace with many drops. The lower tracing, taken one month later, depicts the result of a spontaneous improvement, illustrated by the restoration of the oscillations and the distribution of the drops.

A common finding in psychiatric patients is shown in Fig. 4, which illustrates increased internal inhibition. The upper tracing shows that the base-line secretion was diminished on the application of the positive signal, whereas the application of the negative signal increased the flow, as shown in the lower tracing. This was the typical sign used by Pavlov to demonstrate excess internal inhibition. He called it the "ultraparadoxical phase" and considered it an early manifestation of the onset of the experimental neurosis. Further studies may show that the underlying mechanism of both the spontaneously occurring and the experimentally induced neuroses may be similar.

SUMMARY AND CONCLUSIONS

It is now possible to validate in man Pavlov's observations in animals:

1. By means of the salivary conditional reflex, it is now possible to make a direct comparison of Pavlov's findings in animals with corresponding phenomena in man.

2. Such findings indicate that Pavlov's observations with respect to the experimental neurosis are applicable to emotional disorders in man.

3. The validity of clinical experiments could be enhanced by strict adherence to the conditional reflex technique.

REFERENCES

1. Bykov, K.: Textbook of Physiology, Foreign Languages Publishing House, Moscow, 1958.

2. Sutherland, G. F. and Katz, R.: J. Appl. Physiol., 16(4):740, July, 1961.

CHAPTER 5

The Conditional Psychogalvanic Reflex:
Its Contribution to Psychiatric Diagnosis

By LEO ALEXANDER, M.D.

The absence or a marked diminution and delay of the positive conditional psychogalvanic reflex (PGR) with reduced differentiation between or paradoxical reversal of the responses to excitatory and inhibitory stimuli is an objective positive diagnostic sign of organic or toxic disturbance of the nervous system, chronic schizophrenia, or depression. By contrast, neurotic anxiety states show enhanced responses with poor differentiation and other excitatory generalization phenomena. Acute schizophrenic reactions, however, are characteristically associated with marked, precise responses showing better than average differentiation between excitatory and inhibitory stimuli.

Patients suffering from psychalgic states incidental to depressive illnesses show marked inhibition or abolition of the conditional PGR characteristic of depressive states. Spontaneous PGR fluctuations, if present at all, also tend to be minimal. By contrast, patients suffering from physical pain states show marked spontaneous fluctuations of skin resistance corresponding to the waxing and waning of the physical pain, while the responses to the positive conditional stimuli remain uninhibited. In fact, at times the pain seems to improve responses to the conditional signals, probably because it produces an excitatory state that irradiates and thus facilitates conditional responsiveness.

These differences of response are helpful in the differential diagnosis between psychalgia and obscure organic pain due to undiagnosed physical illness.

Effects of Muscular Exertion and Verbal Stimuli on Heart Rate and Blood Pressure in the Human

By CHRISTIAN ASTRUP, M.D., AND
W. HORSLEY GANTT, M.D.

The purpose of this investigation was to continue the study of the complex problems of schizokinesis [1].

MATERIALS AND METHODS

In the present experiments the effects of maximal muscular exertion on heart rate and blood pressure were studied in 39 normal persons. A visual stimulus of 5 seconds of green light followed by 15 seconds of red light was presented. The persons were instructed to pull as hard as they could when the red light was on. As in a previous study [1], the effects of the verbal stimuli "pull harder" and "take it easy" were investigated. The blood pressure was continuously recorded with the Winston blood pressure follower, the heart rate with a cardiotachometer, and the muscular exertion with a dynamometer. Each person was first given a series of trials without and then a series of trials with verbal stimulation.

RESULTS AND CONCLUSIONS

The results are presented in Fig. 1.

We considered the increases in heart rate and blood pressure during the presentation of green light as conditional and during the presentation of red light as unconditional responses to maximal muscular exertion. For the unconditional responses there was in the first series with no verbal stimulation an average* increase of 11.3 heart beats. The maximum increase was reached during the

*All results cited are averages.

first half of the period of exertion, and a few seconds after exertion the heart rate dropped to its prestimulus level. The blood pressure increased slowly during exertion, and the maximum increase of 11.1 mm was obtained after the persons had stopped pulling the dynamometer.

In the second series of trials, with no verbal stimulation there was an unconditional heart rate increase of 11.2 beats and a blood pressure increase of 11.2 mm, practically the same as in the first series. With the verbal instruction "pull harder" there was an unconditional increase of 14.5 heart beats and 12.8 mm of blood pressure. The instruction "take it easy" produced an increase of 4.9 heart beats and 7.2 mm of blood pressure. This shows that the effect of verbal stimulation is comparatively stronger for heart rate than for blood pressure. In the present study the muscular output was slightly increased by "pull harder" and decreased by "take it easy." The differences in autonomic reactivity are so great that we think our data give evidence of schizokinesis for heart rate as well as for blood pressure [1].

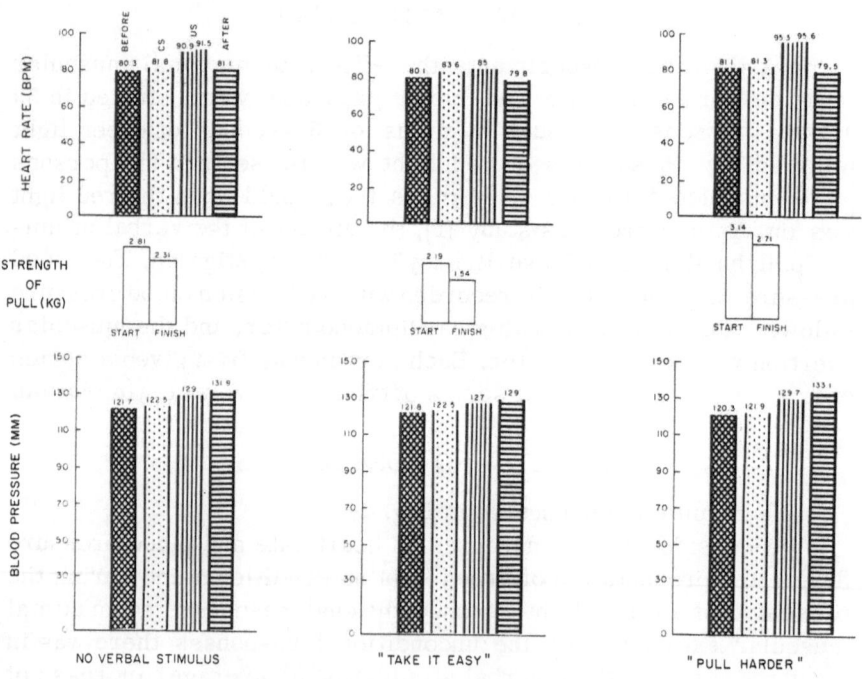

FIG. 1.   Heart rate and blood pressure changes to muscular exertion.

The results in one group of 7 persons with high prestimulus levels of blood pressure (135 mm and higher) and one group of 13 persons with low blood pressure (120 mm and lower) were considered separately. The blood pressure reactions are presented in Fig. 2.

The low-pressure group gave the strongest blood pressure responses and also the strongest increases of heart rate. This might suggest that the high-pressure group has a lowered ability of cardiovascular reactivity to muscular effort.

In the low-pressure group the unconditional increases of blood pressure were only slightly greater with the instruction "pull harder" than with no instruction (13% as compared with 12.2%). For heart rate also, the differences were small (19.9% to "pull harder" and 17.9% without verbal stimuli). "Take it easy" gave unconditional blood pressure increases of 7.1% and heart rate increases of 5%.

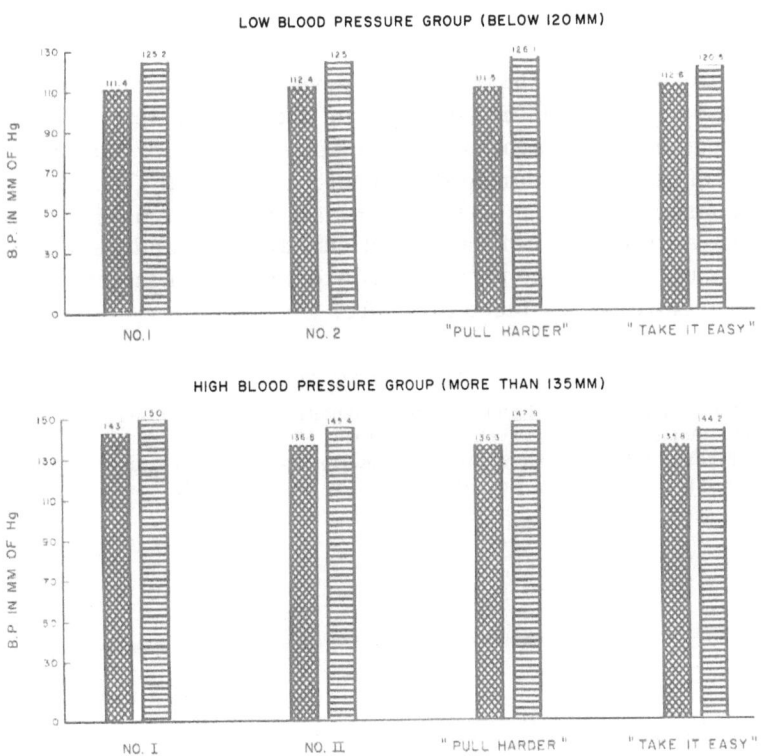

FIG. 2. Blood pressure responses of high and low blood pressure groups.

This verbal stimulation considerably reduces useless visceral overactivity.

In the high-pressure group there was a 6.2% increase of blood pressure and a 11.7% increase of heart rate with no verbal stimuli. "Pull harder" resulted in an 8.6% unconditional increase of blood pressure and a 12.8% increase of heart rate. This verbal stimulus gives markedly stronger increases of blood pressure than no verbal stimulation. "Take it easy" gave a 5.9% increase of blood pressure and a 6.6% increase of heart rate. This means that "take it easy" has comparatively smaller effect in the high-pressure than in the low-pressure group with regard to reducing visceral overactivity. Our data may indicate that schizokinetic blood pressure reactions to psychic stimuli are of importance for high blood pressure. Persons with high blood pressure tend to overreact with blood pressure responses when exerted beyond capacity, and their blood pressure and heart rate cannot "take it easy" in the same way as in persons with low pressure.

During the conditional stimulus the first series with no verbal stimulation gave an increase of 2.5 heart beats and 0.6 mm of blood pressure. For heart rate 8 persons and for blood pressure 12 persons had no increases or even decreases. Peters and Gantt [2] found that 8 persons showed an increase and 3 persons a decrease of heart rate during the signal for exertion. Thus, for heart rate human subjects as well as dogs fall into two types: a majority showing accelerated cardiac conditional reflexes and a few showing decelerated cardiac conditional reflexes. Our data indicate similar reaction patterns for blood pressure.

REFERENCES

1. Gantt, W. H.: Normal and abnormal adaptations in homeostasis, schizokinesis and autokinesis, Dis. Nerv. Syst. 18: July 1957.

2. Peters, J. E., and Gantt, W. H.: Conditioning of human heart to graded degrees of muscular tension, Fed. Proc. 10 (Part 1): Mar. 1951.

CHAPTER 7

Awareness of Stimulus Relationships and Physiological Generality of Response in Autonomic Discrimination

By JAMES D. BLOCK, PH.D.

I should like to describe some data collected in the laboratory of the Psychiatry Department at the Albert Einstein College of Medicine which reflect two phases of our interests in conditioned autonomic discrimination in man. The first phase concerns subjective awareness, or the ability to verbalize essential aspects of the experimental situation. The second concerns the physiological generality, or the amount of spread among organs, of autonomic discrimination in man.

AWARENESS AND CONDITIONING

With reference to subjective awareness, we have posed a specific question, namely, do we find conditioned autonomic discrimination between two stimuli in man in the absence of the awareness of, or the ability to verbalize, the fact that only one of the stimuli may be followed by a painful electric shock? Originally, the aim of our work was to develop a conditioning method for use in investigations of subliminal perception. However, the complexities of the conditioning method that we employed made an initial answer to this question of awareness necessary in order to obtain significant and stable conditioned discrimination in our subjects.

The conditioning situation which we employ can be briefly described. The subject was supine and facing a movie screen and had recording electrodes attached to him. Two stimuli were briefly projected onto the screen: one, a line drawing of a circle, and the other, a line drawing of a hexagon. They were presented singly in random order at random intervals of 20 seconds to a minute. The duration of exposure of each picture was always 0.01 second, but the illumination was systematically varied. A brief electric shock was applied to the subject's leg 10 seconds after one third of the presentations of only one of the two stimuli. We were attempting to create an autonomic discrimination between the stimuli by partial reinforcement of one of them with electric shock.

This basic conditioning method appears to be rather straight-forward. However, by the introduction of ancillary procedures, the procedure was made quite complicated from the subject's point of view. Upon hearing the word "focus" over the intercom, the subject was to look at a small dot on the screen; and then, a few seconds later, one of the two drawings was flashed onto the screen. Within 2 seconds the subject was to press a button to identify which drawing had been presented. Twelve seconds after the stimulus the subject verbally reported the identity of the stimulus; his confidence in this identification by saying "positive," "not sure," or "guess"; and what he actually saw on the screen. This cycle was repeated for the presentation of each stimulus.

This procedure, further complicated by instructions to "lie quietly," "do not close your eyes for any appreciable time," "try not to move," and so on, is apparently so complex even for college students to understand and remember that if they are not informed that the electric shock may follow only one of the two stimuli very few become aware of the fact spontaneously. In fact, when questioned, many of these uninformed subjects may actually report having experienced shock after both stimuli. At first, we found this a bit surprising since we had used only two easily discriminable stimuli and we had not, as others have done, deliberately compli-cated the procedure to obtain lack of awareness or deliberately failed to focus the subjects' attention upon the conditioned or un-conditioned stimuli. Apparently, however, the task of carrying out the peripheral aspects of the experiment had effectively diverted the subjects' attention from the major element of the conditioning situation. If, like Mowrer [1], we view conditioning as a method of communication, we can say that we failed to communicate one aspect of the experiment to the uninformed subject, as judged by the subjects' verbalizations.

In analogous experimental studies a question a number of experimenters have asked is whether the autonomic responses indicate the same lack of discrimination as does the verbal re-sponse. Razran [2] has reported that a salivary response to conditioned stimuli is apparently better learned in the absence of specific instructions concerning the true nature of the experiment. However, his conditioning procedure differed markedly from that of any form of classical conditioning, insofar as the US and UR were present during the presentation of a number of stimuli and apparently were not associated with them under controlled temporal conditions.

The McAllisters [3] have reported that instructions describing the nature of the experiment facilitate eyelid conditioning but that nevertheless conditioning is found to be present in subjects who are not given these specific instructions. However, like many human conditioning experiments, only one stimulus, consistently reinforced, was utilized. In these cases it seems highly unlikely that a human subject can long remain unaware of the CS-US relationship.

Branca [4] has found that autonomic discrimination among a number of stimuli, one of which is reinforced by electric shock, does not occur in the lack of verbal discrimination among the stimuli. Chatterjee and Eriksen [5] have concluded from their findings that autonomic conditioning is no more precise or specific than the subjects' verbalizations.

The results of the following study lead us to a similar conclusion. We have failed to find autonomic discrimination in the lack of conscious discrimination of the specificity of the CS-US relationship, that is, in the lack of a conscious realization that only one of two stimuli may be followed by a painful experience, in this instance, electric shock.

In our experiment we compared the skin resistance, or GSR responses, of a group of six subjects who were uninformed with a similar group who were informed of the CS-US relationship at the beginning of the experiment. All stimuli were presented at illumination levels sufficient for fully conscious, positive recognition of the stimuli.

Figure 1 demonstrates the extent of autonomic discrimination between the shock and the neutral stimulus. For each such series of five shock and five neutral stimulus presentations, the amount by which the responses to the shock stimulus (A) exceeded those to the nonshock stimulus (B) and vice versa for each subject was computed. This was then averaged for each group of subjects. We can see that the informed subjects showed immediate discrimination persisting over 40 stimulus presentations, whereas the uninformed and consequently unaware subjects demonstrated no discrimination over 70 stimulus presentations. The table in Fig. 1 lists, by individual subject, the significance of the difference in GSR magnitude between the two stimuli utilizing the Mann-Whitney "U" test. Discrimination between the stimuli is evident among all six informed subjects at probability levels not exceeding 0.06, whereas the probabilities among the uninformed subjects indicate no significant discrimination for any one of the six subjects.

This latter finding is the most consistent; that is, we do not find autonomic discrimination in the absence of some sort of verbal discrimination of the specific relation of the US to one of the stimuli. The converse, however, is not true. Verbal discrimination in man does not imply the presence of concomitant autonomic discrimination. Simply put, a subject may know that only the circle picture may be followed by shock, but he may or may not show more autonomic mobilization to this picture than to the neutral hexagon picture. In a group of 24 informed subjects who contributed complete records for a subsequent similar experiment in subliminal perception, 15 showed significant GSR discrimination of

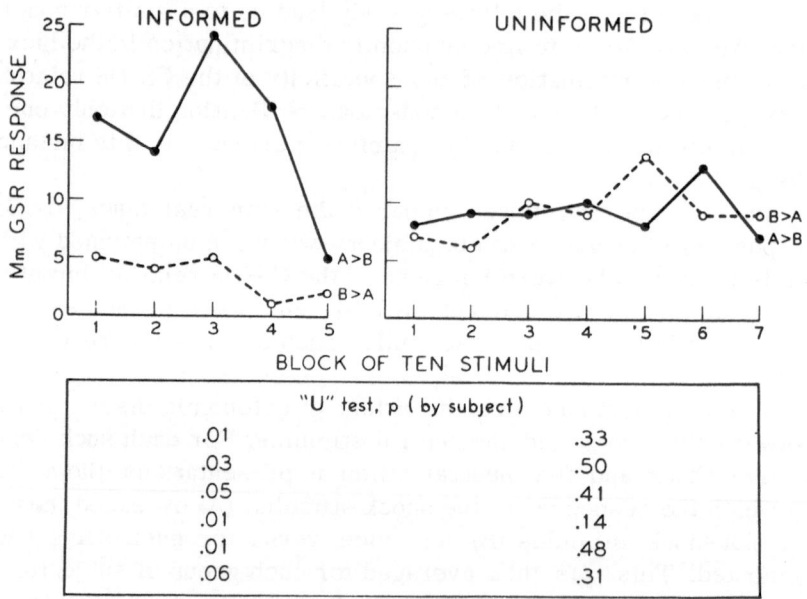

"U" test, p (by subject)	
.01	.33
.03	.50
.05	.41
.01	.14
.01	.48
.06	.31

FIG. 1.   Extent of autonomic discrimination.

easily visible stimuli and the other 9 subjects showed no significant GSR discrimination.

GENERALITY OF AUTONOMIC CONDITIONING

The second finding which I will briefly discuss concerns the physiologic generality of autonomic discrimination in man. The specific question is: How extensive physiologically is autonomic discrimination in man in our discrimination situation? In previous experiments the results were discussed only in terms of the GSR, or skin resistance response. Although the sizable extent of our knowledge of this response is paradoxically often interpreted in a negative manner by some workers, GSR is easy to obtain and measure and can be simple to analyze.

However, the principal reason we have used GSR is simply because it clearly indicates autonomic discrimination between stimuli in cases in which other measures do not do so or do so very poorly. This can be demonstrated in the case of the 24 subjects who participated in a subliminal perception experiment. In this experiment, in addition to GSR, both the heart rate and the respiration rate were obtained from the subjects, thus allowing us to compare the extent of autonomic discrimination among these few physiological measures.

Other than a few details, the subliminal aspects of the experiment need not concern us here. The procedure was similar to that of the previous experiment, except that all the subjects were informed of the specific CS-US relationship and the illumination of the stimuli was varied stepwise above and below a threshold of chance correctness of identification.

The subjects were separated into two groups, one which demonstrated significant GSR conditioning to correctly identified above-threshold stimuli and a group which did not. Fifteen subjects fell into the conditioned GSR group and nine into the nonconditioned GSR group. In the presentation of the data, the subjects were aligned in respect to the illumination level which presented the threshold for chance identification for each subject. Graphs and tests of group data were then prepared for the group at the threshold illumination and for illumination steps above and below it.

In Fig. 2 the mean GSR of both groups of subjects to the shock and to the neutral stimulus are presented as a function of illumination level. In the case of the conditioned subjects, the differences in response to the two stimuli should be noted. This difference is

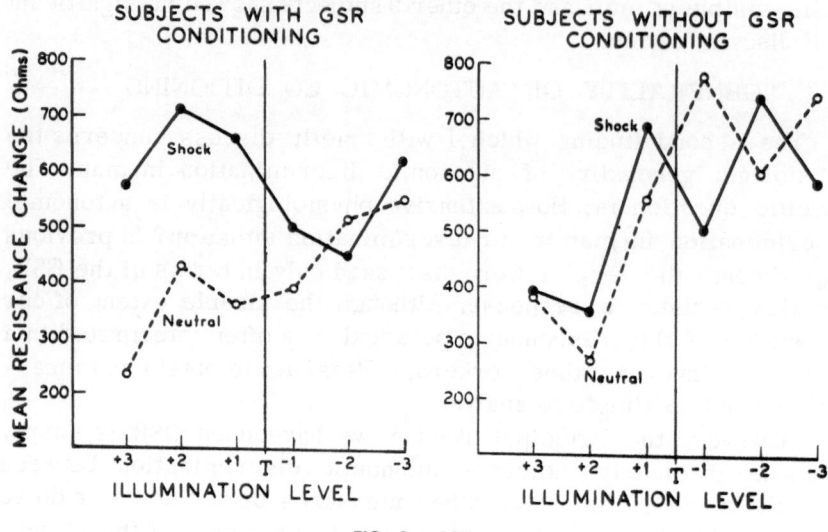

FIG. 2. GSR.

considerable above the threshold but disappears at very low illuminations below thresholds. The difference in the amount of discrimination between the conditioned and nonconditioned groups is, of course, not unexpected since the groups were originally distinguished on the basis of a portion of this data.

The point of interest is that now having established two groups on the basis of GSR, one which evidences autonomic discrimination and one which does not, we may ask how well the heart rate and respiration rate discriminate between the stimuli in these groups.

The heart rate was measured in two ways, either in terms of 5 R-R intervals immediately preceding and following the stimulus or in terms of the average R-R interval during one respiration cycle immediately preceding or following the stimulus. The difference between the shock and the neutral stimulus was explored by using both the poststimulus measure and the difference between pre- and poststimulus measures.

Figure 3 presents the results of the 5 R-R interval analysis. It can be seen that neither group shows appreciable discrimination between the shock and the neutral stimulus, and statistical analysis shows no difference to be significant at any illumination level. The same is true of the heart rate measured in terms of the respiratory cycle (Fig. 4).

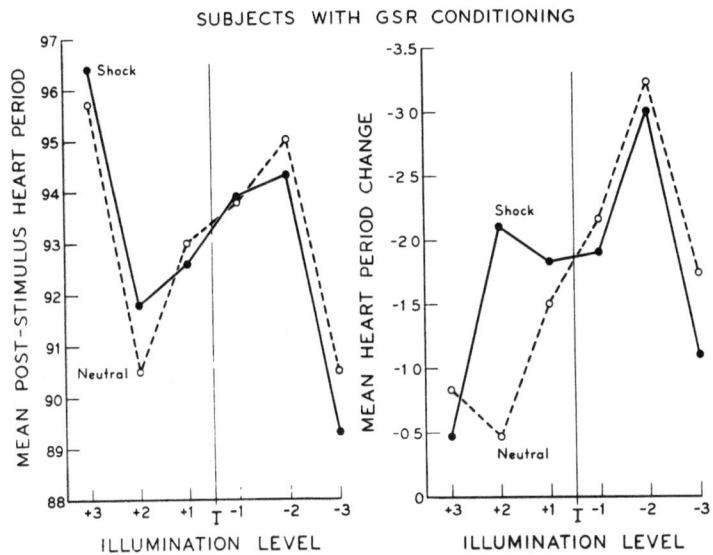

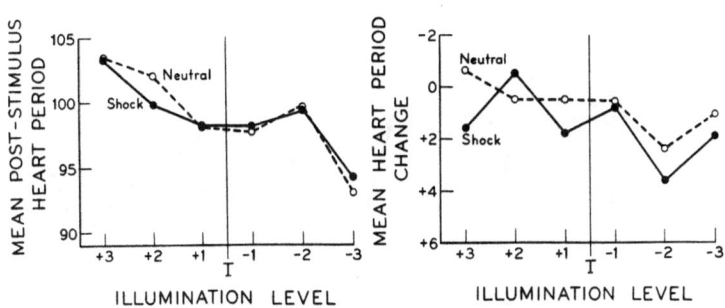

FIG. 3. Heart period (Block 5).

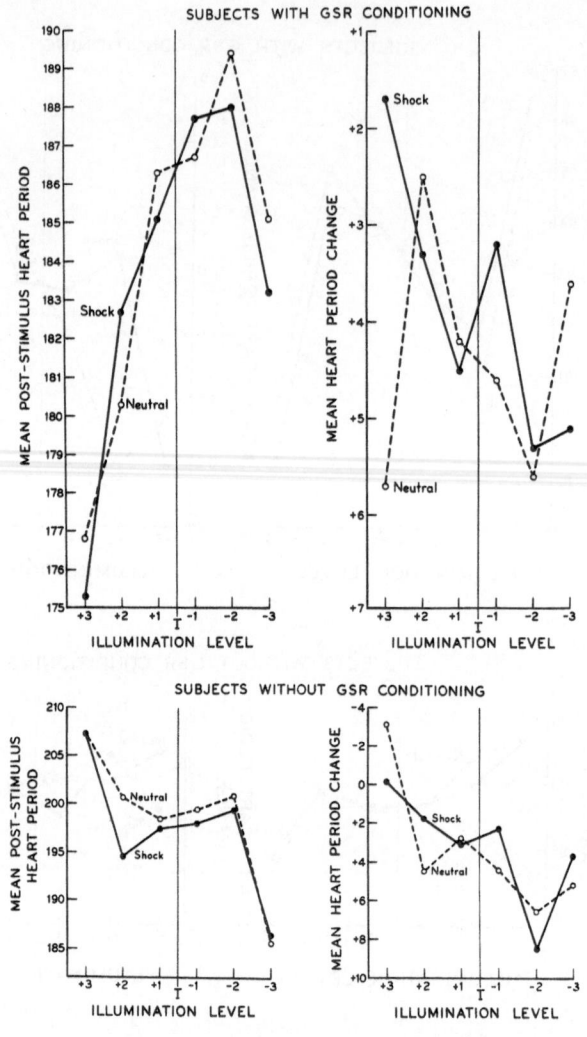

FIG. 4. Heart period (1 respiratory cycle).

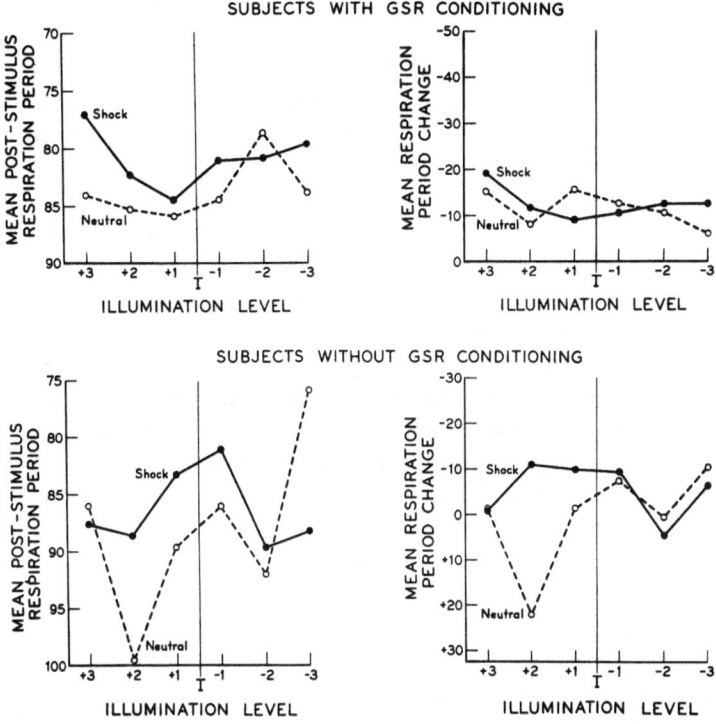

FIG. 5. Respiration.

Figure 5 presents respiratory rate data, for which the basic measurement is the period of one respiratory cycle. Respiration apparently evidences greater discrimination than does heart rate. However, none of the apparent differences are statistically significant.

To take a different approach and simply ask how many of the total of 24 subjects demonstrated significant conditioned discrimination using any heart rate or respiratory measure, the answer is only one or two. This is in marked contrast to the 15 subjects who showed significant GSR discrimination.

CONCLUSIONS

These data offer several tentative conclusions. The first is a very comforting one. Although not all measures may discriminate the effects of stimulation equally clearly, they, at the same time,

do not offer contradictory results. That is, we have found no significant indication that the neutral stimulus causes greater stimulation than does the shock stimulus. Second, it appears that there
are some organs which are more sensitive autonomic indicators
than others for the group as a whole. The GSR appears to measure
the activity of such an organ.

A methodological consequence of this conclusion is that for
many conditioning purposes one should select that measure which
in most individuals sensitively reflects autonomic activation in
man. Also, we may tentatively regard with suspicion the firmness
of negative conclusions based upon the use of a relatively insensitive
autonomic indicator.

Third, the failure of the heart rate, and incidentally the ballistocardiogram in other experiments, to discriminate as clearly
as does GSR is surprising to one who has worked with animals. At
the Cornell Behavior Farm Laboratory I have observed a large
number of goats and sheep on their first day of conditioning. Their
behavior certainly suggests extreme behavioral and physiological
mobilization. Vigilance is so marked that minor environmental
changes which usually provoke merely an ear twitch or a glance
in the barnyard, may produce violent escape movement, extreme
tachycardia, and rapid respiration in the experimental room.

In man we rarely see subjects who react in an extreme manner.
Individuals can be quite confident that the experimenter will not
harm them permanently or pain them considerably. Above all, if
such is the case, they know that they have the option of leaving the
situation. Furthermore, although the unconditioned stimulus of
electric shock arouses much anxious anticipation, upon actually
experiencing it the subjects soon find it to be a fairly innocuous,
nonmeaningful stimulus. In fact, we use partial reinforcement, not
because it has been found to produce stronger conditioning, but
because the more frequent the reinforcement, the more likely that
the intensity of the electric shock that we use will produce minimal
or no autonomic response.

Compared to the goat or sheep, and other animals I suspect,
the relatively low level of man's vigilance in an experimental
situation and the experimenter's natural reluctance to use strong,
highly threatening unconditioned stimuli may both be factors of
considerable value in explaining why evidences of conditioned
autonomic discrimination in animals is found in almost any organ
at which one may care to look whereas in man one tends to find

autonomic discrimination in only a few organ systems, those which apparently reflect minimal autonomic responses to stimulation.

REFERENCES

1. Mowrer, O. H.: The psychologist looks at learning, Amer. Psychol. 9:660, 1954.

2. Razran, G.: A direct laboratory comparison of Pavlovian conditioning and traditional associative learning, J. Abnorm. Soc. Psychol. 51:649, 1955.

3. McAllister, W. R., and McAllister, D. E.: Effect of knowledge of conditioning upon eyelid conditioning, J. Exp. Psychol. 55:579, 1958.

4. Branca, A. A.: Semantic generalization at the level of the conditioning experiment, Am. J. Psychol. 70:541, 1957.

5. Chatterjee, B. B., and Eriksen, C. W.: Conditioning and generalization of GSR as a function of awareness, J. Abnorm. Soc. Psychol. 60:396, 1960.

CHAPTER 8

Application of Conditioning Procedures in the Study of Aging

By JAMES R. WHITMAN, PH.D., CLINTON C. BROWN, PH.D., AND W. HORSLEY GANTT, M.D.

This is a brief report on the results obtained from two studies investigating the changes in conditionability occurring with age. Other investigators have usually selected subjects as representative of contrasting age groups, and they have compared these different groups on the basis of the measures obtained for the purpose of specifying differences which may be associated with increasing age. Responses which have been conditioned have been the eye blink and hand withdrawal, and the findings are to the effect that with increasing age there is some impairment in conditionability. The present studies were concerned mainly with correlation of measures of conditionability with intelligence test scores and clinical findings, and with respect to age the subjects selected represented a homogeneous group.

MATERIALS AND METHODS

The method of conditioning used was that standardized by Gantt as an examination useful in the clinical study of the psychiatric patient. The general procedure consists of presenting to the subject a series of pairs of two different tones, one of which is always followed by a shock to the subject's hand. The subject's task is to learn the relationship between the shock and the tones and to state this in his own words. The subject is also instructed to press a bar or bulb which prevents his receiving a shock.

Normal subjects learn the relationship between the tones and the occurrence of the shock during the first series of trials and are able to verbalize this relationship. Such a performance is given a rating of "A." Subjects who do not learn the relationship with this amount of practice are given additional practice with increasing amounts of information or hints as to what the relationship is. If after 25 pairs of tones, for the last 5 of which the information is given that one tone is always followed by a shock and the other is not, a subject shows no evidence of conditioning, his performance is rated "D." Ratings of "B" and "C" indicate intermediate degrees of difficulty experienced by a subject.

Two different groups of subjects were given this examination. The first group consisted of six patients in a neuropsychiatric hospital who were not capable of conducting their affairs or of taking care of their personal needs. The clinical diagnosis of each of these subjects was chronic brain syndrome. They were selected by the ward psychiatrist as being patients exhibiting the symptoms of senility without other complications. The subjects ranged in age from 60 to 72 years (median age 67.5 age years); and they had been hospitalized for from three to twelve years at the time of the study. There was nothing in a review of their educational or occupational history which indicated that the subjects had been deficient in either of these areas. Intelligence test scores from the Wechsler Adult Intelligence Scale did not reveal gross intellectual deficiencies, except that in one case the score was below the normal range (IQ score 71). In each case the history suggested a gradual onset of the symptoms which led to hospitalization. On admission and at the time of the experiment, an examination revealed no striking deep-tendon reflex abnormalities.

The performance of each of these subjects in the conditioning experiment was rated as "D". That is, after repeated presentations of the tones and the shock with one of these tones, no one in this group was able to anticipate the shock or to state the relationship between the tones and the shock. There was no evidence that any form of conditioning had occurred.

The second group of subjects studied were 24 domiciliary residents without a diagnosis of CNS damage. These subjects were not patients as were those in the first group. They were able to lead a normal life in the domiciliary residence, and all reported for the examination without assistance. In this group over half of the subjects achieved "A" scores; the others either had difficulty with or were unable to form the conditional reflex. Those who failed ("D" scores) gave responses which did not differ from those reported for the first group.

RESULTS AND CONCLUSIONS

The relationships between performance on this examination, IQ scores, and age are shown in Tables I and II. In terms of IQ scores, the group achieving "A" scores did not significantly differ from the group which was not able to do so. High IQ scores were found among both groups, and this result as well as the data from the first group suggests that conditionability is not a direct expression of the type of intellectual function measured by the standard measure of intelligence.

Neurological examinations were completed on most of the subjects. A relationship between the findings of the neurological examination and the performance on the conditioning examination was not evident. It appears that what is being measured is an aspect of human functioning not directly measured by the neurological examination.

TABLE I
Description of Performance Groups According to Age

Performance Group (Score)	Number of Patients	Age Range	Age Median
A	13	40–72	65
B, C, and D	11	62–76	68
Both Groups	24	40–76	65

Note: Difference between groups not significant, $P > 0.05$, median test.

TABLE II
Description of Performance Groups According to IQ Score

Performance Group (Score)	Number of Patients	IQ Score Range	IQ Score Median
A	13	80–121	102
B, C, and D	11	71–126	97
Both Groups	24	71–126	97

Note: Difference between groups not significant, $P > 0.05$, median test.

SUMMARY OF CONCLUSIONS

The results from the conditioning experiment with the two groups of subjects lead to the following conclusions:

1. Age in itself is not always accompanied by an impairment in the ability to form conditional reflexes.

2. The ability to form conditional reflexes is not correlated with intelligence test scores obtained from the standard intelligence test.

3. Impairment in the ability to form conditional reflexes may appear in the absence of neurological findings and therefore may be a precursor of these.

CHAPTER 9

Early Trauma as Revealed by Performance During Initial Conditioning

By A. ULRIC MOORE, Ph.D

This report will be, in effect, a survey of our work at the Behavior Farm Laboratory, at Cornell University, during the period since my last report to this group[1] and will include a brief summary of our most recent experiments.

The Behavior Farm Laboratory is still the only place in this country, so far as we know, where classical conditioned reflex training is being done or ever has been done with an animal free to move about in a room rather than confined in some sort of Pavlov frame.* Several important findings that result from this sort of training are not possible with the animal in a fixed position. For one thing, data can be taken in terms of activity that can be shown to correlate with the amount of emotional stability of the animal. The result is, in fact, an emotionality index similar to that derived from the Hall open-field test used for rats[2] except that the data in our test are taken automatically in terms of precise numbers rather than as observational records. Our data could also be fed directly into tape for computer processing, although to date we have not set up this phase of recording. Since my last report we have refined our methods so that the data obtained are more copious and more precise but do not involve more apparatus so far as the animal is concerned.

---

*Kupalov at the Pavlovian Institute in Leningrad has been doing what he calls "situational conditioning" since before the War, involving conditioning of the dog in a free state (personal communication to H. S. Liddell). The Worcester Foundation for Experimental Biology, Shrewsbury, Massachusetts, has just begun a three-year investigation of the effects of various blood proteins and drugs, including LSD, on emotionality in experimental animals (goats) using our laboratory technique as one of their methods of evaluating differences in response.

A switching system (Figs. 1 and 2) devised to assay pattern as well as amount of movement was added this spring to test mother-deprived bottle-fed kids, inasmuch as our previous experiment with 15 animals (kids and lambs) raised by stepmothers (sheep or goats) showed that the relation of the movement to the walls is at least as important, if not more so, as the amount moved [3-5]. We decided that we needed a more precise measure of this particular wall activity in order to reveal the differences between our experimental and control animals and to correlate with each animal's early experience his characteristic pattern during the conditioning session. We also decided to keep track of the amount of movement per minute by feeding the activity count into recording counters so

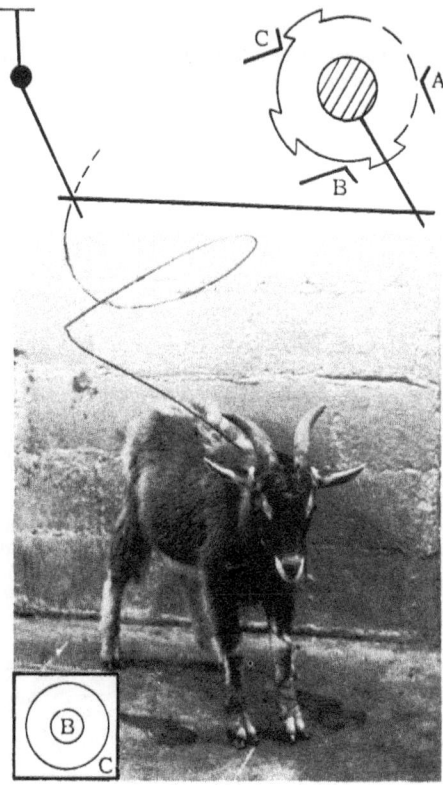

FIG. 1. Goat in the training situation plus a diagram (above) indicating how data are taken through selsyn motors and microswitches. This is a simplified drawing, not a perspective, so that one set of motor and switches is seen head on (right) and the other, which would be seen from the side, is not shown. The stick to the animal's spring attachment hangs from a rod in the center of the ceiling.

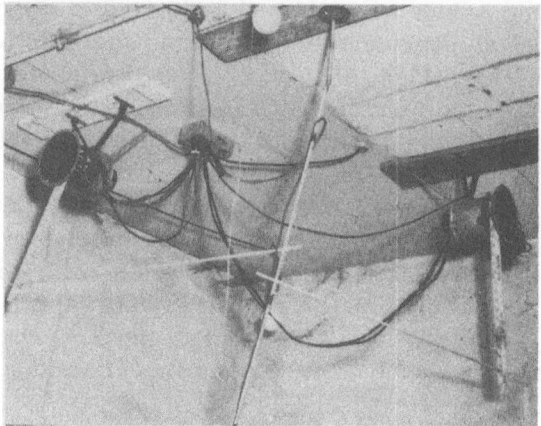

FIG. 2. (A) The motors in the ceiling with their black switching disks and attachment to the center stick hanging from a plate in the ceiling center. (Note: extra switches mentioned previously have not yet been added.)

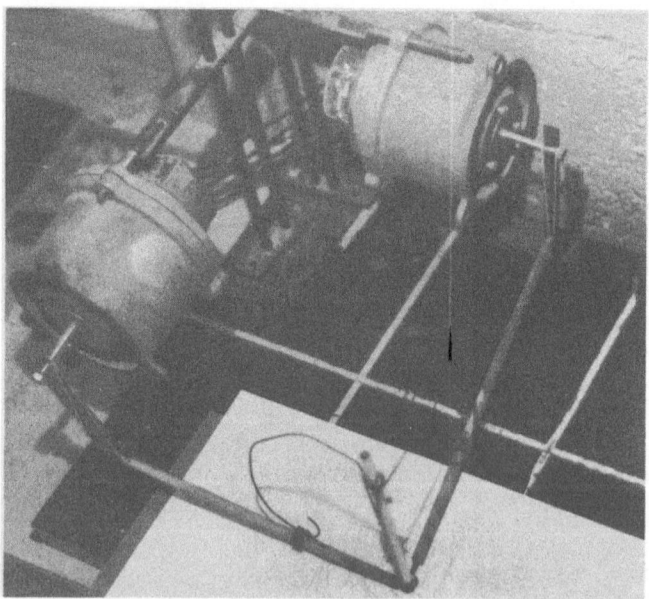

FIG. 2. (B) How the selsyn motors paired with ones activated by the animal (above) can draw a trace of the path the animal follows during any desired period.

that subtotals could be taken at intervals during the "training hour."

Thus, besides the trace of movement during the session (Fig. 3) and the amount the animal moved, we now have a record of the amount moved each minute and the percentage of time spent near the walls or in the center of the room. The five kids normally raised by their mothers and the five raised on bottles by a human attendant were tested in this way. The test proved a valuable adjunct to other tests applied to these animals in our current experimentation, which is part of a continuing joint project between the Behavior Farm Laboratory and the Department of Pediatrics of the New York State Medical College at Syracuse.*

In addition to measurements of dominance and degree of susceptibility to immobilization (animal hypnosis) and other tests reported elsewhere, we included a conditioning session in our Pavlov frame (Fig. 4) during which time we took records of heart and respiration rates and rectal temperature as well as of the conditioned leg flexion response to the signal. Results from the two conditioning sessions, one in the open field (free activity conditioning) and the other in the frame are summarized in Tables I, II, and III. Only the average figures are presented here. The experiments are discussed in much greater detail in other articles [6-8], and all have shown statistically significant differences between our control animals and those with experimentally altered mother-young relationships (mother-deprivation).

The findings presented in the three Tables are interpreted to imply higher emotionality and less stability in the experimental animals. These animals show initial high activity which fades out. Their heart rate is also initially higher and then diminishes somewhat. More important, however, both heart and respiration rates were definitely higher throughout the experiment than those of the controls. Perhaps the most interesting finding, or at least one that ties in with other work being done on emotionality [9], is the clear evidence for greater conditionability of the experimental animals. In all three indices tested, they undoubtedly showed greater plasticity: in speed of conditioning, i.e., how soon the first conditioned response occurred; in vigor of response, i.e., how many times the leg was lifted to any one signal; and in amount, i.e., how many signals were responded to. In this respect they were more

*This project has been supported in part by the Josiah Macy Jr. Foundation (at the Laboratory) and the Ford Foundation (at the Medical College) and is aimed at combining work at the animal and human level with respect to mother-young relationships.

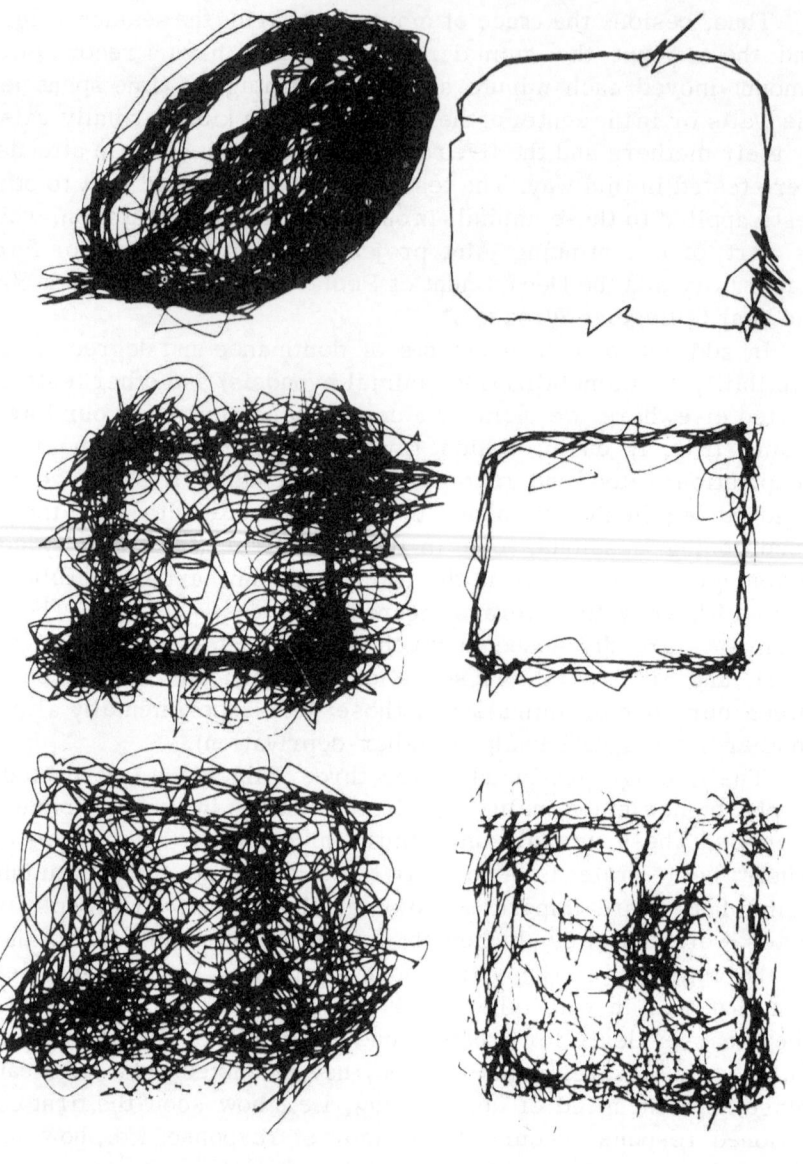

FIG. 3. Path traces of hyper- and hypoactive animals during a standard open-field condition-ing session. (The trace at lower right is closest to the norm.)

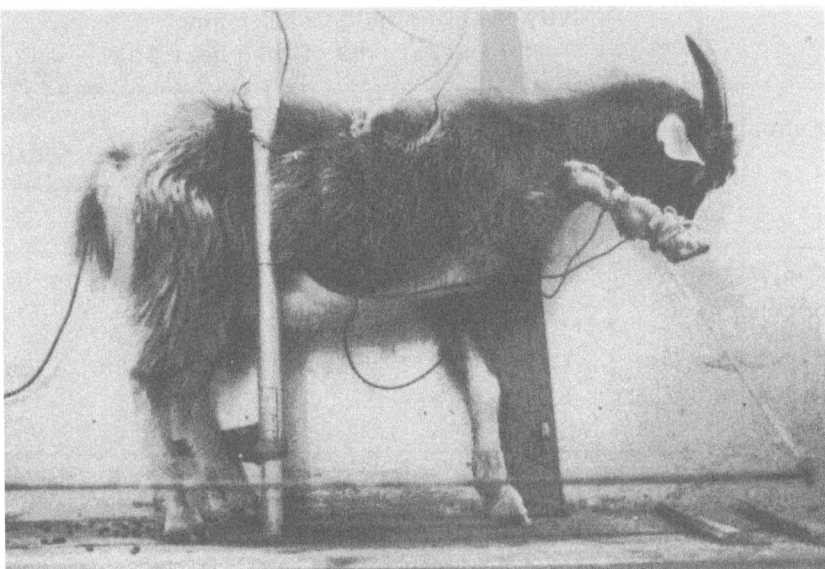

FIG. 4. Goat in Pavlov Frame.

The pipe in front of the goat's "hips" is one side of a narrow "V." The other side is formed by a board hinged to the wall (one of the hinges holding it to the wall can be seen back of the goat's hind-feet). Another tapered board (used for animals in reverse position) can be seen in back of the animal's front feet turned flat against the wall. The taper of this gives an idea of the size of the "V" that fits in front of the animal's hips and back of his rib cage to hold him in position. The pipe part of the "V" can be adjusted for various size animals but actually needs little change as the smaller animals are lower and hence hit the "V" at a narrower part. A bar can be lowered above the back of the animal on the pipe to prevent escape by the animal's rearing upwards. Occasionally a strap around the animal just back of the front legs, fastened to a rod lowered to just above the shoulders, is necessary in early training to prevent rearing or kneeling.

The other attachments are for recording. An electrode for rectal temperature, an electrical pick-up around the chest for respiration, and three electrodes for heart rate clipped back of the shoulders and left front leg are shown; and shock electrodes on the right foreleg are also used. The horizontal bar, seen at the bottom of picture, that angles up and is fastened to the lifted foreleg is for recording time and amount of leg flexion. The two parts are hinged together and the front part is held horizontal by a string to the ceiling, just visible at the right side of picture. The end out of sight at the left is fastened by a universal joint to the axel of a selsyn motor. This means that, though held horizontal by the string, the right end is still free to swing in a horizontal plane nearer or farther from the animal so that as he lifts his leg higher and higher, the horizontal part is turned more and more by the motion of the hinged section fastened to the foreleg and at the same time can move closer to the animal as need be. The turning of the horizontal bar turns the selsyn motor and through the action of its sympathetic twin can be made to move a writing pen or another instrument to record the movement of the animal's leg.

The two features of this arrangement that are unique with us are the frame itself and the hinged horizontal bar for recording leg movement. They are both far more successful in accomplishing their objectives than any other device for this purpose we have ever used. The rigid but not tight hip grip makes possible completely successful conditioning of animals at the very first session. Periods of struggling to escape are few and brief. The same is true of the hinged bar. It places practically no restriction upon the direction, amount, or speed of movement of the animal's foot and can be made to produce an accurate record of any of these indices.

TABLE I
Activity in Open-Field Conditioning
(feet per minute and per cent of time near wall)

Animal Groups	Before Signal Session		During Session		After Session	
	ft	%	ft	%	ft	%
Controls n - 5	4.8	80	8.7	75	0.08	98
Experimentals (bottle-fed) n - 5	18.7	40	11.8	70	3.0	50

Note: A difference between both the amount of movement and percentage of time near the wall exists in the presignal period for the two groups. However, as soon as signals start for the first period, the controls show a rise in amount of activity and the experimentals show a fall, so that the amount now does not significantly differ. Furthermore, the experimentals' percentage of time near the wall rises sharply, whereas the controls' percentage remains about the same, so that in this respect, too, they are now about equal. But as soon as the signal session is over, there is a marked drop in activity for both groups, but the controls' activity drops significantly lower and at the same time the controls spend a higher percentage of time near the wall. All differences mentioned throughout this paper are significant at least at the 5% level, and many as low as 1%. The Kolmogorov-Smirnov two-sample test or Mann-Whitney U test was used in most instances.

TABLE II
Physiological Indices during Conditioning in the Frame
(heart and respiration rates per minute)

Animal Groups	Before Start of Signals (hour session)		During the 2-min Intervals (20 intervals)		During Each 10-sec Signal (20 signals)	
	Heart	Respiration	Heart	Respiration	Heart	Respiration
Controls n - 5	104	48	97	44	99	44
Experimentals (bottle-fed) n - 5	123	87	117	98	114	110

Note: Experimental animals gave higher readings in both indices in all situations. Whereas the onset of signals had little effect on the controls, the respiration rate of the experimentals increased, becoming still faster at each signal, and the heart rate decreased, becoming still slower with the signals. This is true for all the experimental animals, though admittedly the change in each instance is rather slight. The temperature of each animal changed during the session but no correlations were evident.

TABLE III

Specific Conditionability (leg flexion during first 60 signals)

Animal Groups	Speed of Conditioning	Vigor of Conditioning	Amount of Conditioning
	(1st signal responded to)	(number of flexions per signal)	(% of signals responded to)
Controls n - 5	26th	0.35	13
Experimentals (bottle-fed) n - 5	13th	1.33	65

Note: Experimentals exceeded controls in all categories.

like the very young animals conditioned in previous experiments [1] than like normal animals of their own age. It has been shown that in humans those with higher emotionality condition more easily [10]. The animal work is less conclusive [11, 12], but our findings definitely support Pavlov's finding[13] that more excitable animals condition more quickly.

The present trend of the work is continuing along the line so well established by Liddell [14], who showed that all classical conditioning of the animal is stressful, particularly of the immature animal [15], and that such stress may be produced not only in the laboratory situation but also in the animal's natural life by an altered infant relationship to its mother [16]. We have continued to extend the analysis of this stress to the animal's whole life cycle and hope to establish implications at the human level through our joint experimentation with the Pediatrics Department of Syracuse Memorial Hospital headed by Dr. Julius B. Richmond and participated in by Dr. Helen Blauvelt [17] and Dr. Leonard Hersher [18].

REFERENCES

1. Moore, A. U.: Conditioning and stress in the newborn lamb and kid, in Gantt, W. H., Ed.: Physiological Bases of Psychiatry, Thomas, Springfield, 1958.

2. Hall, C. S.: Drive and emotionality: factors associated with adjustment in the rat, J. Comp. Psychol. 17:89, 1934.

3. Moore, A. U., and Amstey, M. S.: Animal hypnosis (tonic immobility) considered as a parameter of behavior in distinguishing between a group of normal and abnormal (experimental) lambs and kids, Anat. Rec. 138:371, 1960.

4. Moore, A. U., and Blauvelt, Helen: Behavior during a conditioned reflex training period used as a measure of early trauma in lamb and kid, ibid. 139: 1961.

5. Blauvelt, Helen, Hersher, L., and Moore, A. U.: The social behavior of goats deprived of maternal and herd care, ibid. 139: 1961.

6. Moore, A. U., and Amstey, M. S.: Tonic immobility: differences in susceptibility of experimental and normal sheep and goats, Science 135:729, 1962.

7. Moore, A. U., and Amstey, M. S.: Mother-neonate separation and tonic immobility in goats, to be published.

8. Amstey, M. S., and Moore, A. U.: Decreased inhibitory activity as a result of three different drugs, to be published.

9. Broadhurst, P. L.: Determinants of emotionality in the rat, Brit. J. Psychol. 48:1, 1957.

10. Runquist, W. N., and Ross, L. E.: The relation between physiological measures of emotionality and performance in eyelid conditioning, J. Exp. Psychol. 57: 329, 1959.

11. Tobach, E. and Schneirla, T. C.: Eliminative responses in mice and rats and the problem of "emotionality," in Bliss, E., Ed.: Roots of Behavior, Hoeber, New York, in press.

12. James, W. T.: Morphological and constitutional factors in conditioning, Ann. N. Y. Acad. Sc. 56:171, 1953.

13. Pavlov, I. P.: Conditioned Reflexes, Oxford University Press, Oxford, 1927. (Anrep, G. V., Trans. and Ed.)

14. Liddell, H. S.: Emotional Hazards in Animals and Man, Thomas, Springfield, 1956.

15. Moore, A. U.: Growth retardation in the goat during periods of conditioned reflex training, Anat. Rec. 134:611, 1959.

16. Hersher, L., Moore, A. U., and Richmond, J. B.: Effect of post-partum separation of mother and kid on maternal care in the domestic goat, Science 128:1342, 1958.

17. Blauvelt, Helen, and McKenna, J.: Capacity of the human newborn for mother-infant interaction. II. The temporal dimensions of a neonate response, Psychiat. Res. Rep. 13:128, 1960.

18. Hersher, L., Richmond, J. B., and Moore, A. U.: Modifiability of the critical period for the development of maternal behavior in sheep and goats. Behaviour, in press.

II SYMPOSIUM ON ETHOLOGY

CHAPTER 10

The Fixed Action Pattern: Empirical Properties and Theoretical Implications

By HOWARD MOLTZ, PH.D.

In a recent article, Lorenz [1, p. 53] wrote, "Like genetics and many other branches of inductive science, ethology started from a real discovery and definitely not from a theory. This is a fact that we do not want to be forgotten." The discovery to which Lorenz referred was made independently at the beginning of the present century by two zoologists, Charles Whitman and Oskar Heinroth. What they discovered was that certain behavior patterns are so typical of particular taxonomic groups as to provide reliable criteria for systematic classification—as reliable, in most cases, as anatomical structures. Behavior patterns having the same or similar properties were subsequently identified in a number of vertebrate and invertebrate forms and were designated as "instinctive movements" (Erbkoordinationen) by Lorenz and as "fixed actions patterns" (FAPs) by most other ethologists.

The concept of the FAP has come to occupy an important position in ethological research as well as in certain areas of ethological theorizing. Indeed, one can hardly discuss the character of contemporary ethology without reference to the empirical and theoretical roles which the FAP currently plays. As part of my contribution to this symposium, I should like to report on both these roles, first by discussing the observable properties of FAPs and then by discussing some hypotheses that have been formulated regarding the physiological events assumed to underlie their development and organization.

This paper was written while the author was in receipt of Research Grant M-3855 from the National Institutes of Health, Public Health Service. It is a pleasure to acknowledge my indebtedness to Dr. Evelyn Raskin for critically reading the manuscript and for offering many important suggestions.

EMPIRICAL PROPERTIES

Despite the attention that has been accorded the FAP, there is no consensus among ethologists in general or among instinct theorists in particular regarding the characteristics considered necessary to distinguish it from all other types of behavior. To be sure, there is widespread agreement that FAPs comprise a unique class of responses, but there is little agreement concerning the criteria requisite for class inclusion. Baerends [2], for example, treats the settling movements involved in incubation as an example of an FAP but declines to regard the form of the movement as independent of extrinsic stimulus control. For Lorenz, however, such independence is one of the primary characteristics of any FAP. Thus it is that the four properties which I shall mention in attempting to describe the empirical character of the FAP would not unanimously be regarded as constituting either unique or necessary differentia. However, I believe that each would generally be considered to have raised rather important theoretical issues. It was on this basis that I have elected to discuss them.

The Stereotypy of the FAP

A reasonably precise distinction is often made by ethologists between appetitive behavior and consummatory acts. The distinction is based on the observation that a behavior sequence frequently consists of two phases, a flexible initial phase and a final, more-or-less sterotyped phase. The hunting behavior of the peregrine falcon, for example, usually begins with unoriented "exploratory" flights within the hunting territory and concludes with the relatively invariable locomotor acts involved in killing, plucking, and eating the captured prey [3].

"Appetitive behavior" is the term used to designate the labile components of such a behavior sequence, while "consummatory act" is the term used to designate the rigid and inflexible components.

Those movement or movement patterns designated as FAPs are classified as consummatory acts since they usually comprise the terminal aspects of a response chain and since they are rigidly stereotyped and constant in form. Theory stereotypy is to be particularly emphasized: indeed, in this respect they have been compared with morphological traits for, as Whitman and Heinroth initially pointed out, FAPs are expressed in a highly invariant manner within a taxonomic group [1].

As an example of this invariance, consider an aspect of the reproductive behavior of the three-spined stickleback. Aeration of the stickleback nest, which is apparently necessary to maintain the oxygen concentration of the surrounding water at a level appropriate for egg development, is accomplished through a movement referred to as "fanning." This consists of using the pectoral fins to exert a forward pressure on the water and simultaneously using the tail and caudal fin to exert a backward pressure equal in intensity to the forward pressure. The result, of course, is that the fish's position remains unchanged while fresh water is moved across the eggs. The invariance of the fanning pattern is evident in the coordination maintained between the pectorals on the one hand and the caudal fin and tail on the other. That is to say, the temporal sequence of movements performed by these structures is the same on each occasion that fanning occurs. Indeed, although the fish may alter the angle between the longitudinal axis of its body and the substrate in response to the experimenter tilting the nest, say 45°, the patterning or coordination of the component response elements remains constant [4]. Even when fanning is performed in the absence of a nest (i.e., when it occurs as a so-called vacuum activity) and the fish, as a consequence, maintains its body parallel to the substrate, the fish still fans in precisely the same manner as it does on those occasions when the nest is present.

Through the use of cinematographic records, Dane, Walcott, and Drury [5] have been able to provide interesting evidence with respect to the stereotypy of several movements exhibited by the goldeneye duck. One of these movements, constant in both form and duration, has been referred to as the "simple head throw." This consists of a rigid extension of the neck, a movement which serves to raise the head about 6 in. above the water. At this height the head is brought back, turned around, and lowered onto the rump. If it is assumed that uniformity in the time taken to perform a response is an index of rigidity, then the simple head throw is indeed rigid. The mean time involved in the performance of this movement is 1.29 seconds with a standard deviation of only 0.08 seconds. (See also [6].)

There are many stereotyped movements that are exhibited not only by a particular species but by taxonomic groups larger than the species. Tinbergen [7], for example, has recently reported on the "display actions" of gulls belonging to the family Laridae. It is maintained that the general function of avian displays is to "release" or elicit selected responses from other members of the species, thus facilitating social and sexual interaction [8, 9]. With respect to the stereotypy of displays throughout the gull family, Tinbergen writes: "In spite of the differences between species, there is for each display, a degree of similarity between species as striking as the morphological similarities" [p. 11]. For example, in the preliminary stages of pair formation, gulls exhibit a movement designated as "head tossing." Depending on the species, this movement may be performed once or it may be repeated several times in rapid succession; it may be performed with the bill closed; or, if the bill is opened, it may be opened slightly or opened wide. But despite this variability, head tossing is readily identifiable, since it consists essentially of pointing the head forward at an oblique angle and then tossing it upwards and backwards with a sharp motion. It is this stable core of response elements to which species' differences have become affixed and which permits head tossing and similarly constituted displays to be classified as FAPs.

It is worth pointing out that there are some movements which exhibit even less interspecific variability than the displays of gulls. Among surface-feeding ducks, for example, many courtship movements have been found to be remarkably stereotyped, although exhibited by species strikingly different in external appearance [10, 11]. What is particularly interesting here is that these highly invariant movements are combined or coupled differently in each species, so that the courtship configuration is interspecifically variable while the constituent elements are interspecifically constant. Thus in the mallard, the "head-up tail-up" courtship movement is followed by the "nod-swim" one, while in the gadwall it is followed by the "down-up" movement. In the European teal, "head-up tail-up" is followed by a movement designated as "turn-toward-female," while in the Bahama pintail it is not followed immediately by any distinctive movement.

Occasionally, an FAP is found among members of a systematic group even larger than the family. For example, the "wing-leg" and "double-wing-neck stretch" movements are distributed throughout the class Aves [12], and the scratching movement, which is performed with the hindlimb crossed over the forelimb, is common to most amniotes [11]. These examples are especially dramatic in view of the morphological diversity of the species involved.

On the basis of what has been said thus far, it should be apparent that the stereotyped movements which ethologists have designated as FAPs are quite different from the instinctive action systems of which McDougall spoke. For him the distinguishing feature of such a system was its plasticity and lability. McDougall was concerned neither with the temporal sequence of muscular contractions comprising a response nor indeed with individual responses as such. His emphasis was on the "appetitive quality" of behavior: the variable initial aspect that terminates in goal attainment. He would have found the stereotyped and particulate nature of the FAP quite alien.

Independence from Immediate External Control

What I mean by "independence from external control" can best be illustrated by contrasting the FAP with those movements or movement patterns which have been termed "taxes." In most cases the distinction between a taxis and an FAP can easily be drawn, since the taxis is often more variable in form than the FAP. However, some taxes are performed from one occasion to the next in a comparatively rigid manner, making stereotypy in itself insufficient for classifying a movement as an FAP. Additional criteria must obviously be invoked. One such criterion, relevant specifically to the distinction between the taxis and the FAP, is freedom from immediate external control. That is, if a movement pattern is to be classified as an FAP, the temporal sequence of muscle contractions comprising the pattern must be independent of afferent regulation. Such independence is evidenced by the fact that the movement will often continue to completion irrespective of changes in external conditions. A taxis does not possess this property, for, in contrast to the FAP, it is continuously directed by events external to the animal. Once elicited, it remains oriented with respect to its eliciting stimulus, ceasing to occur when these stimuli are removed. The following behavior pattern, described in detail by Lorenz and Tinbergen [13], illustrates the difference between the taxis and the FAP:

A brooding graylag goose that sees an egg that has rolled out of its nest reacts in a characteristic manner. After alternately glancing toward and away from the egg, the goose stretches its neck and begins to stare intently. It then slowly rises from the nest and approaches the displaced egg. Upon the goose's reaching it, the neck is extended downwards and forwards so that the undersurface of the bill comes to rest against the far side of the egg. Two distinct movements are then employed which serve to roll the displaced egg in the direction of the nest: a sagittal movement that keeps the egg rolling in the bird's median plane and a lateral, or side-to-side, movement that keeps it from deviating too far either to the right or to the left. The sagittal movement has been classified as an FAP, the lateral movement as a taxis.

Consider the characteristics of the sagittal movement. Its form remains constant despite the irregularities of the terrain over which the egg is rolled and despite differences in the shape of those objects that have been experimentally substituted for the egg. Furthermore, if the egg rolls away from the bill, as occasionally happens in the natural situation, the sagittal movement does not usually cease. Instead, the goose will often continue to perform this movement in the same manner it did when the egg was present, indicating that once elicited, the movement is no longer under extrinsic control.

The lateral, or side-to-side, movement, in contrast, is both evoked and continuously directed by contact of the egg with the undersurface of the bill. If the egg deviates slightly from the birds median plane, a compensatory movement either to the right or to the left immediately restores it to its path. If an object that is unlikely to deviate (e.g., a cylinder or light wooden cube) is substituted for the displaced egg, few or no lateral movements are performed. And lastly, if the egg happens to roll completely free of the bill, the lateral movement ceases while the sagittal movement continues until the goose reaches the nest.

The head-turning response of the human infant can also be used to illustrate the difference between a taxis and an FAP. The neonate performs a rhythmical side-to-side movement of the head, the axis of which runs through the vertebral column. This movement can be evoked by tactile stimulation of a large, undifferentiated area around the mouth and occasionally by tactile stimulation of other parts of the body [14]. Once elicited, the movement is not only stereotyped but independent of its eliciting stimulus. It is worth noting that at two or three weeks postpartum (but considerably longer in premature babies) the rhythmical side-to-side movement develops into a spatially oriented response. Unlike the side-to-side movement, this response is variable in form and is specifically directed toward a particular locus of stimulation. Prechtl [14, p. 238] concludes that "it is obvious that the side-to-side movement is an Erbkoordination [FAP] in the sense of Lorenz and directed head turning a taxis."

Egg rolling by the graylag goose and head turning by the human infant offer clear examples of the distinction between taxis and FAP. It should not be concluded, however, that this distinction can always be drawn so easily. In many cases it is difficult to determine whether a particular movement is directed by external events or is simply released by such events and consequently whether it is to be classified as a taxis or as an FAP [15]. Furthermore, the taxis and the FAP frequently occur either simultaneously or in close succession, such "interlocking" making differentiation additionally difficult [9]. But despite these difficulties, independence from immediate external control serves as an important criterion for classifying a movement pattern as an FAP.

At this point it is appropriate to emphasize what has thus far been implicit in our discussion, viz., that the FAP does not possess the characteristics of a chain reaction. Although it may involve a relatively complex pattern of muscle contractions, the FAP cannot be fractionized into successive response links through the manipulation of "qualitatively different external stimuli ..." [16, p. 574]. Each element of an FAP, in other words, can be elicited only by the same stimulus or stimulus complex as that which elicits the entire FAP. Consequently, in referring to a particular movement pattern as an FAP, the word "pattern" is to be thought of as an amalgam of behavioral elements that cannot be further analyzed into parts having different stimulus factors responsible for their evocation.

Spontaneity

A third property of the FAP is its alleged spontaneity. I use the word "spontaneity" here to indicate fluctuations in threshold that are independent of changes in external conditions. The general rule observed to apply to such fluctuations is that an organism's readiness to perform a particular FAP and the intensity with which that performance occurs are a positive function of the time elapsing since the movement was last evoked.

Lorenz and Tinbergen [13] pointed out that it was much easier to reelicit the egg rolling of the graylag goose, particularly the sagittal component, the longer one waited before presenting the animal with a displaced egg. Van Iersel [17] demonstrated that when a male stickleback is prevented from fanning for several minutes, a significant increase in the intensity of this activity will occur after the fish is allowed to return to its nest. It has been shown that such extrinsic conditions as the accumulation of carbon dioxide and other gases released by the eggs in the fish's absence were not involved by repeating the experiment and keeping the nest completely covered.

Fatigue has also been ruled out as a factor contributing to the fluctuations in the occurrence and intensity of FAPs. If one keeps a cichlid in close confinement with conspecifics so that stimuli evoking fighting are continuously present, the thresholds of such "agonistic" movements as lateral tail beating, spreading the gill membrane, and erecting the median fins are raised [1]. That this is not due to general fatigue is evidenced by the fact that the fish will at the same time perform other activities that involve the same effectors and that appear to require just as much effort.

The most dramatic bit of evidence regarding the spontaneity of the FAP is its tendency under certain circumstances to "go off of itself without any outward stimulus" [18]. That is, when an FAP has been prevented from occurring for a considerable period by the withholding of the external stimulus normally responsible for its "release," it will sometimes be performed in the absence of that stimulus. An FAP that occurs under such conditions is referred to as having occurred in vacuo and is an extreme example of the extent to which the readiness to perform an FAP can fluctuate.

The most frequently cited instance of in-vacuo performance is provided by Lorenz's [9] description of fly catching by a well-fed hand-reared starling that had been deprived of the opportunity to catch flies for a considerable time. Lorenz reports that the starling suddenly flew up, searched the ceiling of the room for insects, snapped at nothing discernible, returned to its perch, performed the tossing movements by which many insectivorous birds kill their prey, and finally swallowed several times.

A more appropriate example of the in-vacuo performance of a particular FAP is provided by van Iersel [17] who reports that fanning is occasionally exhibited in perfect detail by the stickleback in the absence of a nest. Similarly, Prechtl [14] found that the side-to-side head turning of the infant will frequently occur without benefit of an external eliciting stimulus. And finally, Lorenz [19] has called attention to the fact that the complex motor pattern involved in the weaver bird weaving strands for its nest is sometimes performed in the absence of plant fibers that normally serve as the functional object.

Vacuum activities are performed infrequently and under abnormal conditions. However, as has already been mentioned, the tendency for less extreme variations in elicitability to occur as a function of the time elapsing since previous performance is considered to be characteristic of all FAPs. Moreover, this characteristic is often emphasized in the attempt to distinguish the FAP from reflexes or reflex-like movements [12, 13, 18, 20]. Activation of the patellar reflex, for example, does not occur more easily if it has not been elicited for a long period of time. And while it is of course possible to "exhaust" this reflex by repeated stimulation, what is exhausted is not the patellar reflex, as such, but the effectors involved in its execution. Repeated evocation of an FAP, on the other hand, is considered to result in a specific type of exhaustion, as evidenced by the fact that the same effectors can be used in the performance of other motor activities. Lorenz [18, p. 247] puts it succinctly in stating that under repeated attempts to evoke an FAP it will "cease to be at the disposal of the organism long before the organism as a whole or its effectors are tired out."

Independence from Individual Learning

"Unless the changes of environment impinging on the animal during its development are so radical as to impair its physical health in appreciable degree, no changes in instinctive movements can be noticed at all" [1, p. 54]. That is to say, the form or coordination of an FAP will be performed in species-typical fashion despite wide fluctuations in environmental conditions during ontogeny. This is considered by many ethologists to indicate that, among other things, FAPs are not learned, that is, that they are neither influenced by nor in any way dependent upon conditioning, imitation, or other processes usually designated as learning. Accordingly, we may specify a fourth criterion for membership in the class of fixed action patterns: exclusion of the possibility that the movement or movement pattern has been specifically learned prior to its first occurrence.

The isolation technique is frequently regarded as the critical method for assessing the influence of learning. In its simplest form, this technique consists of removing an animal at the time of birth or hatching from members of its own species and then determining whether the response in which the experimenter is interested is subsequently performed in a manner identical to that shown by animals raised with conspecifics.

Tinbergen [21] reports that male sticklebacks reared in isolation performed a typical zigzag dance before they had ever seen another stickleback; in fact, it was performed on the first occasion that they were introduced to a cardboard model of a gravid female. Cullen [22] recently obtained the same results using a larger number of animals in a more carefully controlled experimental situation.

Frequently the conditions of isolation are such as to prevent the isolates from practicing the response. Grohmann [23], for example, raised pigeons in individual cages that were so small that the birds were unable to make any wing-beat movements. They nevertheless flew upon release in a manner indistinguishable from controls. Grohmann's experiment has been cited [e.g., 12] as evidence that the wing-beat movements used in flying are not learned, since they appear in perfect detail in animals deprived of the opportunity either to observe or practice them.

However, the isolation technique is not the only means of excluding the possibility that a movement pattern has been learned. Thus, the side-to-side head movement of the human infant is present at birth [14] and the gaping response of the thrush is present at hatching [24]. The fact that these and many other movements designated as FAPs occur so early in ontogeny is taken to indicate that they could not have been learned in any ordinary sense of that term.

Occasionally, rather dramatic examples are adduced to illustrate the independence of the FAP from individual learning. In one species of surface-feeding ducks, courtship involves a preening movement by which the drake exposes a brilliantly colored tertiary feather that it wriggles in a striking manner. Lorenz [19, p. 171] reports the case of a drake that had, for unknown reasons, failed to develop this feather but which nonetheless persisted in performing this preening movement "an inch above his back where the feather should have been." It was argued that since the movement occurred independently of the feather structure, the form that it initially exhibited could not have been due to previous specific practice.

The fighting behavior of the goose is also cited as a dramatic example [21]. The goose holds its adversary with its bill and "beats" it with a sharp forward motion of its wing. Now, a young gosling in an aggressive encounter holds its adversary in exactly the same position in space and uses exactly the same beating movement despite the fact that its wings are not large enough to touch its opponent. This has been regarded as an example of a movement appearing in ontogeny long before it possesses functional utility and hence long before a (presumably) necessary condition for learning is present.

A final point regarding learning can be conveniently made here. I refer to the conception entertained by some ethologists that learning necessarily involves reinforcement, the implication, of course, being that if no source of reinforcement can be identified in connection with a particular response, then that response is perforce not learned. Eibl-Eibesfeldt and Kramer [12, p. 184] are quite explicit on this point. They write that "experiments with animals have ... shown that those fixed patterns may develop independently of a specific pattern of previous reinforcement, i.e., learning" (also see [19]). Most of us, of course, need hardly be reminded that the issue of whether reinforcement is necessary for the acquisition of conditioned responses is still quite controversial. But despite their tendency to regard the absence of reinforcement as evidence of the absence of learning, there is no doubt that ethologists have pointed to many complex aspects of animal behavior which are certainly not learned. This is not to say that they have thereby demonstrated the reality of behavior elements that are uninfluenced during ontogeny by extrinsic stimulus conditions, or by what may be more succinctly labeled "experience." It is important to note in this connection that learning and experience are not equivalent agents in the determination of behavior, the influence of experience being much broader and more pervasive than that which is usually regarded as learning or habit acquisition. Thus, while most ethologists would agree that learning does not enter into the development of the FAP, not all would agree that the FAP thereby develops without experimential regulation.

THEORETICAL IMPLICATIONS

Up to this point I have treated the FAP as a descriptive concept in the attempt to delineate its empirical characteristics. I assiduously avoided using such terms as "preformed" or "inherited," since I was concerned, not with inferred events, but with observable properties. Now, however, I should like to examine some of the mechanisms or processes that have been assumed by instinct theorists to underlie the development and organization of the FAP.

Genetic Encoding

Instinct theorists refer to the FAP as being "innate," "genetically determined," "part of the original constitution of the organism," etc. Eibl-Eibesfeldt and Kramer [12, p. 184], for example, state that "just as the mallard duck inherits its green head... it also inherits its grunting whistle." And Lorenz maintains that behavioral traits of this kind "are not something which animals may do or not do, or do in different ways according to the requirements of the occasion, but something which animals of a given species 'have got' exactly in the same manner as they 'have got' claws or teeth of a definite morphological structure" [25, p. 238].

Now it should be pointed out that such statements are not to be interpreted as implying that instinct theorists believe that FAPs develop independently of a specific embryogenic environment. They are well aware that there is no trait, either behavioral or organic, that could possibly do so; all organismic traits obviously develop in response to both genotypic and environmental factors. What then is controversial about the statements we quoted? Broadly stated, it is the implication that the genic constitution participates in or contributes to the FAP in a direct and specific manner. Indeed, it is often more than just implied. Lorenz and others are quite explicit in maintaining that each FAP is genetically encoded and that such encoding is expressed in the organization of neural centers which function to control and coordinate the sequence of muscle actions involved in performance. In other words, they conceive FAP's to be centrally preformed in the sense that a genotypically fixed correspondence or isomorphism is assumed to exist between the details of a particular FAP and the anatomical and physiological characteristics of the neural mechanism underlying it. Bullock [26, p. 55] has stated that instinct theorists' position on this point quite clearly: "It seems at present highly likely that for many complex behavioral actions the nervous system contains not only genetically determined circuits but also genetically determined physiological properties of their components so that the complete act is presented in coded form and awaits only an adequate trigger, either internal or external."

There is, of course, no longer any doubt that certain brain areas function in the integration of certain types of behavior. As examples, one need recall only the recent research of Miller [27], Andersson [28], and Harris [29] to realize the close association that has been demonstrated between neural loci and specific responses.

But instinct theorists go much further, for they speak of the FAP as being, not only centrally integrated, but also centrally itemized— itemization that is directly provided for in the growth process itself. And they contend that it is by virtue of this intrinsically established itemization that the FAP, as a temporally patterned system of response elements, can appear without having been onto-genetically organized. Indeed, since such systems are considered to be genetically specified down to the smallest detail, the influence of extrinsic factors in determining their configuration is held to be not only unnecessary but ineffective [9].

In view, then, of the highly specific encoding that is postulated, it is understandable that instinct theorists speak of the FAP as being "innate" in much the same sense that skull structure, for example, is spoken of as innate. Not that either one is conceived to develop during embryogeny without environmental participation, but in each case the extent to which experiential events are re-sponsible for organizing and modulating phenotypic expression is "held to be inconsiderable to the point of being negligible" [1, p. 53]. And it is also understandable, again granting the specific encoding, that they speak of FAPs as constituting the nucleus of an animal's response repertoire, a nucleus that is overlaid with acquired elements during ontogeny but that can nonetheless be identified in the behavior of the adult organism.

Action-Specific Energy

Instinct theorists have been particularly impressed with the spontaneity of the FAP, often regarding it as that property which renders the FAP a unique type of behavioral event. Its fluctuation in threshold, its independence of external stimulation, and its tendency to go off in vacuo have been referred to as constituting the "main completely unsolved problem regarding instinctive movements ..." [12, p. 185].

To Lorenz, this spontaneity suggested the operation of intrinsic mechanisms of excitation. More specifically, it suggested that each FAP possesses its own source of energy which accumulates in that locus of the central nervous system responsible for its co-ordination. This accumulation is assumed to occur while the par-ticular movement is quiescent and to be expended when the movement is discharged. In other words, a reservoir-type model of motivation was proposed: response-specific energy flows away in action and is subsequently replenished during rest.

An additional aspect worth mentioning is that the energy is

conceived to arouse appetitive behavior which presumably continues until the animal attains the stimulus situation necessary to release the FAP (and thus consume the energy) or until the energy reaches a level sufficient to cause the FAP to erupt in vacuo. As Lorenz [25, p. 248] puts it: "Any one of these particular innate behavior patterns, however small and unimportant it may seem in itself, develops into an active source of excitation which influences the whole of the organism whenever it finds its outlet blocked. In this case the undischarged activity becomes a motive in the literal and original sense of the word, derived from *movere*, 'to move.'"

Tinbergen [31] has also used an essentially similar model, except that he incorporated it in a somewhat different framework. Tinbergen proposed a hierarchically organized system of neural centers responsible for the activation of a chain of functionally related activities (e.g., those involved in reproduction). Such a chain was conceived to begin with appetitive behavior of a very general nature and to terminate in a discrete and particulate con-summatory act. Each center except the uppermost was assumed to receive motivational impulses from the one above it as well as to be "loaded from within" by its own excitatory mechanism.

What is of particular theoretical interest with respect to the reservoir-type model of motivation is the assumption that energy not only accumulates in a specific center but that it is generated by that center, and what is more, generated in an organized fashion. In other words, the instinct theorist assumes that motor impulses are endogenously produced and that the basic pattern of production not only occurs independently of afferent inflow but is in fact re-fractory to modulation by such inflow.

In maintaining that the spontaneity of the FAP is a manifestation of a purely central automaticity, the instinct theorist points to cardiac and respiratory activities, as well as other basic functions, and considers evidence regarding their spontaneity as providing clues for understanding the neurological basis of complex be-havioral spontaneity. In this connection, the studies of Adrian [30], von Holst [31], Maynard [32] and others are frequently cited. Adrian and Buytendijk [33], for example, concluded that respiratory activity is endogenously generated after they found that potential changes recorded from the isolated brain stem of the goldfish exhibit the same frequency as that of normal breathing movements. And Maynard [32] found that when the factors which influence heart beat in the lobster are held constant, a complex, periodic pattern of impulses is still generated by the cardiac ganglion.

It is important to note in this context that one can never be certain, even when working with isolated nerve-cell preparations, that the environment is not partly responsible for the pattern of excitation that is present [30]. All that one can be sure of is that a particular neural rhythm is not the result of a corresponding afferent rhythm. However, let us concede that the rhythmically recurring activities that we have just mentioned are in fact endogenously generated—that neither phasic nor nonphasic sensory input is necessary for their production. Even so, it obviously requires a considerably long inductive leap to go from the comparatively simple functioning evidenced by an isolated segment of the nervous system to the temporally organized behavior of the intact animal. But it is precisely this leap that the instinct theorist has taken. And although it shows boldness and imagination, it must be emphasized that there is no evidence presently available to suggest that the spontaneity of the FAP is neurologically akin to the spontaneity of a deafferented ganglion. Although the possibility of such a relationship should not be summarily dismissed, it should be considered speculative in the extreme.

CONCLUSION

If one considers the empirical properties of the FAP as well as the theoretical correlates that have been deduced therefrom, it should be apparent that the FAP is not at all similar to response patterns that have been traditionally regarded as "instinctive" and which have usually been given such global designations as "maternal behavior," "filial behavior," "migratory behavior," etc. What must be emphasized is that each of these labels refers to a complex of functionally related activities of which only a few might be both empirically and conceptually identical to the FAP. Recall the properties of the FAP—stereotypy, resistance to external control, spontaneity, independence from individual learning; recall the mechanisms that have been assumed by instinct theorists to be causally related to these properties—genetic encoding and endogenous generation; now think of the potpourri of activities that comprise the maternal behavior of the rat—nest building, devouring the placenta, licking and cleaning the young, huddling, nursing, retrieving, etc. Few, if any, of these activities possess the empirical properties of the FAP. And to my knowledge, no contemporary instinct theorist ever considered maternal behavior, as such, to be innate in the same sense that the FAP is considered to be innate. Certainly, it is manifestly irrelevant to criticize either the reality or the significance of the FAP by showing that patterns like maternal behavior, or any pattern of such heterogeneous composition, is experientially organized and consequently could be neither genetically encoded nor endogenously generated. The tendency to identify the FAP with traditional instincts—a tendency that has been all too prevalent—has led to a good deal of confusion and to several inappropriate evaluations.

One final point. Since I considered my task at this symposium to be that of simply reporting on the empirical and conceptual status of the FAP, I largely refrained from criticizing certain aspects of it. I must say that this required a measure of self-control, for I believe that there is much that warrants criticizm. Perhaps in the discussion that is to follow some of these criticisms will be considered without, I hope, losing sight of the importance of this contribution.

REFERENCES

1. Lorenz, K.: The objective theory of instinct. in L'Instinct dans le Comportement des Animaux et de l'Homme, Masson et Cie, Paris, 1956.

2. Baerends, G. P.: The ethological analysis of incubation behaviour, Ibis 101:357, 1959.

3. Tinbergen, N.: The Study of Instinct, Oxford Univ. Oxford Press, 1951.

4. Baerends, G. P.: The ethological analysis of fish behavior. in Brown, M. E., Ed.: The Physiology of Fishes, Vol. II, Academic Press, New York, 1957.

5. Dane, B., Walcott, C., and Drury, W. H.: The form and duration of the display actions of the goldeneye *(Bucephala clangula)* Behaviour 14:265, 1959.

6. Morris, D.: 'Typical intensity' and its relation to the problem of ritualisation, ibid. 11:1, 1957.

7. Tinbergen, N. Comparative study of the behaviour of gulls (Laridae): A progress report, Behaviour 15:1, 1959.

8. Lorenz, K.: Der Kumpan in der Umwelt des Vogels, J. Orn. Lpz. 83:137, 289, 1935. in Schiller, C., Ed. Instinctive Behavior, International Univ. Press, New York, 1957.

9. Lorenz, K.: Ueber die Bildung des Instinktbegriffes, Naturwissenschaften 25:289, 307, 324, 1937. in Schiller, C., Ed.: Instinctive Behavior, International Univ. Press, New York, 1957.

10. Lorenz, K.: Vergleichende Bewegungsstudien an Anatinen, J. Ornithol. 89: Sonderheft 19, 194, 1941.

11. Lorenz, K.: The evolution of behavior, Sci. Am. 199 (6): 67, 1958.

12. Eibl-Eibesfeldt, I., and Kramer, S.: Ethology, the comparative study of animal behavior, Quart. Rev. Biol. 33:181, 1958.

13. Lorenz, K., and Tinbergen, N.: Taxis und Instinkthandlung in der Eirollbewegung der Graugans, Z. Tierpsychol. 2:1, 1938. in Schiller, C., Ed.: Instinctive Behavior, International Univer. Press, New York, 1957.

14. Prechtl, H. F. R.: The directed head turning response and allied movements of the human baby, Behaviour 13:212, 1958.

15. Baerends, D. P., and Baerends-van Roon, J. M.: An introduction to the study of the ethology of cichlid fishes, ibid., suppl. I, 1950.

16. Hinde, R. A.: Some recent trands in ethology. in Koch, S., Ed.: Psychology: A Study of a Science. Vol. II. McGraw-Hill, New York, 1959.

17. Iersel, J. J. A. van: An analysis of the parental behaviour of the male three-spined stickleback, Behaviour, Suppl. III, 1953.

18. Lorenz, K.: Vergleichende Verhaltenforschung, Zool. Anz. Suppl. 12:69, 1939. in Schiller, C., Ed.: Instinctive Behavior, International Univ. Press, New York, 1957.

19. Lorenz, K.: Morphology and behavior patterns in closely allied species. in Schaffner, B., Ed.: Group Processes, Josiah Macy, Fund. 1955.

20. Thorpe, W. H.: Some concepts of ethology, Nature 174:101, 1954.

21. Tinbergen, N.: An objectivistic study of the innate behaviour of animals, Biblioth. biotheor. 1:39, 1942.

22. Cullen, E.: Experiment on the effect of social isolation on reproductive behaviour in the three-spined stickleback. Anim. Behav. 8:235, 1960. (Abs.)

23. Grohmann, J.: Modifikation oder Funktionsreifung? Z. Tierpsychol. 2:132, 1939.

24. Tinbergen, N., and Kuenen, D. J.: Ueber die ausloesenden und die richtungge-benden Reizsituationen der Sperrbewegung von jungen Drosseln (Turdus m. merula L und T.e. ericetorum Turton), ibid. 3:37, 1939. in Schiller, C., Ed.: Instinctive Behavior, International Univ. Press, New York, 1957.

25. Lorenz, K.: The comparative method in studying innate behaviour patterns, Symp. Soc. Exp. Biol. 4:221, 1950.

26. Bullock, T. H.: The origins of patterned nervous discharge, Behaviour 17:48, 1961.

27. Miller, N. E.: Experiments on motivation: studies concerning psychological, physiological, and pharmacological techniques, Science 126:1271, 1957.

28. Andersson, B., Jewell, P. A., and Larsson, S.: An appraisal of the effects of diencephalic stimulation of conscious animals in terms of normal behavior. Neurological Basis of Behaviour (Ciba Symposium), Churchill, London, 1958.

29. Harris, G. W., Michael, R. P., and Schott, P. P.: Neurological site of stilbesterol in eliciting sexual behaviour, Neurological Basis of Behaviour (Ciba Symposium), Churchill, London, 1958.

30. Adrian, E. D.: The control of nerve-cell activity, Symp. Soc. Exp. Biol. 4:85, 1950.

31. Holst, E. von.: Studien ueber Reflexe und Rhythmen beim Goldfisch (Carassius auratus), Z. vergleich. Physiol. 20:582, 1934.

32. Maynard, D. M.: Activity in a crustacean ganglion. II. Pattern and interaction in burst formation. Biol. Bull. 109:420, 1955.

33. Adrian, E. D., and Buytendijk, F. J. J.: Potential changes in the isolated brain of the goldfish, J. Physiol. (Brit.) 71:121, 1931.

CHAPTER 11

Ethology and Psychology

By DANIEL S. LEHRMAN, PH.D.

INTRODUCTION

The study of animal behavior has, in recent years, developed along two different lines representing, for the most part, the activities of two different groups of scientists, formulating problems in somewhat different ways, and deriving their interest in animal behavior from somewhat different sources. Psychologists use the term "comparative psychology" to designate those of their number, mostly in the United States, whose primary interest is in the study of the behavior of animals, rather than that of human beings. "Ethology" is the term used primarily by zoologists to designate those of their number, mostly in Europe, whose primary interest is in the study of the behavior of animals, rather than in the other aspects of their biology. While it is not possible to make absolutely sharp distinctions between these two groups of workers, with their respective activities, it is the purpose of this paper to describe the general characteristics of ethology and to point out some similarities and differences between it and comparative psychology.

THE BACKGROUND OF ETHOLOGY

Present-day ethology has its roots in the interest in animal behavior which was displayed early in this century by a number of naturalists, bird-watchers, zoo directors, and other amateur and professional zoologists whose interest in living animals led them to their study of naturally-occurring behavior patterns. The American zoologist C. O. Whitman, of the University of Chicago, who was interested primarily in the study of evolution, kept and bred doves of many different species in order to study the inheritance of various characteristics of interspecies hybrids. In the course of this work, he became aware that the different species of doves were different from each other not only in their structure, but equally predictably in their behavior, and that many details of their social and sexual behavior were just as useful in finding and studying similarities and differences between species as were details of their structure and plumage. Simultaneously, O. Heinroth, observing various species of ducks in the Berlin zoo, independently noticed that the evolutionary relationships among different species and genera of these birds could be demonstrated just as well by the similarity and differences in courtship behavior patterns as by those of their plumage. The work of these men helped to lay the foundation for the present widespread use of behavior charac- teristics in the study of evolution [1]. Meanwhile, zoologists such as Julian Huxley and Eliot Howard, observing birds in the field, studied the behavior of a variety of species of birds in detail, and developed a number of generalizations to describe the characteristic features and development of the main patterns of social, sexual, and parental behavior. Birds have always been the principal object of interest of field observers of animal behavior, partly because of the readiness with which they may be observed, and partly because of the wide appeal that bird-watching has had for many kinds of professional and amateur observers.

Many of these disparate types of observers and students of animal behavior found a sharp focus, during the 1930s, in the work of Konrad Lorenz and Niko Tinbergen. In a series of theoretical papers, Lorenz [2] provided an account of various aspects of in- stinctive behavior, and a schematic theory of instinctive behavior, both based upon his studies of the behavior of captive and semiwild birds in his institute near Vienna, and later in Germany. These ideas attracted a great deal of attention, and became a focus for the development of intensive and varied work on many aspects of animal behavior, and indeed for the very existence of the groups of scientists who recognize themselves as belonging to a common dis- cipline which can be denoted by the term "ethology." Meanwhile, Tinbergen published a number of papers based on studies of the behavior of various animals in their natural environment, with a more experimental approach than Lorenz's early papers, but with a similar general orientation. A paper jointly written by Lorenz and Tinbergen [3] in 1938, presenting an experimental demonstra- tion, mostly by Tinbergen, of the theoretical ideas which had been expounded by Lorenz during the preceding years, may be regarded as an important event in the modern history of ethology.

Today, ethological work flourishes in a number of European

universities and research institutes. In England, the universities of Oxford and Cambridge both have substantial groups of workers on ethological problems in their zoology departments. In the Netherlands, work on animal behavior is a major part of the effort of the zoology departments of Groningen and Leiden. In Germany, the universities of Freiburg, Göttingen, and others, and several laboratories of the Max Planck Institute, are centers of ethological work.

SURVEY OF BEHAVIOR REPERTOIRES IN NATURE

One of the most interesting and characteristic trends in ethological work has been the incorporation into the scientific literature of detailed descriptive studies of the over-all behavior patterns of a wide variety of species of animals. Tinbergen's studies [4, 5] of the behavior of herring gulls and of sticklebacks and Baerends' monograph [6] on the digger wasp are excellent examples.

Observations of behavior in the field often suggest problems for more detailed analysis, which might not appear at all to the worker who merely keeps animals in cages in the laboratory. For example, many species of pigeons and doves can breed perfectly well in the laboratory, without displaying the complicated aerial flights which are a part of their breeding behavior in their natural environment. Descriptions of the behavior of such animals, based entirely on observations of successful breeding in the laboratory, will of course be lacking in important details. Even when studies are being carried out entirely in the field, lack of knowledge of the over-all behavior pattern may often lead to misinterpretations and blind spots in the analysis of any particular part of the pattern. For example, the courtship behavior of some species of birds includes elements derived from preening behavior, sleeping attitudes, etc. In other cases, courtship may include feeding of one mate by the other, using patterns derived from the feeding of the young by the parents; in sticklebacks, some fighting movements appear to be similar to nest-building movements. In any of these cases, attempts to analyze the origin and the dynamics of either of the types of behavior would necessarily be unsuccessful in the hands of an observer who did not know enough about the pattern of the animal's behavior to recognize the similar elements of different behaviors of the same species.

A further point is that the behavior and breeding arrangements of animals in captivity may often be different from animals in the wild because some of the conditions necessary for parts of the naturally occurring behavior pattern may be lacking in the cage situation. In such cases, analyses of behavior based solely on the behavior of captive animals may represent important distortions of the actual ways in which the animals relate to their natural environment [7].

For all of these reasons, ethologists characteristically regard thorough study of the natural behavior patterns of a species, either in nature or in an artificially provided environment which is as close to the natural one as possible, as an indispensable prerequisite to the analysis of any part of the behavior.

BEHAVIOR AND EVOLUTION

The study of the naturally occurring behavior patterns of animals has made clear that different species of animals, even closely related ones, differ in the details of their behavior just as consistently and reliably as they differ in the details of their structure. Indeed, one of the major tendencies of ethological work has been the study of the evolution and "comparative anatomy" of behavior, and studies of the role which behavioral mechanisms have played in evolution.

Numerous studies have shown that analysis of the similarities and differences in the social behavior patterns of different kinds of animals may be just as useful as studies of their structure in determining the degree of phylogenetic relationship between species. Indeed, in some cases behavior may be a better indicator of evolutionary relationship than any simple set of structural characteristics. Lorenz [8] points out that all members of the order Columbiformes (pigeons, doves, and sand grouse) drink by immersing the bill in water and pumping water into the esophagus until they are satiated. All other birds drink by taking a mouthful of water, lifting the head, and letting the water run down the throat. This one behavioral characteristic is characteristic of all members of this order, and of no members of any other order. There is no single structural characteristic which is thus capable of defining this entire group of birds.

In some cases, behavior characteristics have actually been used by taxonomists in defining specific relationships. For example, Mayr and Bond [9] pointed out that the types of nest built by the various species of swallows are capable of separating this family of birds into a number of very distinct genera, although the structural differences among the genera, while consistent, are not nearly so striking as are those in nest-building behavior. Some species of animals may resemble each other so closely that it does not even become clear that the naturally existing populations belong to two separate species until it is discovered that there are consistent differences in the behavior of the different populations. For example, Adriaanse [10] discovered a hitherto unsuspected new species of digger wasp solely by observing that the wasps in one locality consistently built nests in a different manner than those in another locality.

In addition to constituting a criterion for the relationships among species, behavior may actually play a role in the formation of species. As pointed out by Mayr [11], an essential step in the splitting of a species into two species in the course of evolution occurs when the original species becomes divided into two populations which, for one reason or another, do not interbreed. In many cases, it is clear that a primary factor preventing interbreeding between incipient or recently separated species is incompatibility of the reproductive behavior patterns, so that animals of the two species do not breed with each other even though opportunity arises [12]. A great deal of attention has been paid by geneticists recently to this problem of "reproductive isolation" among closely related species [13].

The interest of ethologists in the variation of behavior patterns from species to species is thus rooted in a biological conception of behavior as being part of the nature of the species, developed through evolution, and of the fact that behavioral mechanisms actually play a role in the dynamics of evolution.

EXPERIMENTATION IN THE FIELD AND LABORATORY

Experimental work in ethology is characterized by the fact that the problems selected for experimental analysis are, in general, those suggested by observation of the animal's natural behavior pattern. No attempt will be made here to discuss the types of theory of behavior toward the elaboration of which such experiments are directed, but merely to give some idea of the type of behavior characteristically studied by ethologists, and the characteristic method used.

A typical example of the kind of experiment possible in field studies of animal behavior is the analysis of Tinbergen and Perdeck [14] of the behavior of newly hatched herring gulls. These young birds get food by pecking at the bill of the parent, which regurgitates the food for the chick. By using models which resembled the bill of the parent herring gull in various ways, and varying different features of the model, such as size, color, shape, etc., these workers were able to show which aspects of the parent's bill were responsible for the direction of the chick's pecking.

Artificial models resembling the "natural" object of a behavior have been widely used by ethologists as a means of investigating the stimuli in the natural environment which normally elicit various parts of an animal's behavior pattern.

Studies of the variations in the form and intensity of "instinctive" behavior patterns under different conditions of elicitation have been used as background for the development of Lorenz's characteristic theory of instinctive behavior. A good example is a study by Prechtl [15] of the way in which the food-begging behavior of young thrushes, in their nests, varied in intensity and in ease of elicitation as a function of the frequency and recency of the performance.

Recently, von Holst and his co-workers [16] have studied the elicitation of various species-specific behavior patterns in the domestic chicken by means of brain stimulation through implanted electrodes, as a means of analyzing the physiological organization of such behavior. Such work may be expected to become increasingly important.

These cursory remarks about a variety of types of ethological experimentation were not intended to be an exhaustive survey, but merely to indicate that the kinds of experiments characteristically performed by ethological workers are suggested by, and directed toward the explanation of, the naturally occurring species-specific behavior patterns.

ETHOLOGY AND PSYCHOLOGY

This brief description of the mood and method of ethology makes clear a major difference between "ethology" and what is usually called "comparative psychology" in the United States. The principal emphasis of ethological work is upon the behavior of the animal, considered as a part of nature, which the investigator wishes to understand. The research is oriented primarily toward gaining understanding of the origin and nature of the behavior patterns which characterize an animal's normal life in its normal environment.

By contrast, most work in animal psychology in this country is not based upon the researcher's interest in the animal as an object of investigation, but rather on the use of an animal, such as the laboratory rat, as a tool for the investigation of a problem which the investigator considers to be a problem of "general" psychology, rather than an aspect of the life of the rat. Indeed, there is an unspoken assumption in much of "rat psychology" that the justification for the work, and our conception of its significance, depend upon the extent to which we think the behavior of the animal being used in the experiment is representative of the behavior of animals in general, including human beings. A trivial but illuminating consequence of this difference in attitude is to be found in the fact that the titles of papers in American psychological journals often fail to state what species of animal was the experimental subject—an omission which one would not find in an ethological journal!

American comparative psychology is now a highly developed science, from the technical point of view. Its graduate students are trained in all pertinent statistical techniques, are educated to high and rigid standards of experimental procedure, are exposed to the problems of scientific philosophy and method, and in general are introduced into a discipline of considerable sophistication. A good deal of ethological work is still in what might be called an earlier stage of systematic description, extended use of anecdotal evidence, and casual admixture of experimental demonstrations in essentially descriptive projects. This is not, of course, the only content of ethological work, as will be clear from my earlier remarks, but the continuous contact of ethological work with the problems of naturally occurring species-specific behavior patterns is reflected in the continuing concern with descriptive studies of the behavior of animals in nature. Ethology is a rapidly changing and growing field of work which gives an impression of great vitality.

One ought not to overestimate the sharpness of the differences between "ethologists" and "comparative psychologists." The term and the concept of "ethology" originally developed within a small group of workers all fairly intimately associated with each other and all consciously and actively identified with the set of theoretical ideas originated by Lorenz and Tinbergen during the 1930s and the 1940s. At that time it would have been quite proper to say that an ethologist was somebody who believed in Lorenz's theory of instinct. Trends toward the differentiation of groups of ideas among European ethologists (e.g., Hinde [17]), as well as increasing communication and mutual exchange of influences between and among ethologists and comparative psychologists, now make such definitions, and such sharp distinctions, seem archaic and unnecessary. In addition, it must be pointed out that many of the characteristics I have described as being specific to ethology have also, from time to time, been found among American psychologists who are in no way influenced by the European trends described in this lecture. The files of such journals as the "Journal of Animal Behavior," "Journal of Comparative Neurology," and the early "Journal of Comparative Psychology" contain ample evidence that such psychologists as Watson, Lashley, Yerkes, and others were truly concerned about the analysis of the characteristic behavior patterns of animals, viewed as problems in their own right. More recently, the work of Schneirla and his students has constituted a trend in American comparative psychology which pays careful attention to the problems of evolution, and of the biological adaptiveness of behavior, and which expresses concern for the physiological basis of behavior and for the ways in which behavior expresses the biological nature of the species [18]. These trends are expressed in a different way in the work of Schneirla and that of the European ethologists, but the difference certainly does not consist of any less concern on the part of the comparative psychologist than on that of the ethologist for the problems of evolutionary biology or of the analysis of the naturally occurring patterns of animal behavior.

During recent years, attendance of American students of behavior at the international conferences of ethology, held at various European universities, has provided a means of communication and of mutual modification of attitudes which will make possible constructive changes in many areas. There has been a growing American interest in the work of European ethologists and a growing openness on the part of European ethologists to consideration of problems raised by American work. Some differences in viewpoint and in language stem from the fact that most comparative psychologists are primarily interested in the comparative psychology of learning, while most ethologists are primarily interested in species-specific behavior patterns which do not appear to owe anything to the kind of learning studied by psychologists watching rats in mazes.

No attempts have been made in these remarks to consider actual attitudes or ideas of either ethologists or comparative psychologists. I have merely tried to suggest the general background, mood, and interest of ethological workers in such a way as to make plain the main characteristics of this trend and some of the ways in which it differs from traditional American ways of studying animal behavior.

REFERENCES

1. Roe, A., and Simpson, G. G., eds.: Behavior and Evolution, Yale University Press, New Haven, 1958.

2. Lorenz, K. Z.: Ueber die Bildung des Instinktbegriffes, Naturwissenschaften 25:289, 307, 324, 1937.

3. Lorenz, K. Z., and Tinbergen, N.: Taxis und Instinkthandlung in der Eiroll-bewegung der Graugans, I., Z. Tierpsychol. 2:1, 1938.

4. Tinbergen, N.: An objectivistic study of the innate behaviour of animals. Bibl. biotheor., Leiden, D 1:39, 1942.

5. Tinbergen, N.: The Herring Gull's World, Collins, London, 1953.

6. Baerends, G. P.: Fortpflanzungsverhalten und Orientierung der Grabwespe *Ammophila campestris* Jr., Tijdschr. Ent. 84:68, 1941.

7. Hediger, H.: Wild Animals in Captivity, Butterworths, London, 1950.

8. Lorenz, K. Z.: Vergleichende Verhaltensforschung, Zool. Anz. 12 (Suppl. Vol.):69, 1939.

9. Mayr, E., and Bond, C. R.: Notes on the generic classification of the swallows, Hirundinidae, Ibis 85:334, 1943.

10. Adriaanse, M. S. C.: *Ammophila campestris* Latr. und *Ammophila adriaansei* Wilcke. Ein Beitrag zur vergleichenden Verhaltensforschung, Behaviour 1:1, 1947.

11. Mayr, E.: Systematics and the Origin of Species, Columbia University Press, New York, 1942.

12. Hinde, R. A.: Behaviour and speciation in birds and lower vertebrates, Biol. Rev. 34:85, 1959.

13. Dobzhansky, T.: Genetics and the Origin of Species, Columbia University Press, New York, 1951.

14. Tinbergen, N., and Perdeck: On the stimulus situation releasing the begging response in the newly hatched herring gull chick (*Larus argentatus argentatus* Pont.), Behaviour 3:1, 1950.

15. Prechtl, H. F. R.: Zur Physiologie der angeborenen ausloesenden Mechanismen, I. Quantitative Untersuchungen ueber die Sperrbewegung junger Singvoegel, Behaviour 5:32, 1953.

16. Holst, E. von, and St. Paul., U.: Vom Wirkungsgefuege der Triebe, Naturwissenschaften 47:409, 1960.

17. Hinde, R. A.: Changes in responsiveness to a constant stimulus, Brit. J. Anim. Behaviour 2:41, 1954.

18. Schneirla, T. C.: Levels in the psychological capacities of animals. in Sellars, R. W., ed., Philosophy for the Future, Macmillan, New York, 1949, pp. 243-286.

Ethological Concepts and Human Development

By WAGNER H. BRIDGER, M.D.

In this paper I shall first present a general discussion of the relationship between ethology and human development, then describe a comparative psychophysiological approach, and finally give an account of some of my own research.

One can deal with ethological concepts from two viewpoints—from inside the field of the study of animal behavior or from outside that field. This discrepancy of viewpoints probably exists in most theoretical problems. Thus, psychoanalysis is considered by people outside the field to have a definite point of view related to Freudian concepts and its various revisions. Among the psychoanalysts there are those whose concepts are completely alien to Freud, but their ideas in no way represent the role psychoanalysis plays in human affairs.

The same situation is true in respect to ethology. There are ethologists whose ideas are at variance with Lorenz's original postulates [1] in many basic ways. And even Lorenz will modify his basic concepts to meet specific objections [2]. However, when he presents his ideas to workers from other fields, his basic viewpoint prevails; and we hear again of his own father's hugging instinct, of innate releasing mechanisms that govern human sexual behavior, of the innate reaction of little boys to imitate their fathers and little girls their mothers [3].

The ethological concepts that I am discussing are those that are identified with the Lorenz-Tinbergen school of instinct theory [4, 5], since it is this theory that affects the thinking of psychiatrists and psychologists outside the field of animal behavior. The word "ethology" no longer signifies the study of animal behavior in the natural habitat with the utilization of specific behavioral patterns

This investigation was supported in part by the U. S. Public Health Service, Mental Health Career Investigator Grant M-2249.

for the purpose of taxonomic classification. It now stands for a series of specific postulates related to instinct theory. Some of these postulates are no longer supported by their original proponents. Some ethologists question the instinct concept in toto. However, regardless of the protestations of ethologists and other students of animal behavior, the concepts that are called to mind when ethology is mentioned remain the same—the classic Lorenz-Tinbergen instinct theory. It is the application of this theory to human development that I want to deal with.

ETHOLOGY AND HUMAN DEVELOPMENT

A short listing of these ethological concepts is in order. Ethology views instincts or instinctual acts as innate patterns of behavior whose mechanisms are built into the central nervous system. These patterns are innately related to the satisfaction of certain basic needs, such as sex, food getting, and child rearing. These a-priori neurally organized behavioral patterns are released by specific external sign stimuli which trigger an innate releasing mechanism and lead to the specific action. For each of these innate patterns there is a reaction-specific energy which builds up and can manifest itself in vacuum activity. Internal stimuli, such as hormones, the level of blood glucose, etc., influence these behavioral patterns through specific actions on these built-in central nervous system mechanisms. While most of the specific sign stimuli that release these instincts are innate, there are some that are acquired through an irreversible process called "imprinting." The occurrence of behavioral patterns governed by one instinct during a different instinct activity is explained by the displacement of the reaction specific energy from one center to the next.

All these concepts name and describe problems, but there is no evidence at all that they either explain or solve them. There is no positive evidence that instincts are innately preformed in the nervous system, that there is such a thing as reaction-specific energy, or that the central nervous system is innately set to react to specific gestalt perceptions. Ascribing the source of a behavioral pattern to a neurally organized center is based upon the elimination of specific external factors but not on the discovery of the neural center itself. Displacement and imprinting describe but do not explain certain forms of behavior. While there is no solid evidence to confirm these instinct concepts, many other students of animal behavior have supplied experimental evidence that replaces these hypothetical constructs with causal mechanisms. The work of Lehrman [6], Moltz [7], Schneirla [8], Birch [9], Rosenblatt and Aronson [10], Toback [11], Hebb [12], Bindra [13], and Hinde [14] are good examples. Rather than repeat their critiques, I would prefer to discuss the relationship of these ethological concepts to human development.

There are at least two ways of evaluating a scientific concept. One is from the standpoint of its intrinsic truth and the other from the standpoint of the role it plays in the advance of scientific knowledge. In respect to intrinsic truth, none of the previously mentioned postulates has proven true by the methods of experimental verification. However, the role that these ethological concepts are playing in elucidating problems of human behavior is more complicated and is, in a sense, a dialectical contradiction. The main school of thought in the field of human development that has reacted to and utilized ethological concepts is psychoanalysis.

Psychoanalysis ascribes the basic source of human behavior to innate instincts or drives. However, psychoanalytical instinct theory is a metapsychological construct and in no way identical with the biological instinctual behavioral patterns postulated by ethology. Psychoanalytic instinct concepts are rather global and presented as Eros, life force, or libido; and Thanatos, death instinct, or aggressive drive. Such metapsychological constructs, regardless of their clinically descriptive usefulness, are akin to vitalism and thus untestable by experimental investigation. However, there is an affinity between these concepts and ethology in that both essentially view the sources of behavior as residing in the organism and projecting out into the external world, which modifies but does not essentially change the instinctual core of the behavior. This affinity has led some psychoanalysts to rely on ethological examples in order to buttress their metapsychological argument. An example is a report by Mortimer Ostow [15] at a panel on ethology and psychoanalysis at the December, 1959, meeting of the American Psychoanalytic Association. He states:

> ...What is the value of ethology for psychoanalysis? First, ethology confirms the biological soundness of Freud's original assumption that motivation is internal and that motivational impulse is displaceable. Second, ethology demonstrates the primitive nature of some forms of human behavior which we tend to consider the results of "higher" mental

processes, for example, defense of territory, courtship maneuvers, and parent-young activities. Third, ethology demonstrates in the overt performance of animals, behavior corresponding to psychoanalytically inferred unconscious impulses in humans, for example, the triggering power of crucial, often innately determined configurational patterns.

In this way psychoanalysts use ethology as support for their metapsychology. Of course, they state that these ethological concepts apply primarily to the instinctive core of human behavior, the id, and that overlying this and manifesting itself in all human functioning are various kinds of learning patterns and ego adaptations.

Another example of the relationship between analysis and ethology comes from the writings of the noted psychoanalyst John Bowlby [16]. He criticizes the emphasis on the role of orality in the development of the mother-child relationship and tries to replace metapsychological constructs with specific, discrete instinctive acts. Among the specific instances of behavior that he feels become integrated into the mother-child relationship he includes smiling, sucking, clinging, crying, and following. While he considers these instinctive acts as innately given and governed by the concepts previously described, by focusing on specific observable phenomena instead of on the more general stages of libido theory he has presented a conceptual model that is possible to test experimentally. Recently the analysts themselves have become aware of this experimental threat to their metapsychological edifice and have started to attack the relevance of ethological concepts to psychoanalytic problems.

For example, Max Schur [17,18], a well-known analyst, has written a series of articles criticizing the application of ethological concepts to psychoanalysis. In his criticism he utilizes the writings of Lehrman, Birch, and Schneirla. However, he does not apply their critical approach to psychoanalysis itself. His main additional point is that the Freudian concept of instinctual drive is a psychological concept and that the biological roots of this concept are rather vague and not in any way specified by psychoanalytic theory. Some psychoanalysts thus utilize ethological concepts in the belief that it will support their metapsychological theories, while others reject these concepts because of a concern that a reliance on ethology opens the door to the scientific elucidation of specific causal mechanisms and the possible demise of instinct theory in general.

COMPARATIVE PSYCHOPHYSIOLOGY

The approach in this paper is based on the personal belief that ethological concepts are not intrinsically true or applicable to the problems of human development. The question remains, what can the comparative psychophysiological study of animal behavior tell us about problems in human development? Ethologists deal with those forms of behavior in animals that they call "instinctive" or "motivated." These behavioral patterns have one thing in common—they appear to be goal directed. These goal-directed behavior patterns are related to basic biological needs, such as sex, hunger, child rearing, and nest building.

It would appear to me that, in trying to understand the mechanisms and modes of functioning of specific goal-directed, or motivated, patterns of behavior for each species, we should delineate the potential adaptive capacity of the species for all its functions. That is, the mechanisms and modes that underlie all of an animal's adaptive functioning are also the kinds of mechanisms that underlie its food-getting and reproductive activities. For example, Schneirla [19] has shown that the ant's maze-learning capacity is rather stereotyped. Whatever enables the ant to link together certain partial behavior patterns into a full-blown maze-running phenomenon would appear to be the same kind of mechanisms that govern its natural food-getting and reproductive activities. This would also be true with rats, cats, and monkeys. Their food-getting, maternal, and reproductive behavior seems to be governed by nervous-system mechanisms that are more mobile and less rigid than those in other animals. The partial responses or reflexes that become integrated to produce this maternal and food-getting behavior become integrated by mechanisms that by their very nature are mobile and variable. Plasticity in all aspects of behavior increases as one ascends the ladder of phylogenetic development. Rosenblatt and Aronson [10] and Beach [20] have shown that the sexual behavior of the cat as compared to the rat is somewhat less dependent on specific hormonal stimuli and more dependent on previous experimental integrations. In order to understand the mechanisms underlying motivated, or goal-directed, behavior, one should look at the adaptive potential and capacity of the species that govern all forms of its behavior. In man, the same would hold true. I believe that man's capacity for general adaptation is primarily dependent on his social experiences and on the capacity of his nervous system for symbolic thinking. Thus, in order to understand his maternal, reproductive, and food-getting behavior one should look for the mechanisms underlying all his adaptive behavior. It is in man's social or cultural existence that we will find the key factors that govern his biologically motivated behavior.

As Money and the Hampsons [21] have demonstrated in their work on pseudohermaphrodites, sex behavior and gender role of humans are products, not of genes, gonads, or hormones, but of the gender role assigned them at birth, usually on the basis of the perceptual features of their external genitals. This in no way negates the fact that hormones and their interaction with the genitals will influence human sexual activity.

It has also been shown that with increased emotional arousal the nature of the learned behavior becomes more stereotyped, that is, it is less easily disrupted or extinguished [22]. Thus, in human motivated behavior it would not be surprising to find that certain so-called basic behavioral patterns are not as easily extinguished or as plastic and variable as certain adaptations that are less emotionally meaningful. However, as we well know, the emotional significance of the behavior in man is in no way necessarily correlated with its biological relevance. In man many socially crucial forms of behavior are more emotionally significant and in a sense sometimes more stereotyped. It appears that the stronger the stimulus or the lower the threshold for reaction to the stimulus, the more difficult the discrimination and the less the plasticity or variability of the response. This in no way means that the response was invariable in origin but rather that, owing to its intensity, it becomes more rigid in its maintenance.

The concept of increased plasticity with phylogenetic development does not imply that lower forms are governed by instincts and higher forms by learning. Rather, the integrating mechanisms responsible for the behavior are different in the various species. These differences, however, are not necessarily qualitative for each species: Recent Soviet investigators, using conditioned reflexes as a reflection of central nervous system processes, have demonstrated that inhibition gradually increases in both ontogenetic and phylogenetic development [23]. While central nervous system connections or integrations are readily formed in almost all species, the inhibitory processes that underly the extinction of the conditioned responses increase with development. Furthermore, connections made between internal stimuli are more resistant to extinction than connections between external stimuli. It would appear that the differences in the rigidity of so-called instinctive acts depends, not on the presence of innate instinct centers, but perhaps on quantitative differences in basic physiological processes.

However, I would consider these theoretical considerations merely guide lines as to what would seem to be the relevant questions to ask. They tell us where to look for the mechanisms coordinating and underlying certain forms of behavior, that is, to look for chemical mechanisms in lower forms, hormonal mechanisms in somewhat higher forms, conditioned reflexes in even higher forms, and the social milieu and symbolic thinking in man. But these theoretical considerations are in no way a substitute for careful, analytical scientific investigation at all levels.

RESEARCH REPORT

I would now like to present an example of such an analytical approach from our own laboratory at the Albert Einstein College of Medicine. The problem we chose to study, the oral activity of human infants, has been a source of considerable interest and controversy for behavioral scientists. Both the interest and controversy seem to stem from the widespread use of the concept "drive" to describe and explain this oral activity. Psychoanalytical theory postulates that sucking is a manifestation of a primary inborn drive whose vicissitudes play an important part in personality development. Experiments by psychologists conducted from the learning theory point of view have presented evidence that sucking is a learned or secondary drive [24]. This problem is particularly emphasized by Harlow's statement [25] that the sucking activity of hungry human neonates demonstrates the goal directedness of inborn drives.

It is our feeling that the everyday observation of babies sucking most frequently when they are hungry is not sufficiently explained by the term "hunger drive," which merely names the gains of the activity without clarifying the processes involved. The term "drive" is used to explain many different phenomena which do not necessarily have the same underlying causal mechanism. One important variation in the use of the drive concept is its identification with nonspecific arousal as measured by behavioral and physiological indices. However, even the term "arousal" cannot be automatically used as an explanation for specific behavioral patterns. This general arousal must be analyzed into its various components and conditions. We know from observations that babies are aroused when hungry. Thus, the question is: Does this arousal itself explain the increase of sucking of hungry babies or, if not, how does hunger-induced arousal differ from states of arousal elicited by other stimuli?

In order to deal with this problem we decided to undertake an exploratory study* to see whether we could experimentally induce babies to suck as much when satiated as when hungry by artifically increasing their level of arousal through external stimulation. The subjects for this study were 12 two- to three-day-old normal full-term babies from the newborn nursery at the Bronx Municipal Hospital Center. These babies, who were on a 4-hour feeding schedule, were studied 15 minutes after feeding and then $3\frac{1}{2}$ hours after the same feeding, during which time there was no fluid intake. During the experimental session their heart rates were measured continuously with a direct-writing standard electrocardiograph utilizing two precordial leads. A standard pacifier was kept in the babies' mouths throughout the experimental session. The pacifier was connected by an air-filled tube to a capacitance pressure transducer, and the pressure changes caused by each sucking movement were directly recorded on a polygraph. Three independent observers made notes throughout the experiment as to the total behavior and activity of the infant.

Each baby was studied during the two prefeeding and two postfeeding states, and the experimental procedure in both states was identical. This procedure involved keeping a pacifier in the baby's mouth and inserting the baby's right foot in water 6 to 8 C for 8 seconds. This arousing stimulus was applied three times per session with an interval of 3 minutes between stimulations. A fourth stimulation consisted of an attempt to elicit a standard grasp response from the right hand.

The data were recorded and analyzed in the following manner: Because of technical considerations, we measured only the frequency of sucking, ignoring the intensity and other qualitative aspects. We measured the number of sucks as expressed in sucks per minute during the 45 seconds prior to stimulation and during

*A detailed report of this study was presented at the biennial meeting of the Society for Research in Child Development, March 16, 1961, State College, Pennsylvania.

the 90 seconds after stimulation. The heart rate in beats per minute was measured for the same period of time.

We analyzed the relation between the level of arousal as measured by heart rate and the amount of sucking in both the hungry and satiated states. As we have shown in a previous study [26], the heart rate level correlates closely with the behavioral assessment of arousal in the individual baby but not across the population. Thus, with a heart rate of 150 beats per minute some babies cry while other babies sleep. Any correlation experiment using heart rate as one of the parameters must be performed on the individual baby and not across the population. Since our behavioral observations had shown us that when the babies become very aroused they cease sucking and start crying, we made the same arbitrary cut-off point for each baby in both the hungry and satiated states. This cut-off point was the heart rate at which the baby became disrupted and ceased sucking. Using both the heart rate and sucking data below this level, we did Pearson product-moment correlations for each baby in the two states. All the correlations in the satiated states were then averaged and found to be significant at the 0.0001 level of confidence. The average correlation in the hungry state was significant at the 0.0004 level of confidence. Thus, regardless of whether the baby was hungry or satiated, there was a highly significant positive correlation between sucking and heart rate level with disruption of sucking at high levels of arousal. The question still remained, did this nonspecific arousal, which clearly facilitated sucking independently of hunger, fully account for the sucking seen during the hungry state?

Since we had found that the amount of sucking was positively correlated with heart rate level, we decided that the only way we could meaningfully compare sucking in the hungry and satiated states was to make the comparison only when the individual baby had the same level of heart rate in both states. After equating for heart rate, we found that in the beginning of the experiment the hungry babies sucked more than the satiated ones, 29.8 sucks per minute to 20.7 sucks per minute, significant at the 0.02 level of confidence. At the end of the session they sucked the same amount, 38 sucks per minute and 37.9 sucks per minute, respectively. It was also evident that the satiated babies at the end of the experimental session sucked significantly more than the hungry babies did at the beginning. The hungry babies also increased their sucking from the beginning to the end of the experimental session without changes in heart rates.

Thus, the experimental procedure itself, which lasted 10 to 15 minutes, facilitated the sucking activity in both hungry and satiated babies. However, the effect was more pronounced in the satiated baby in that it brought the satiated baby up to the level of the hungry baby.

To summarize our data: We found two main factors influencing sucking: (1) the general level of arousal as measured by heart rate and (2) the history of this arousal, i.e., the specific events occurring prior to and during the experimental procedure.

The second factor needs further discussion. We found that our behavioral observations gave us certain leads. A behavioral comparison of the babies at the onset of the experiment—when seen in their bassinet in the nursery—revealed that the hungry babies were awake and active while the satiated babies were asleep. The activity of the hungry babies included spontaneous sucking, hand-mouth contacts, and various head-turning, rooting responses. When the satiated babies were first aroused with ice water, they cried but tended to quickly drop off to sleep again. After the second or third arousal they remained awake.

Thus, after equating for arousal as measured by heart rate level, two additional factors were present in the hungry baby and absent in the satiated baby at the beginning of the experiment. The first was the longer length of time of arousal and the second, an accompaniment of the first, the oral activity that occurred with long-activity arousal. In respect to this oral activity, we found in another pilot experiment that sucking was increased with increased oral stimulation. In that experiment we compared a thin-based pacifier with a wide-based pacifier and found that with the increased labial stimulation produced by the wide-based pacifier there was increased sucking.

Our conclusion is that satiated babies could be artificially induced to suck as much as hungry babies if three factors are taken into account: (1) the nonspecific arousal level as measured by heart rate, (2) the duration of the arousal, and (3) the amount of specific oral stimulation and sucking which facilitates subsequent sucking. It would seem then that the increased sucking seen in hungry babies can be explained by these three factors without having to involve as an explanation the goal directedness of an inborn drive.

As a further commentary on the relation between hunger and

sucking, we would like to point out that Peiper [27] has stated that neonatal stepping, climbing, grasping, and swimming responses are most easily demonstrated in the hungry baby, suggesting that arousal increases all basic reflexes including sucking.

This brings us back to the concept of drive as nonspecific energy or arousal. In our experiment there were specificities involved in the behavioral pattern not fully explained by the level of arousal itself. This arousal appeared to be a discontinuous function. As the quantity of arousal increased, there appeared qualitative changes in behavior. These specific qualities depended on the stimulus and self-stimulating conditions and were not explained by the inference of a causal drive which did little more than restate the facts to be explained.

I feel that our experimental evidence contradicts the ethological concept that views instinctive or drive behavior as innately organized. Instead, our data indicate that such behavior develops through coordination of the many organic resources in the organism interacting with the developmental milieu. These results also indicate that in the human neonate one should not assume any built-in connection between metabolic lacks and the specific behavioral patterns that ultimately remedy these lacks. In addition, it would appear that the sucking of the baby may not only alleviate hunger but also inhibit the baby's response to other external stressful stimuli.

In our laboratory Beverly Birns [28] has compared the effects of cold stress on the autonomic and behavioral activities of neonates with and without a pacifier. The babies with the pacifier showed significantly less arousal with stress than those without the pacifier. The former primarily increased their sucking. Birns also described the inhibiting or soothing effects of loud sounds and other stimuli. Perhaps the nonnutritional sucking seen in older babies develops because sucking happens to be the main soothing device used by the mother. Babies who are soothed by stimulation through other modalities may in the course of development seek auditory or kinesthetic stimulation rather than oral activity. These questions are open to investigation, and any a-priori definition of the object or stimulus need would be misleading and incorrect.

CONCLUSION

In conclusion, I would propose that we replace ethological concepts with a developmental attitude that emphasizes the quest for psychophysiological mechanisms that deal with the continuous interaction of organism and environment at all levels of functioning.

REFERENCES

1. Lorenz, K.: The comparative method in studying innate behavior patterns. in Symposium of the Society for Experimental Biology, Vol. IV, Academic Press, Inc., New York, 1950.

2. Lorenz, K.: [The objectivistic theory of instinct]. In L'Instinct dans le Comportement des Animaux et de l'Homme, Masson & Cie, Paris, 1956.

3. Lorenz, K.: in Discussion on child development. In World Health Organization Study Group on Psychobiological Development of the Child, 1953–1956, International Univ. Press, New York.

4. Lorenz, K.: King Solomon's Ring, Crowell, New York, 1952.

5. Tinbergen, N.: The Study of Instincts, Oxford Univ. Press, New York, 1951.

6. Lehrman, D.: A critique of Konrad Lorenz's theory of instinctive behavior, Quart. Rev. Biol. 28:337, 1953.

7. Moltz, H. Imprinting: empirical basis and theoretical significance, Psychol. Bull. 57:291, 1960.

8. Schneirla, T. C.: The concept of development in comparative psychology. in Harris, D., Ed: The Concept of Development, Univ. Minnesota Press, Minneapolis, 1957.

9. Birch, H.: The pertinence of animal investigations for a science of human behavior, Am. J. Orthopsychiat. 31:267, 1961.

10. Rosenblatt, J. S., and Aronson, L. R.: The decline of sexual behavior in male cats after castration with special reference to the role of prior sexual experience, Behavior 12:285, 1958.

11. Toback, Ethel: Eliminative responses in mice and rats and the problem of "emotionality." In Bliss, E. Ed.: Roots of Behavior, Paul B. Hoeber, Inc., New York, in press.

12. Hebb, D. O.: Drives and the C.N.S., Psychol. Rev. 62:243, 1955.

13. Bindra, D.: Motivation, Ronald Press, New York, 1959.

14. Hinde, R.: Concept of drives. In Brazier, M., Ed: The Central Nervous System and Behavior, Trans. Third Conf., Josiah Macy, Jr. Found., New York, 1960.

15. Ostow, M.: Psychoanalysis and ethology, J. Am. Psychoanal. Assoc. 7:533, 1960.

16. Bowlby, J.: Nature of the child's tie to its mother, Internat. J. Psycho-Anal. 39:350, 1958.

17. Schur, M.: Animal research: psychoanalyst's comments, Am. J. Orthopsychiat. 31:276, 1961.

18. Schur, M.: Discussion of Dr. John Bowlby's Paper, Psychoanal. Study Child 15:63, 1960.

19. Schneirla, T. C.: Ant learning as a problem in comparative psychology. in Harrisman, P., Ed.: Twentieth Century Psychology, Philosophical Library, New York, 1945.

20. Beach, F.: A review of physiological and psychological studies of sexual behavior in mammals, Physiol. Rev. 27:240, 1947.

21. Money, J., Hampson, Joan G., and Hampson, J. L.: An examination of some basic sexual concepts: the evidence of human hermaphroditism, Bull. Johns Hopkins Hosp. 97:30, 1955.

22. Bridger, W.: Signal systems in the development of cognitive functions. In Brazier, M., Ed.: Central Nervous System and Behavior, Trans. Third Conf. Josiah Macy, Jr. Found., New York, 1960.

23. Razran, G.: The observable unconscious and the inferable conscious in current Soviet psychophysiology, Psychol. Rev. 68:81, 1961.

24. Davis, H. V., Sears, R., Miller, H. C., and Brodbeck, A. J.: Effects of cup, bottle, and breast feeding on oral activities of children, Pediatrics 2:549, 1948.

25. Harlow, H.: in Current Theory and Research in Motivation: A Symposium, Univ. and Nebraska Press, Lincoln, 1953.

26. Bridger, W and Reiser, M.: Psychophysiologic studies of the neonate, Psychosom. Med. 21:265, 1959.

27. Peiper, A.: Die Eigenart der kindlichen Hirntaetigkeit, Leipzig, 1956.

28. Birns, Beverly: ref. in Bridger, W.: Sensory and autonomic function of the neonate, J. Acad. Child Psychiat., in press.

III DRUGS AND SOMATIC APPROACHES IN PSYCHIATRY

CHAPTER 13

Psychotropic Drugs and Experimental Psychiatry
ACADEMIC ADDRESS

By JEAN DELAY, M.D.

Progress in psychopharmacology has made available to clinicians a whole series of psychotropic drugs capable of influencing behavior in different directions. The word "psychotropic" is useful since it identifies in a general fashion a whole group of natural or artificially occurring substances that modify behavior. Whether they depress, stimulate, or deviate the mental energies or produce a state of stimulation, relaxation, or delusion, it is possible to classify them clinically in a rather simple fashion, at least until a more scientific classification becomes possible which will allow one to correlate psychological changes with chemical formulas and to selectively localize their site of action in the brain and their intracerebral metabolism.

Psychopharmacology has opened up new areas which hold promise for investigation of problems in human psychology and experimental psychiatry. I will limit my presentation to three aspects: (1) variations of psychological "tonus," (2) induction of the neuroleptic syndrome, and (3) experimentally induced states of abnormal behavior.

EXPERIMENTAL VARIATIONS OF PSYCHOLOGICAL "TONUS"

Just as muscle tonus depends on whether there is a state of contraction, semicontraction, or rest, there exists a state of mental "tonus" which varies according to the intellectual effort expended and is thereby a function of the level of cerebral activity. In the psychological as in the muscle systems there are oscillations between the states of contraction that can be called concentration and relaxation whether we use physiological or psychological terms.

The Annual Academic Address is supported by a grant from the Manfred Sakel Foundation. The address was delivered in French; the translation is by Dr. H. C. B. Denber.

Pierre Janet was the first to conceptualize the mind's function in a dynamic sense based on the "psychological tension" and its oscillations. The hierarchy of activity that he described rested on the opposition of "involuntary and synthetic activity," the former referring to low-tension states which allow fantasies to take place and the latter referring to states of heightened tension and implying a voluntary act of concentration. Each human being experiences both of these states. We all feel the effects of our psychological tension, depending upon whether we are awake or drowsy, attentive or distracted, tense or relaxed, stimulated or depressed. The organism's needs for dynamic adaptability to the complexities of daily life are far more exhausting than when the activities are involuntary. Involuntary activities require no conscious attentive effort, no matter whether we are dealing with an act learned by rote or with free association as in daydreams. What we call "fantasies" today were described years ago by Maine de Biran when he drew the analogy to dreamy meditation, which referred to the decrease in the synthetic and adaptive functions of the mind leaving the inner self submerged by a succession of images, like waves beating against the shore. Moreau de Tours felt that ego flexibility permitted the individual's reality adaptation. Janet developed his dynamic concept of the levels of psychological tension based, among others, on these lines of thinking.

For Pierre Janet, psychological readiness depended on the state of nervous tension which was comparable to an electric potential. This assumes more than metaphoric importance if we think of comparing the brain to an electronic unit functioning according to the laws of cybernetics.

In describing psychasthenia Janet wrote, "We are unaware of the causes that inhibit the brain's reactivity; if there is a special center that produces or regulates this tension; if this center is cortical, subcortical, or located in an endocrine gland." One of the principal contributions of modern neurophysiology has been to recognize the regulation of psychological activity by the brain through the cortical and subcortical circuits. It would be foolhardy to attempt to localize the center regulating the state of psychological tension. The problem is worthy of discussion, nevertheless, in view of the center's dependence on the set and mood of the organism and their regulation by cerebral mechanisms.

There is a gross analogy between oscillations of the psychological tonus and the state of "vigilance." Janet considered the highest degree of psychological tension to be the state of awareness (of past, present, and future), an intellectualized function. On the other hand, he felt that fantasy resulted from liberation of the subconscious, as tensions decreased and consciousness was less sharp. If one goes a step further, it could be said that the opposite of psychological tension could be considered as sleep, a periodic loss of consciousness in which the mental faculties are inoperative and the dream becomes master.

Most physiologists today define "sleep" as a cortical inhibition originating in the diencephalon. The oscillations between the waking and sleeping states appear closely linked to the sympathetic nucleus of the diencephalic portion of the reticular activating system. Sympathomimetic substances stimulate this formation, leading to insomnia, while sedatives are depressant agents leading to sleep. The state of psychological tonus depends on the cerebral centers regulating the states of consciousness or sleep. To a degree, this state of tension is related to the oscillations of the state of alertness.

The basic emotional disposition of the individual is intimately linked to the state of psychological tension. The former is a function of oscillations in emotional tonus between vigilance and apathy. These mood swings, which exist in all people, show characteristic periodic exaggerations in the affective disorders. In 1946, I attempted in my book, "Disorders of the Affect" [1], to unify neurophysiological, neurosurgical, and neuropsychiatric observations, indicating that mood is regulated by the central nervous system. Since then, many similar observations have been made. The cortico-subcortical circuits are related to this complex in a fashion similar to the state of vigilance. However, some of the key areas are localized in the hippocampus and diencephalon. The variations in psychological tonus and mood changes are related to the same cerebral centers insofar as the former is dependent upon the latter.

Psychopharmacology has shed new light on the neurophysiological concepts of psychological tonus. Through the experimental use of psychotropic drugs, which act directly on the central cerebral regulating mechanisms, it has been possible to experimentally lower or heighten the psychological tonus by decreasing or increasing either the state of alertness or mood or both.

Lowering of the psychological tension was described by Pierre Janet as "psycholepsy," an interesting word derived from the Greek. It would be, perhaps, more appropriate to speak of "psychocatalepsy," the "cata" signifying "down." It would seem to me of more than passing interest to conserve the meaning that Janet gave to the word "psycholepsy." Thus, "psycholeptics" would be drugs that diminish the psychological tonus, while those that produce the reverse effect would be called "psychoanaleptics" (the Greek "ana" meaning "up").

The compounds that depress psychological tension are called "psycholeptics," whether the result is a decrease in consciousness or of the intellectual forces or the sedation of psychic tension. One may subdivide this large group into two categories: (1) hypnotics— those drugs that decrease states of consciousness—and (2) tranquil- izers or mood depressants. All hypnotics comprise those drugs capable of depressing consciousness, and when used correctly can achieve different levels between the waking and sleeping states. In the first (hypnoid) stage, there is a decrease of the cognitive functions undetectable by the electroencephalogram. The second stage shows slight alterations of the electroencephalogram, usually considered to be the desirable level for hypno- or narcoanalysis. The third (hypnotic) stage shows clinical and electroencephalographic signs of sleep; this is the state used for the sleep cure.

Tranquilizers are those drugs that depress the emotions, and their action is to substitute a state of torpor for agitation. They are sometimes called "ataractics," since ataraxia is by definition a state free of emotional problems in an individual unperturbed by external stimuli. The tranquilizers produce an experimental ataraxia, just as the barbiturates produce an experimental sleep.

In 1952, Deniker and I described the first results with chlor- promazine in the treatment of mental illness and noted its psycho- logical action as follows: "The psychological syndrome resulting from treatment with chlorpromazine consists of an apparent in- difference, increased reaction time, flattened affect, decrease of initiative and self-preoccupation, without alteration of consciousness or the intellectual faculties."

The experimental production of a state of ataraxia with psycho- tropic drugs is not new if we think of the fact that the Greeks used "nepenthes." May I cite in this regard a passage from Homer's "Odyssey":

>...Telemachus has described the siege of Troy and the unhappiness in his country, as his compatriots began to cry. Helen, daughter of Zeus, poured some "nepenthes," a balm, into their glasses, making them forget their problems. He who drank this potion could not cry all day, even if his

parents or beloved son were killed before his very eyes. This excellent liqueur was given to Helen by Polydamna, wife of Phebus, born in Egypt whose fertile land produced many balms, some healthy and some deadly.

Nepenthes is in a way the ancestor of the ever-growing list of modern tranquilizers.

It is necessary to distinguish between the minor and major tranquilizers (neuroleptics). The latter differ from the former by virtue of a greater degree of psychologic activity and through the induction of a neurological syndrome. The reduction of emotional tonus by the neuroleptics lends itself to many applications in psychiatric and psychosomatic medicine. The continued barking of aggressive dogs will induce a Basedow disease in the rabbit. But, prior treatment with neuroleptics will block the thyroid reaction and there will be no signs of Schreck-Basedow disease.

All the psychoanaleptics stimulate the psychological tonus no matter if this be owing to a more intense state of wakefulness, which can lead to insomnia and an increase of the intellectual functions, or to a heightening of the psychic tension, which can lead to euphoria or anxiety. Compounds that make the individual more alert stimulate the thinking processes (psychotonic effect) and produce insomnia (antihypnotic).The amphetamines (methylamphetamine) best characterize this group, whose effects are antagonistic to the barbiturates. Other compounds in the amphetamine group are: methylphenidate (Ritalin), oxazimedin (Preludin), pipradol (Meratran). Centrophenoxine derived from the acid growth factors of vegetables has been found to be particularly effective in the treatment of alterations of consciousness resulting from organic cerebral damage on a traumatic, vascular, or neoplastic basis. It can be used in comas as well, where it tends to awaken the patient, although it is not actually a stimulant like the amphetamines.

Mood-elevating drugs affect psychological tonus, either by giving rise to euphoria by direct action, as cocaine would, or by influencing a depression, as the antidepressant drugs do. These compounds are effective chemotherapeutic agents in depression and can replace electroconvulsive treatment. The monamine oxidase inhibitors (iproniazid) are good examples of such activity but more important is imipramine, which is not an inhibitor of this enzyme. Imipramine has been described as a thymoleptic, but it is really a thymoanaleptic since it heightens the mood and increases emotional reactivity.

The classification of psychotropic drugs in relation to psychological tonus has value only to clinicians, in that it allows them to categorize each group according to its major effects. Although the division between psycholeptic and psychoanaleptic is generally clear, the subdivisions of these groups are not so sharp. Barbiturates depress the state of wakefulness and to a lesser degree the mood as well. The phenothiazines, on the other hand, are mood depressants and do the same to the state of wakefulness, although to a lesser degree. The amphetamines alert and to a lesser degree elevate the mood. Imipramine lifts the mood and to a lesser degree makes the individual more "vigilant." Although the hypnotic and antihypnotic drugs are antagonistic, the difference between tranquilizers and mood-elevating drugs is not clear. This can be shown in studying benactyzine or the potentiating effect of levomepromazine on the antidepressant effects of imipramine.

A classification based on the drug's psychological activity is essentially of clinical interest and must be compared to others being developed by psychopharmacologists. Bovet uses the electro-encephalogram to distinguish between those substances that depress or activate the reticular activating substance, while Monnier distinguishes between trophotropic and ergotropic drugs.

Experimental study of psychological tonus and psychological tension (in Janet's sense of the terms) has been made possible by the use of psychopharmacological agents through an analysis of the variations in these states under the effects of drugs that either stimulate or depress the emotions or the state of consciousness. Since it has been shown that the psychotropic drugs tend to localize in various subcortical centers, particularly the reticular-activating system and its cerebral projections, the suggestion is made that consciousness and mood are regulated by central cerebral mechanisms. The use of sulfur-tagged chlorpromazine can give useful evidence in this area. Variations in different neurohumors (adrenalin, noradrenalin, serotonin, etc.) and other chemical mediators of central nervous system activity have brought forth evidence of the biochemical mechanisms underlying depression and agitation. The discovery of these chemical mediators and their psychophysiological implications cannot help but recall the old Cartesian doctrine of "the animal spirits."

THE NEUROLEPTIC SYNDROMES

Since 1954, we have used the term "neuroleptic" when referring to that subgroup of psycholeptic drugs which are highly effective in the treatment of acute and chronic psychoses. Chlorpromazine and other phenothiazines were the major compounds in use with reserpine. To these have been added a whole new series of non-phenothiazine and nonreserpine drugs, of which haloperidol is a good example. What criteria justify the separation of neuroleptics as a group, as opposed to the hypnotic agents and other tranquilizers?

In humans, as well as in animals, the syndrome produced by drug saturation of the tissues* can be accompanied by somnolence, but drug-induced sleep is not seen at the therapeutic doses used. It is always possible with these doses to awaken the animal by simple stimulation if the drug produces a hypnotic effect. It would appear as if the indifference and inertia produced by neuroleptics facilitates sleep without a real hypnotic effect. As Bergson said, "Sleep is a form of indifference." Neuroleptics cannot be considered as a variant of sleep treatment, since at equal doses the patients treated with neuroleptics do not fall asleep.

The neuroleptics, like the other tranquilizing drugs, reduce the mood tone until a state of emotional indifference and flatness is achieved. The neuroleptics to a greater degree than the others have diminished agitation and aggression, as a result of which special services for the disturbed and the need for restraints have been eliminated in psychiatric wards. This has led to a transformation of the atmosphere in psychiatric hospitals, so that in the future they will not be much different from general hospitals.

The unusual sedative action of tranquilizers has been demonstrated in laboratory experiments on naturally aggressive animals (*Macaca rhesus* and the fighting fish). Other work has been done with the sham rage of decorticated preparations, and animals in whom agitation is experimentally induced (Thuillier worked with 3-amino-diproprionitrile, which causes rats to move in circles endlessly). The neuroleptics not only are effective against various acute and chronic psychiatric syndromes, but they can abruptly stop an artificially induced state ("model psychosis") or even present it through prior administration. The principal criteria which allow their differentiation from other tranquilizers is the production of a neurological syndrome (from which the word is derived).

There are several varieties of this syndrome or group of syndromes which have in common an extrapyramidal reaction, and they depend to a degree on the particular compound. Their characteristics are different with prochlorperazine, as opposed to the sulfonamide

*"imprégnation médicamenteuse."

phenothiazine-thioproperazine. But the clinical syndrome also depends on the individual's sensitivity, for catalepsy and the experimentally induced hysteroid states are seen much more frequently in subjects with a hysterical personality and in those prone to cataleptic phenomena. Even though the symptoms are polymorphous in type, they can be separated into three general groups: (1) the hypokinetic or akinetic syndrome, characterized by a reduction in motor activity and initiative, (2) hypertonic syndromes, characterized by muscle hypertonus, and (3) the hyperkinetic or dyskinetic syndrome, characterized by abnormal movements.

Frequently, if a minimal neurological syndrome due to neuroleptic medication develops, it can pass by unnoticed if one is unaware of what treatment the patient is receiving. Actually, there is a whole series of gradations from the most minor neurological symptoms to the major clinical syndromes. We have approached the problem through a minute study of the sequential changes in the facial features of patients being treated with neuroleptics. A slight change in facial expression resulting from hypertonia of the facial muscles can always be demonstrated. This often precedes the hypertonia of the body musculature and appears in a determined order: palpebral and lateral nasal muscles, then frontal and periorbital muscles, and finally the peribuccal and mandibular musculature. It is thus possible to follow the tissue drug saturation as well as the regression of anatomical changes, which take place in reverse order. In correlating these tonic changes of the facial musculature and expression with modern neurophysiology, one can ask what role the temporal amygdaloid nucleus plays. This formation has projections to most of the cerebral centers that have been implicated as sites of action for the neuroleptics.

The signs and symptoms of the akinetic syndrome are relatively constant and some cases can exhibit the picture of catalepsy, while the hypertonic syndrome resembles parkinsonian rigidity. On the other hand, the hyperkinetic or dyskinetic syndromes are polymorphous in appearance and a whole series of abnormal movements can be produced by the neuroleptics: parkinsonian tremor, which with akinesia and hypertonia produce an experimental parkinsonian state; paradoxical kinetic movements with latero- and retropulsion; choreiform bradykinesias; tasikinesia and akathisia; cervical, facial, and buccal-laryngeal dystonic seizures; and finally the major hysteroid crises.

There are a number of problems inherent in the consideration of the neurologic syndromes produced by neuroleptics: (1) their analogy to the epidemic encephalitic syndrome, (2) the meaning of the hyperkinetic syndrome, (3) the relationship of hysteroid states to hysteria, (4) the linkage of psychological and motor changes, (5) the effectiveness of chemotherapy in the psychoses as related to the intensity of the neurologic manifestations, and finally (6) the prevention or blocking of the neurologic changes by other psychotropic drugs, which are antagonistic in nature. Even though we cannot pretend to offer a solution to these difficult problems, there is a certain usefulness in considering them.

Deniker and I have compared the transitory and reversible neurological syndromes due to drugs with those observed during or after the von Economo encephalitis: the akinetic syndrome of Lhermitte, the hypertonic Parkinson syndrome (Steck), and the excitomotor syndrome of Marie and Levy. These entities are not only analogous but identical. It would seem as if the neuroleptics have the same neurotropism as the virus of von Economo's encephalitis, leading to a sort of therapeutic encephalitis by the saturation of the meso-diencephalic centers with drugs in a selective but transitory fashion. This concept is corroborated by an analysis of the autonomic, endocrine, and metabolic changes resulting from neuroleptic treatment.

Pierre Marie made very clear that his description of the abnormal movements seen after epidemic encephalitis (excitomotor syndrome) was purely clinical and unrelated to pathogenesis. It was not indicated if there was focal excitation of the central nervous system or only a liberation of these centers with respect to the normal inhibition exerted by subcortical centers according to the Jacksonian concept of "escape from control." We believe that the hyperkinetic or, more correctly, the dyskinetic syndrome produced by the neuroleptics should be considered in the light of the latter hypothesis.

The neuroleptics depress without stimulating nervous activity, and the inhibition of the superior centers is the prime condition for the escape of activity from the lower involuntary centers giving rise to the different abnormal movements. These apparently new ("positive") reintegrative aspects of the latter symptoms are conditioned by the negative* aspects which in Jacksonian terms would be equated to a return to a less complex function.

Early investigators classified some of the symptoms of the

*A direct effect of the pathological process.

hyperkinetic syndrome (particularly severe with prochlorperazine and thioperazine) as hysteria or a hysteroid state. The same problem arose earlier with epidemic encephalitis when a whole sequence of symptoms of obviously organic nature appeared—choreiform movements, torsion spasms, cervicofacial and buccal-laryngeal dystonias, opisthotonos, and the entire Charcot's syndrome. As a result of these observations, Marinesco and van Bogaert developed their diencephalic theory of hysterical symptoms.

The neuroleptic-induced hysteroid states are particularly important because the acute neurological manifestations are paired with psychological changes: suggestibility, psychomotor variations, and the narrowing of the field of consciousness. These symptoms can be eliminated by suggestion without a loss of any of the drug's activity. As noted previously, these reactions appear, above all, in those patients who seem predisposed to them, particularly those patients in the paranoid and paraphrenic states.

Even though this tendency to suggestibility exists in the hyperkinetic syndrome, indifference is the rule in the akinetic group and a tendency to depression is relatively frequent in the parkinsonian hypertonia. While one may discuss at length the relationship between psychological changes and motor phenomena, the essential problem still remains to determine whether or not a relationship exists between the neurological syndrome and the therapeutic effects. There is much evidence to show that the results have often been directly related to the intensity of the neurological effect, but this remains to be demonstrated conclusively. Briefly stated, our view is that there is no such relationship but rather that the neurological syndrome offers evidence of a generalized drug diffusion and penetration to the subcortical centers, where those centers regulating mood and consciousness are found. According to this concept, the centers related to the mental syndrome are anatomically contiguous to those producing the neurological syndromes. Thus, the induction of the latter has a "spill-over" effect and favorably influences the former.

One could eventually consider the possibility that a selective localization of the drugs might be dissociated from any therapeutic activity. As noted before, the whole problem is still unclear, and it would seem reasonable to analyze the effects of the neurological syndrome on the mental symptoms by studying the influence of the compounds capable of blocking the former syndrome. The akinetic syndrome is blocked by antidepressants and other drugs that increase alertness; the hypertonic syndrome is affected by the various anti-Parkinson drugs; and the autonomic syndrome is affected by sedatives. At present there does not exist any drug capable of annulling all three syndromes at one time.

My collaborators and I have studied the effects of adenosine triphosphate (ATP), since it appears to protect laboratory animals against experimental diencephalic lesions produced by reserpine. When given by intravenous drip in man, adenosine triphosphate can annul the hyperkinesia, hypertonia, and autonomic nervous symptoms produced by neuroleptics but akinesia and somnolence are accentuated. This would seem to demonstrate how difficult it is to eliminate all symptoms of the drug-induced neurological syndrome simultaneously and thus be able to determine if the elimination had any effect on the therapeutic process. On the other hand, it is possible to correlate the action of adenosine triphosphate on the neuroleptic-induced syndrome with the very important role it plays in neuromuscular metabolism. This has served as a point of departure for some of our current investigations.

It can be said in a general way that the major biological treatments used in psychiatry have a common point of reference with regard to the drug-induced neurological reactions in that the neurological syndrome they induce suggests involvement of the subcortical centers and the cortico-subcortical pathways. This is obvious with electroconvulsive treatment and cardiazol shock. Both act on the diencephalon and implicate the cortico-subcortical pathways as well. Some antidepressant drugs lower the convulsive threshold and may trigger a dormant epilepsy. The sleep cure and insulin coma are similar, for both sleep and coma imply participation of the basilar portions of the brain; the same can be said for cerebral pneumotherapy and prefrontal lobotomy. Chemotherapy and the shock therapies, insulin coma, and psychosurgery indicate that the biological treatments in psychiatry are essentially acting on and modifying the brain function. These different findings offer strong evidence that mental illness represents an organic brain change, more often functional, with changes in the dynamic equilibrium between the different cerebral centers. Those who espouse a purely psychogenetic view of the neuroses and psychoses have frequently lost sight of these facts.

EXPERIMENTALLY INDUCED STATES
OF ABNORMAL BEHAVIOR

Up to this point we have been considering only those drugs that elevate or lower the psychological tonus and that exercise a stimu-

lating or depressing action. The psychodysleptic* compounds are
the most interesting for experimental psychiatry since they produce
an artificial or "model" psychosis. The substances that can be
considered in this group are those that disturb the functioning of
the mental apparatus, confuse thinking processes, and distort the
individual's perception of reality. They produce dreamlike and confusional states, hallucinations, depersonalization, and in a general
way a complete mental disorganization.† Lewin has called these
drugs "phantastica," since they give rise to dreamy states with
visual and mental disturbances. Hashish, cocaine, mescaline,
LSD-25, and psilocybin are some of the more important drugs in
this group.

The psychodysleptic drugs are antagonized by the psycholeptic
agents, which diminish the intensity of or inhibit the drug-induced
states of abnormal behavior. Yet, comparison with the psychoanaleptics is more difficult. Cocaine, which stimulates at high
doses, will, if the dose is pushed high enough, produce a delusional-
hallucinatory syndrome. The psychodysleptic drugs unquestionably
stimulate the mood and appear at times to stimulate the intellectual
activity as well. However, these newly apparent "positive"‡ effects
are in reality the result of negative factors. In other words, the
drug's psychological effects must be considered in the Jacksonian
frame of reference as an "escape from control," a regression and
liberation of the mental functions.

The relationship of drug-induced states to toxic deliria, stuporous conditions, and apparently spontaneous mental disturbances
was noted in antiquity, but the first real experimental study dates
to the nineteenth century with the report by Moreau de Tours. His
publication on "Hashish and Mental Illness" appeared in 1845 and
was based on self-observations with the drug and on studies with
normal subjects and highly gifted individuals. He concluded that by
using hashish it is possible to reproduce the primary aspects of
mental illness: splitting apart of the different components of the
mind and a hallucinatory syndrome which he compared to the
structure of a dream. Today one speaks of the psychotic-like
characteristics of a dream.§ In following Kant's definition ("the
insane person is like the dreamer in a waking state"), Moreau de

---

*The "dys" means "distortion of."
†"Délire" in the etymological sense (de lira) means "out of line."
‡ As used in the Jacksonian sense.
§"structure onirique."

Tours not only felt that psychoses and dreams are analogous but that they are one and the same. While this concept can be criticized, it is correct when applied to the visual hallucinations resembling a dream state ("onirisme").

Hashish is a hallucinogen, as are most of the drugs used to produce artificial psychoses where the delusional state seems to depend both on a localized irritation of the sensorial analyzers (particularly those concerned with visual perception) and on a general reduction in the level of consciousness. I would like to insist on the fact that visual hallucinations are often absent and may only represent an illusory phenomenon even with mescaline and psilocybin. They are but one element of an extremely complicated clinical state which corresponds to the dream life of the mental apparatus. These drugs are not only hallucinogenic but can produce delusions, fantasies, dream states, etc.* They give rise to a state best defined as one in which the synthetic powers of the mind no longer function, in addition to which there is a release of the unconscious.**

In a Jacksonian frame of reference, we can speak of regression as suggested by the loss of the frames of reference for perception and memory, distortions in time and space, disturbances in body image and personality (ego), as well as a disruption of the philosophical unity and direction of the individual. These processes lead to a disruption of the normal mental stream. There is, running parallel to this, a loss of control, a liberation of the fantasy life, a projection of the esthetic aspects of the subconscious, and a reorganization of the apparently anarchic quality of the thought processes according to the needs of the instinctual life rather than to the demands of reality.

In the light of these facts, the experimental endogenous states of abnormal behavior can bring to light latent personality traits, since we dream or hallucinate in accordance with what we have and what we are. Long before psychoanalysis emphasized the meaning of the unconscious projections, of symbolism in dreams and hallucinations, Moreau de Tours had noted with interest the importance of a psychodynamic analysis of the hashish-induced state. One of our patients dreamed of killing his mother while under the effects of this drug; this feeling reflected a severe reality conflict. The drug-induced experience was so overpowering that, feeling it to

*"onirogène."
**"régime onirique."

be true, he surrendered to the police for the ostensible crime he imagined he had committed. Nevertheless, in general the projection of underlying conflicts during the artificial drug-induced state is not frequent, at least as seen in our studies with 40 patients who received mescaline, 75 who received LSD, and 100 who received psilocybin. The general tenor of the projections during the experimental psychosis was nonspecific, varying with many factors and ofttimes was purely fortuitous. In our experience, psilocybin is one of the most interesting drugs used to induce an experimental abnormal state of behavior.

I would now like to discuss some self-observations with psilocybin, carried out in the presence of two of my collaborators, one of whom noted the somatic and the other the psychological reactions. The sequences of this personal experiment could be divided into three phases: (1) hallucinations with colors predominating, (2) a resurgence of highly charged emotions, and (3) a veritable cascade of various psychomotor phenomena. I will now describe some of these findings.

The first phase was marked by visions of a kaleidoscopic nature with many colors, giving rise to much feeling, particularly the reds and violets. A sentence was noted in the protocol which under ordinary circumstances I could never have said, "If I were a painter, I would like to color this violet, which would make the whole world happy." The colors were very bright, present with eyes closed, and disappearing with eyes opened.

The phase in which previous memories returned began with an auditory illusion. I confused the noise of an airplane passing over the hospital for the noise of a train. This produced a memory recall, in which I found myself back in 1917. At that time I lived with my family in the country in a house whose property was traversed by a railroad. This house surged forth before my eyes in an unmistakable fashion, but, curiously enough, it had neither doors nor windows. Certain of the details suddenly stood out with extraordinary clarity: a magnolia leaf in front of the door, a shawl left on one of the pieces of garden furniture, the empty bird cage whose door had been torn off. Although no human figures appeared in these visions, I was wracked with tense emotion and, losing all self-control, began to cry, not paying any attention to the presence of my two assistants. One of them took my blood pressure, which had risen from 150/90 mm Hg to 210/100 mm Hg, probably a result of the strong emotional reaction rather than a direct effect of psilocybin. I wondered why the hallucination of this old house, whose name was Saint Bernard,* provoked such strong emotions in me. This was linked both to significant memories of my childhood and to fortuitous circumstances. Actually, I had learned several days before the experiment that the house, which had been rented for the past thirty years, was to be sold. I had learned this with no apparent conscious reaction, but subconsciously there must have been some telling effect. I must at this point note another memory triggered by a kinesthetic stimulus. As my knees were pressed against my desk, I had the same feeling as years ago when I was a child and leaned against the window sill of our house in Bayonne; here in the Basque country I could look at the wharfs along the Nive River which meandered below the window. And again, the eerie magic lantern of my childhood lit up the apartment in a sort of halo, yet in a very exacting manner showing different pieces of furniture whose existence I had forgotten about long ago.

Next, there was a relative logorrhea which gave the observers an impression of confusion and incoherence. Body image defects appeared which I recalled afterwards, as well as a tendency to perseveration. At the end of three hours, the experiment was ended. I was able to go about my regular work that afternoon without any trouble but nevertheless noted that my mood was somewhat quickened and that colors appeared brighter than usual; this disappeared several days later. It is of interest to report Volmat's studies in our department of psychopathological art at Saint Anne. He observed that some painters not only had a modification in their color sense after psilocybin but in their technique as well.

In London this past March, Pichot, Lemperiere, and I presented our results concerning the somatic and psychological effects of psilocybin in 101 abnormal and 52 normal patients. We observed changes in (1) emotional, volitional, and intellectual spheres, (2) perception of the body image, (3) contact with the surroundings, (4) mood, and (5) time and space. Analysis of these parameters with psilocybin offers an advantage over mescaline because of the time factor—the whole experiment lasts about four hours. Systematic analysis of these changes can be very useful for experimental psychiatry. Thus, data become available on the differences between hallucinations and hallucinosis, the changes in self, and the individual's relations in time and space. Outside these particular problems, the technique is of value for analysis of the individual's

*It had formerly been a monastery.

psychological state and psychopathological condition since each entity has its own particular way of reacting to psilocybin.

One may ask, what is the relation between the experimental psychoses and the endogenous psychoses? Do these relationships offer any argument in favor of the biochemical origin of the psychoses? Do they have any importance insofar as diagnosis and treatment of mental illness is concerned?

The artificially induced psychoses produced by the psychodysleptic drugs are acute exogenous states whose symptomatology is variable, depending upon the drug and the patient as well as on the interaction between both, oscillating between a depersonalized state and one in which there is a complete loss of the associative processes with confusion, delusions, hallucinations, temporal-spatial disorientation, etc. The acute experimental exogenous psychoses are the same as the hallucinatory psychotic states seen in the wards whether the latter are endogenous or exogenous in origin. These drugs can produce a whole gamut of syndromes which can be suggestive of different diagnoses. Even a psychiatrist with considerable experience, when asked to examine blindly patients under the effects of LSD or psilocybin, will not fail in some cases to question the possibility that these may be cases of early schizophrenia.

The psychodysleptic drugs can produce a hallucinatory psychosis but cannot reproduce the characteristics of schizophrenic process. However, if one takes into account the polymorphic characteristics of the artificial psychoses and the early schizophrenic syndromes and if one compares one acute state with another (not an acute with a chronic condition), certain similarities become apparent. Depersonalization and confusion with loosening of the associative processes can resemble the schizophrenic dissociation. Régis certainly had this in mind when he separated the condition called "chronic mental confusion" or "postconfusional schizophrenia." The experimentally induced drug states are, of necessity, short lasting, but chronic states are known, as with hashish. Uzman described the latter clinical condition as analogous to a schizophrenic dissociation. The drug-induced state differs from the paranoid syndrome because of the preponderance of visual hallucinations and the confusional state. But, between the hallucinatory dreamy states* and autistic thought, there is a strong structural similarity, as suggested by an analysis of the symptoms, the psychodynamics, and the Rorschach material.

*"pensée onirique."

In addition, certain schizophrenic conditions begin with an acute delusional state, periodic attacks of visual hallucinations, or a dream state with clouded consciousness and frequently lead to chronic schizophrenia. It would not seem necessary to give these a special name ("oneirophrenia," according to Meduna), since they are probably all varieties of the same fundamental schizophrenic process. The symptoms of paranoid schizophrenia respond very well to chemotherapy, just as the drug-induced states, provided that in the former sufficiently high doses are given for a considerable period of time, as one would do in the chronic psychoses. Is it not possible, then, that there might be some pathogenetic similarity between both conditions? Hippocrates said, "Treatment will reveal the nature of the illness."

Inappropriate affect and laughter (noted previously by Moreau de Tours with hashish), dysphoria, ecstatic states, bizarre behavior, feelings of being "far away," strangeness in the immediate environment, and inexplicable changes in relationship of self to the world have been noted in some of the experimental psychoses. All of these symptoms are observable in early schizophrenia, as Morcelli indicated with regard to mescaline. Some of the chronic schizophrenic patients can relive their earlier acute psychotic symptoms under the effects of these drugs, particularly psilocybin. The relationship of the catatonic syndrome observed during an early acute exogenous psychosis with catatonic schizophrenia has already been discussed by Baruk and de Jong, as well as Buscaino, and more recently by Gjessing in his studies of periodic catatonia. Taking into strict account the problem of nosology in the group of schizophrenias as well as our limited experiences with the psychotropic drugs (which, nevertheless, increases and even changes directions with time), it can be said that there are some similarities between certain forms of the artificially induced psychoses and certain schizophrenic syndromes; to be analogous does not, of course, mean being identical to. This analogy has given new impetus to the biochemical theories of psychoses.

The organic concept of mental illness is strongly opposed by those favoring the psychodynamic etiological approach. Yet, the apparent dissimilarity between the opposing view is more apparent than real. In any case, the psychopharmacologic studies are aimed at the pathogenetic mechanisms of the mental syndromes so that there really is no conflict with the psychodynamic hypotheses.

Is it not possible that emotional tension of either an acute or

chronic variety can give rise to metabolic disorders via the mechanisms of the alarm and exhaustion syndromes? Thus, the psychodynamic pathogenesis could still be considered even though their
effects theoretically were produced by biochemical mechanisms.
There is even more. The human emotions are capable of inducing
symptoms that are as intense and variable as those induced by
psychotropic drugs (whose action can be depressing, stimulating,
or disorganizing) with disorders in the intellectual, emotional,
visceral, and motor spheres. In addition, it has·been known for a
long time that an emotional shock is not only symptom producing
but symptom removing as well, perhaps by the alarm-reaction
mechanism acting through the diencephalic-pituitary axis. In all
probability, there is reason to believe that symptoms of the various
psychoses are organic in nature, resulting from the organization
and integration of different central cerebral pathways. The psychophysiological mechanisms described can also be precipitated by
somatic and psychological factors as well as by psychotropic drugs.
Their effects are felt via the intermediary of the central physico-
chemical changes in the brain; this can be considered one of the
bases of mental life but not necessarily the only one.

Experimental studies with psychotropic drugs in the light of
their selective central action have elicited a wealth of information
on the topographic etiological localization of the different mental
syndromes. One of the central problems of psychopharmacological
research today is the relationship between the cortical and subcortical structures: consideration could be given to the diencephalon
and reticular-activating substance in relation to the regulation of
sleep and waking states, the influence of hypothalamic and limbic
structures in the regulation of mood and emotional tone, the relation
of the mammillary bodies and their projection tracts to the psycho-
pathology of time relation and memory, and the cortico-infracortical
pathways in respect to psychomotor activity. Everything that we can
learn about the localization of action of psychotropic drugs will
help in understanding the specific central pathological component
of mental illness.

The importance of pinpointing the topographic localization of
these syndromes is self-evident, but yet more important is a
knowledge of the biochemical mechanisms. Much has been written
about the many contributions of neuropathology to neurology and
the sterility of such findings in the psychoses. It would, indeed, be
tempting to conclude that with no neuropathologic changes in the

psychoses, consideration of an organic cause would be fruitless. However, the problem is of such importance that it could be considered from another angle—the functional biochemical disturbance. This would not be a matter of an anatomical lesion but of physiological changes revealed through the use of biochemical techniques.

The concept of the functional biochemical disturbance, conceived from neurochemical evidence suggesting metabolic changes of central neurohumoral substances and their enzymes, represents one of the most heuristic orientations in biological psychiatric research. This is particularly true in so far as the problems of enzymatic inhibition are concerned. Certain drugs, for example, act by inhibiting the enzyme that normally destroys a mediator (monamine oxidase and iproniazid). Other drugs do the contrary—inhibit an enzyme whose role is in synthesis. Enzymatic control, thus, can act in two ways: inhibition or activation of a mediator. It is only recently that the biochemical mechanisms of action of mediators has been elucidated. Thus, some of the pharmacological activity of catechol amines (e.g., hyperglycemia) can be explained by the activation of a phosphorylytic enzyme necessary to break glycogen down to glucose. In this regard, may I point out that psilocybin is not only the first naturally occurring phosphorylated indole but that the phosphorylation of this nucleus is probably unrelated to the drug's action, since psilocin (a dephosphorylated psilocybin) has the same properties as psilocybin.

A study of the antagonism between psychotropic drugs can yield much interesting information. Thus, psychoanaleptic states induced by amphetamines are neutralized by psycholeptic states induced by barbiturates and vice versa. The psychodysleptic states can be terminated or even blocked by the neuroleptics. One can even go further. Studies of the antagonism between LSD-25 and serotonin have opened new horizons as well as stimulated research concerning central variations in serotonin and noradrenalin content resulting from reserpine and neutralized by antireserpine compounds. The indole nucleus, present in some substances capable of inducing an abnormal state of behavior, has stimulated other studies. The structural analogy between LSD-25 and psilocybin is clear, since both possess a 4-substituted indole nucleus.

In spite of all these theoretical considerations of experimental psychoses, the clinical use of psychodysleptic drugs does not seem to be justified as a general procedure. They should not be used clinically without specific indications, either diagnostic or therapeutic. This, of course, does not relate to experimental studies by volunteers or physicians.

PSYCHODYSLEPTIC DRUGS AS AIDS
IN DIAGNOSIS AND TREATMENT

Psilocybin offers diagnostic possibilities. A psychodynamic analysis of the material revealed during the .drug study period permitted one to understand the unconscious material much better; it could almost be called a chemical psychoanalysis. I will come back to the possible therapeutic aspects later.

Since psilocybin exaggerates the underlying neurotic or psychotic trends, it can clarify many problems and help in the diagnoses of clinical problems that are unclear. For example, an atypical anorexia nervosa showed a frank hebephrenic reaction, which was then treated with neuroleptic medication. There was, on the other hand, an atypical depression treated unsuccessfully for one year with psychotherapy. Psilocybin produced a frank melancholic reaction. Subsequent electroconvulsive treatment eliminated all the symptoms of depression, and the patient was well. Hebephrenic patients show an atypical excitement or cataleptic state, with the only signs of emotional involvement being inappropriate laughter. The paranoid or chronic delusional psychotic individual shows a depersonalization and derealization resembling the earlier phases of the illness, a hallucinatory delusional state, the reappearance of significant psychotic symptoms, or an anxiety syndrome with agitation and combativeness. The psychoneurotic patients show a fairly constant picture with anxiety and dysphoria predominating. The type of reaction will differ according to the significant character traits—hysterical, phobic, obsessive, or others. The neurotic subject generally lives through the drug-induced experience much more intensely than normal subjects, focusing upon and abreacting the traumatic events and past significant conflicts.

The interest in using psilocybin, as well as other pharmacologic substances, in the traumatic neuroses is obvious, in view of the possibility of producing, almost at will, an abreaction of past events. Besides these rather infrequent cases, one can consider the drug's therapeutic action from two points of view.

There is first a direct biological mood-stimulating effect on the organism. This is very clear in neurasthenic conditions and some depressions. In depression there can at times be a mood reversal under the effects of the drug. Second, there is the psycho-dynamic action I have already mentioned. The physician can use this material to great advantage in terms of the patient-physician relationship during the experimental period. The patient can play a dual role—the observer and the observed. He thus can be close to the symbolism inherent in the drug-induced state and yet observe it at a distance. Since this all takes place in clear consciousness, a detailed analysis is possible at a later time, since it is only in the hours and days that follow that the analytic work becomes more meaningful. The patient can bring together his past and drug-induced present, and with the therapist arrive at a synthesis—a "psychobiography."

One frequently observes changes in the patient-physician re-lationship as a result of the emotional changes in the patient. The transference which is often very strong during the experimental period continues afterwards as well. This can be used psycho-therapeutically, since the analysis can now proceed without the transference resistance.

This leads me to state a concept of fundamental importance in psychiatry—the reciprocal relationship between chemotherapy and psychotherapy. The neuroleptic drugs have facilitated the psycho-therapeutic process by removing those symptoms that have blocked the patient's efforts in relating to others. Actually, they have not decreased the need for social therapy, psychotherapy, and other modalities but have facilitated their application and extended their use to patients hitherto unreceptive to such treatments. In addition, it has been possible to introduce new techniques in psychotherapy through the use of leptic, analeptic, and dysleptic drugs. I refer here to narcoanalysis, amphetamine shock, and the drug-induced states of abnormal behavior produced with LSD and psilocybin; and, in all probability, new drugs and new techniques will appear in the years to come. In one of his last works, Freud wrote, "Only psychodynamically oriented treatment is of interest to us, since this is all we have at the present. In the future, we will probably learn to influence the libido directly and the mental life as well through the use of chemical compounds." This perspective, which to him seemed so distant, has in reality arrived, for in fact pharmacologic agents are· capable of influencing psychological activity in a psychodynamic frame of reference.

Psychoanalysts and others have tended to identify psychiatry as a discipline based on philosophical, moral, and ethical values, as well as the psychotherapy of mental illness. But, there has developed in a parallel fashion a biological approach based on neurophysiological research aided by the contributions of neurochemistry, endocrinology, and psychopharmacology. Yet, psychiatry cannot be reduced to a sort of pharmacologic medicine, no more than it can be reduced to the mere status of psychological medicine. The ancient opposition between psyche and soma has given rise to a holistic approach, a global concept. The physician can now view the personality as a totality in which biological, social, and psychological processes are only artificially separated for study. In this concept of the individual, psychiatry today is striving to remove its prejudices and its clashing doctrines so as to integrate the use of all techniques, physical or psychological, in its continued fight against the scourge of mental illness.

REFERENCES

1. Delay, Jean: Les dérèglements de l'humeur, Presses universitaires de France, Paris, 1946.

CHAPTER 14

On a Proposed Theory for the Mechanism of Action of Serotonin in Brain

By M. H. APRISON, PH.D.

Because it was difficult to explain the diverse effects of centrally acting drugs on the basis of the single neurohumoral agent acetylcholine (ACh), Brodie and Shore [1, 2] proposed in an interesting hypothesis that 5-hydroxytryptamine (serotonin or 5-HT) and norepinephrine might act as the main neurohumors of the trophotropic and ergotropic systems in brain. Much of the recent data from Brodie's laboratories have been explained in terms of this theory [3-6]. The theory was based on the concepts of Hess [7, 8], namely, that there is a functional integration of the autonomic nervous system with the rest of the brain and that a subcortical system exists which consists of separate and antagonistic divisions, the ergotrophic and trophotropic. These ideas completely omit from discussion any reference to the ACh-cholinesterase (ChE) system. Data in the literature suggest that ACh is an important link in the chain of biochemical events associated with excitation of brain neurons, and in the author's opinion ACh should be included in any theory of neurohumoral action [9-11]. Furthermore, the criteria necessary for a neurohumoral classification as used for serotonin and norepinephrine—such as (1) stored in an inactive form, (2) easily changed to a free or active form, (3) localized in different parts of the brain at varying concentration levels, (4) an enzyme present for its synthesis, and (5) an enzyme present for its destruction—apply equally well for ACh. In addition, when one compares the activities of cholinesterase and monoamine oxidase (MAO), the enzymes which keep ACh and 5-HT at physiological levels, it is

The investigations reported in this paper were supported by a research grant MY-3225 from the National Institute of Mental Health, U. S. Public Health Service.

interesting that in the brain the ratio is approximately 100 in favor of ChE activity, whereas in the peripheral organs, such as the liver, it is a small fraction of this value [12, 13]. Even if one suggests that ChE is normally present in great excess, a comparison of ACh content with 5-HT in the brain of some species from which data is available indicates that the former is present in amounts about ten times higher [see ref. 14, 15 for comparison in the rat, ref. 16 for rabbit midbrain]. Such data, taken together with the other facts, suggested to the author that ACh rather than 5-HT could be the more important neurohumoral agent in brain. If a trophotropic division exists in brain, then ACh could take the role suggested originally for 5-HT. One would then be left to explain the role of serotonin.

The following two assumptions can be made: (1) Hess is correct in his idea of the presence of two opposing divisions in brain, and (2) ACh is the neurohormone for the trophotropic division. It is not difficult to understand how a "coarse" control of behavior can result in an organism by either the activation or depression of one of the two antagonistic divisions. However, what is difficult to understand is how such a mechanism would result in "fine" or subtle behavioral control. This line of reasoning led the author to wonder whether there did not exist a second system within each division that had the role of regulating (via a negative chemical feedback mechanism) or modulating the output of the main division. That is, could 5-HT inhibit ChE activity in such a way as to produce a biphasic effect via the action of the resulting level of ACh? Furthermore, if 5-HT had such an effect on the trophotropic division, what biochemical compound was the counterpart of 5-HT for the ergotropic division? Is it also 5-HT [17]?

Our experiments to date in this area of research have involved only the study of the interaction of 5-HT on the ACh-ChE system. Data from several experiments are presented in this paper. In addition, a theory for the mechanism of action of 5-HT is presented in which it is possible to explain its biphasic action in brain and possibly in other organs in terms of the ACh-ChE system.

EXPERIMENTAL

Brain cholinesterase assays were made employing the Difunctional Recording Titrator and using the conditions previously described [18]. All titrations were made under nitrogen. Acetylcholine determinations were made employing a bioassay technique previously described [19].

Cholinesterase assays were also run at five different substrate concentrations and at two 5-HT concentrations in order that sufficient data be obtained to construct the Lineweaver-Burk plot; this reciprocal plot of enzyme activity and substrate is used to provide information about the type of inhibition present. Substrate levels higher than that permitting maximum enzyme activity were not employed.

The following chemicals and drugs were used: (1) serotonin creatinine $\cdot H_2SO_4 \cdot H_2O$ and D,L-5-hydroxytryptophan hydrate (California Corporation for Biochemical Research); (2) serotonin bioxolate* and 5-methoxytryptamine (The Regis Chemical Company); (3) acetylcholine chloride (Merck vials, 100 mg; (4) trans-dl-2-phenylcyclopropylamine hydrochloride (SKF 385, kindly donated by Smith, Kline and French); and iproniazid (Marsilid, a gift from Hoffmann-LaRoche, Inc.).

RESULTS

The data in Table I show that rabbit brain (caudate nucleus) cholinesterase activity at pH 7.8 and 37 C is inhibited in the presence of 5-HT. The final ACh concentration in the reaction vessel was $3 \cdot 10^{-3}$ M. As the inhibitor concentration approached that of the substrate, the ChE activity was reduced to approximately

*Specially prepared for the author and supported by a special contract from the Psychopharmacology Service Center, National Institute of Mental Health.

TABLE I

Effect of 5-Hydroxytryptamine on Rabbit Brain Cholinesterase

5-HT Conc. (final M)	ChE Activity (% normal)	% Inhibition
0	100	0
$9.0 \cdot 10^{-4}$	70	30
$2.2 \cdot 10^{-3}$	57	43
$4.5 \cdot 10^{-3}$	37	63
$9.0 \cdot 10^{-3}$	0	100

50%. When the 5-HT concentration was doubled ($2.2 \cdot 10^{-3}$ to $4.5 \cdot 10^{-3}$) the ChE activity decreased below a critical level (Fig. 2). If the assay is carried out at decreasing pHs (10 to 6), it is found that the same concentration of serotonin results in more inhibition. However, if a comparable amount of 5-methoxytryptamine is sub-

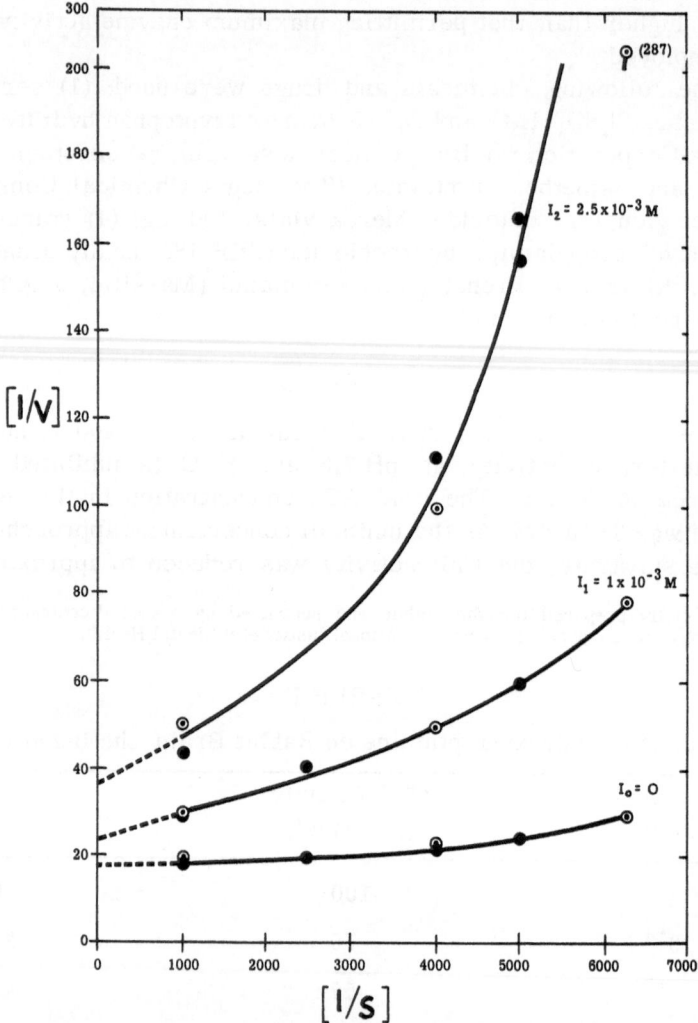

FIG. 1.   Double reciprocal plot demonstrating "mixed" inhibition of cholinesterase activity by serotonin. (pH of the reaction mixture was 7.8.) The black and white circles (mean of three determinations) represent two separate experiments.

stituted for 5-HT, varying the pH over the same range does not markedly change the percent of inhibition.

In Fig. 1, data in the form of a Lineweaver-Burk plot are presented to show the effect of varying both the ACh (below that required for V_{max}) and 5-HT concentrations on brain ChE activity. Apparently the equilibrium constant for the combination of serotonin with free enzyme and the enzyme-substrate complex are not equal, resulting in a more complicated inhibition. The latter is sometimes referred to as "mixed," i.e., it has some of the characteristics of competitive inhibition and some of noncompetitive inhibition [20, 21].

In vivo experiments were designed to determine if ChE inhibition occurs when brain 5-HT levels are elevated. Rabbits (white, albino adults) were injected intravenously with the serotonin precursor, 5-hydroxytryptophan (10 to 20 mg/kg), with and without iproniazid (100 mg/kg) or SKF-385 (2 mg/kg) pretreatment. One hour after the last injection, the animals were sacrificed by injecting air into the marginal ear vein. Samples (approximately 100 mg) of cortex, caudate nucleus, thalamus, and medulla were taken and analyzed for ChE activity. Inhibition of *in vivo* ChE activity in the tissue samples taken could not be demonstrated consistently in these brain parts. The rabbits exhibited marked behavioral patterns. In addition to the usual signs of elevated 5-HT levels, many of the rabbits tended to move backwards.

In order to determine if the *in vitro* inhibition of ChE activity by 5-HT is reversible or not, brain homogenates with and without this inhibitor were dialyzed against 0.11 M NaCl for fifteen hours. Aliquots from these dialysis bags were measured for ChE activity. In addition, samples similarly made up but not dialyzed were also assayed for ChE activity. The data from this experiment are summarized in Table II. The inhibition of ChE by 5-HT was completely reversible.

It became important to determine whether 5-HT inhibits ChE immediately or if an incubation period is necessary for complete inhibition to occur. The data in Table III show that after incubating 5-HT with brain homogenates for different lengths of time, the percent of inhibition was essentially the same. When these data are extrapolated to zero time, it appears that the inhibition is instantaneous.

Several years ago Aprison and co-workers [22, 23] reported in separate studies the ChE activity and free ACh content in the right and left cerebral cortices and caudate nuclei from albino

TABLE II

Effect of Dialysis on ChE Inhibition by 5-Hydroxytryptamine

Length of Dialysis Against 0.11 M NaCl (hr)	5-HT Conc. (final M)	ChE Activity (ml 0.005 N NaOH to keep pH 7.8 for 200 sec pS 3)
0	0	0.078
0	$3 \cdot 10^{-3}$	0.025
15	0	0.078
15	$3 \cdot 10^{-3}$	0.076

rabbits exhibiting compulsive turning movements (to the left) after receiving a unilateral (right) intracarotid injection of 0.1 mg/kg of diisopropyl fluorophosphate (DFP), a potent anticholinesterase drug. Although the ChE and ACh data were obtained from two different series of albino rabbits, it is now instructive to compare these data since both groups received the same dose of DFP under the same experimental conditions. These data (the mean of six to eight animals per part) are shown in Fig. 2. There was no change in the free ACh content in either the cortex or caudate nucleus when the ChE activity was reduced to approximately 40 to 50% of normal by DFP. However, when the inhibition of ChE activity fell below some critical value near this range, the free ACh content

TABLE III

Effect of Incubation Time on Cholinesterase Inhibition by 5-Hydroxytryptamine

ChE Activity without 5-HT (ml 0.005 N NaOH to keep reaction pH at 7.8 for 200 sec) pS 2.5	ChE Activity with 5-HT (final conc. $9 \cdot 10^{-4}$M)	Incubation Time (min)	% Inhibition
0.153	0.098	3	36
0.145	0.099	13	32
0.149	0.094	30	37

rose to over 200% of normal, indicating the loss of physiological control of the enzyme for its substrate.

Normally ACh is destroyed when it is hydrolyzed by ChE. However, ACh probably produces its physiological effect at a receptor protein different from the protein ChE. On the other hand, because the electrical charge distribution on the ACh molecule at pH 7.35 remains unchanged, it is highly possible that the site on the receptor protein and the enzymatic site on ChE are essentially the same or identical. Consequently, if 5-HT molecules inhibit the enzyme action of ChE on ACh, they should also be able to compete with the ACh molecules at the ACh-receptor protein.

THEORY

Based on *in vitro* data, Aprison [24] suggested in a preliminary report in 1960 that a biphasic 5-HT effect could be explained in terms of the cholinergic system depending only on the levels of 5-HT present at the receptor protein and ChE sites. It is suggested

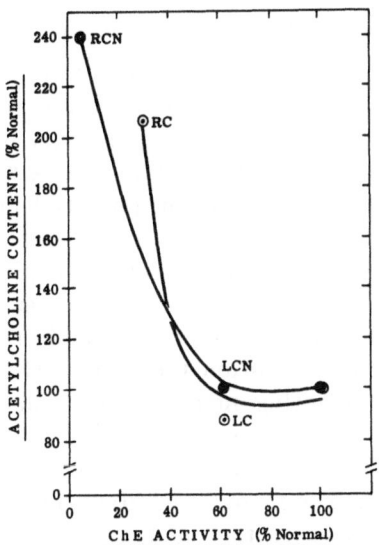

FIG. 2. Correlation of cholinesterase activity and free ACh content in the right and left cerebral cortices (RC, LC) and caudate nuclei (RCN, LCN) from rabbits given a 0.1mg/kg DFP injection into the right common carotid artery. Each point is the mean of six to eight animals and is expressed as percent of normal.

that when the free 5-HT content rises to levels "slightly" higher than normal, sedation would result owing to the competition of free 5-HT molecules with ACh molecules at the appropriate sites in brain and possibly at other organs (but not on smooth muscle where these compounds apparently either act at independent sites or through some unknown mechanism [25]). Note the resemblance of these molecules at pH 7.35 (also compare with norepinephrine).

$$\underset{CH_3}{\overset{O}{\nearrow}}C\text{-}O\text{-}CH_2\text{-}CH_2\text{-}\overset{+}{N}\equiv(CH_3)_3 \qquad \text{ACETYLCHOLINE}$$

$$HO\text{-}\overset{}{\underset{N}{\boxed{}}}\text{-}CH_2\text{-}CH_2\text{-}\overset{+}{N}\equiv H_3 \qquad \text{SEROTONIN}$$

$$\underset{HO\text{-}}{HO\text{-}}\boxed{}\text{-}\underset{OH}{CH}\text{-}CH_2\text{-}\overset{+}{N}\equiv H_3 \qquad \text{NOREPINEPHRINE}$$

At these 5-HT levels, some inhibition of ChE would occur but not enough to reduce the enzyme activity below a critical value; hence, ACh levels would either remain the same or tend to rise slightly. ChE is present in excess, since the activity of this enzyme must be reduced to levels below 40% before its effects are noted both on ACh levels in brain and the action potential in nerve [26]. On the other hand, when high free 5-HT levels occur in brain, such as after reserpine administration to animals pretreated with MAO inhibitors, the resulting excitation might be caused by a significant accumulation of ACh due to the greater inhibition of ChE by serotonin. During such a situation the ChE activity should be below the critical level, resulting in a rise in ACh content. This state of excitation caused by excess ACh might then result from direct stimulation of excitation centers or opposing inhibition centers (yielding an unbalance in favor of excitation centers). These ideas suggest that in addition to the mechanism mediated via norepinephrine to produce excitation in an animal [2, 27] still another is available, namely, that which is due to an accumulation of ACh at appropriate centers. One need only recall the forced or compulsive circling in animals produced by the unilateral intracarotid injection of DFP to see that excessive levels of brain ACh are correlated with an active animal [9, 22, 23].

DISCUSSION

The data presented in this paper suggest that serotonin at a physiological pH level competes with ACh for the latter's receptor site in the CNS. Friess and McCarville [28] have concluded from their studies of certain inhibitors on ChE activity that a "good" inhibitor should have a charged nitrogen and a properly situated locus of high electron density. Investigators in this field feel that the positively charged nitrogen would be attached to the negatively charged anionic site of the enzyme surface (or a particular charged membrane) while the point of high electron density in the substrate or inhibitor would be attached to the esteratic site. Krupka and Laidler [21] have shown that in cases in which a mixed type of inhibition occurs (such as in the case of 5-HT acting on ChE) it is still possible for an inhibitor and substrate to combine with the enzyme at the same site. Their work is important because classical enzymatic theory suggests that only in the case of competitive inhibition do substrate and inhibitor compete for the same site on the enzyme surface.

Although *in vitro* inhibition of ChE is easily demonstrated, this was not so in the case of *in vivo* inhibition. In the experiments reported in this study, it is possible that in the process of homogenizing the brain samples any excess 5-HT that was present in sufficient amounts to inhibit ChE would have been diluted out to noninhibitory levels. This is due to the fact that the inhibition has been shown to be completely reversible. Therefore, other types of experiments must be designed to show the action of 5-HT on ChE and the ACh-receptor protein in the presence of ACh. These are in progress.

It is now possible to explain some of the data in the literature by means of the theory suggested in this paper. It is well documented that sedation occurs after reserpine treatment. This result is explained by the fact that after such treatment the capacity of the brain to store serotonin is impaired and that initially there is a rise in free 5-HT, which then falls to some equilibrium value determined by the activities of the synthesizing and destroying enzymes, namely, 5-hydroxytryptophan decarboxylase and monoamine oxidase respectively. This equilibrium value for free 5-HT is probably higher than that present in the normal nontreated animal. The free 5-HT then competes with ACh for the sites on both the ChE surface and the receptor protein where ACh normally produces its physiological effect in brain. The result should be a reduction in the usual ACh effect and, as a consequence, the sedated animal might have an initially elevated total ACh content, since the rate of utilization could conceivably be associated with its release from storage sites. In 1959, Malhotra and Pundlik [29] demonstrated that the total ACh content in five CNS parts from dogs rose after the animals received 0.5 mg/kg of reserpine iv, whereas in the case of the hippocampus there was a significant fall. Pepeu and Giarman [30] reported that in rats given reserpine in a dose of 0.5 mg/kg daily, total brain ACh was elevated on the second day but that no change was noted in subsequent days (up to eight days).

The suggestion by Brodie and co-workers that the reserpine effects, namely, sedation, hypothermia, ptosis, and the blocking of a previously established avoidance-escape conditioned reflex, are due to a loss of 5-HT is weakened by the data of Canal and Maffei-Facciolo [31]. These authors have shown that after injecting 5 mg/kg of reserpine into rats, the further administration of iproniazid (100 mg/kg) 6 hours before killing the animals doubled the serotonin level of brain (over that of the control animal which had received reserpine alone) and that yet the animals still exhibited the usual reserpine signs. Also, Aprison and co-workers [32] have recently found that 5-HT levels in specific pigeon brain areas were high during the behavioral effect produced by the administration of the precursor 5-HTP. When the 5-HT returned to normal values in these parts, the behavioral effect ceased. During the behavioral effect, the birds were not able to perform the learned task, namely, working on a multiple fixed ratio-fixed interval schedule of reinforcement [33,34], and the performance resembled that of birds given reserpine or reserpine-like compounds [35].

Pretreatment with a monoamine oxidase inhibitor, such as iproniazid, antagonizes the behavioral depression induced by reserpine [36]. The "stimulation" or "excitement" usually observed in the animal after such treatment could now be explained as being due to the higher levels of free 5-HT in brain, since the enzyme which destroys 5-HT is inhibited. These higher serotonin levels are probably capable of inhibiting ChE below its critical value. The net result of this reaction could be a large excess of free ACh. Because of the competition of ACh and 5-HT molecules at the appropriate receptor sites, it is possible, as in the case of competitive inhibition, for excess substrate to overcome the competition of the natural inhibitor molecules. This action would result in excessive stimulation due to high ACh levels at appropriate sites. This does not rule out any reaction due to elevated norepinephrine levels within its own system.

With MAO inhibitors given to animals after reserpine, instead of before, a reversal of the reserpine effect was not observed in the earlier studies [37, 38]. From the theory presented in this paper, it is possible to predict that this finding is true only for a short period of time after the MAO inhibitor injections. Depending on the dose of the MAO inhibitor injected, 5-HT would accumulate slowly since it is constantly being synthesized by the enzyme 5-hydroxytryptophan decarboxylase and not being destroyed as rapidly as in the normal animal. Therefore, this action should result within a finite length of time in a situation that approaches the case in which the MAO inhibitor is injected prior to reserpine administration. Recently, Stein and Ray [39] demonstrated in their behavioral studies on rats that there was indeed an accelerated recovery from reserpine depression by MAO inhibitors. However, these authors feel the delayed reserpine reversal by the MAO inhibitors is due to the recovery of norepinephrine rather than of serotonin. They base their conclusions on data from the brain stem of reserpinized rabbits from another laboratory [40]. Future studies on the same species and of many brain areas are necessary for further clarification of this point.

Recently, Gertner [41] reported in an interesting paper the ability of several MAO inhibitors to block superior cervical ganglionic transmission in the cat. When using β-phenylisopropyl hydrazine (JB-516), he found that during the block in transmission ACh release from the preganglionic nerve endings was unaffected. On the other hand, if during this block an injection of ACh was made into the ganglion, it was still effective in stimulating the ganglion cells. However, Gertner points out that the dose of ACh necessary to stimulate the ganglion cell above is of the order of 1000 times greater than that released on nerve stimulation. He asks, "How then do the monoamine oxidase inhibitors block transmission if they are not working on the classical acetylcholine-cholinesterase system?" An explanation can be made in terms of the theory presented in this paper. First, it is probable that MAO activity is inhibited since 5-HT has been demonstrated in the perfusate from similar preparations [42, 43]. However, it is possible that the latter might be released through some other mechanism.

Therefore, free 5-HT is present in sufficient amounts to block normal ACh released (mμg). However, when a large excess of ACh (10 μg) is injected into the perfusion stream, there are sufficient ACh molecules available to reverse the 5-HT blocking effect. One should now do the critical experiment with this preparation, namely, inject solutions of ACh plus varying amounts of 5-HT into the perfusion fluid, to note what level of 5-HT, if any, blocks ACh action. The theory predicts such a concentration will be found.

Much work remains to be done. It is becoming increasingly evident that new microchemical methods are necessary in order that free and bound 5-HT, ACh, and norepinephrine can be simultaneously determined in extremely small amounts of nervous tissue. The measurement of total ACh, 5-HT, and norepinephrine in large amounts of tissue, such as the whole brain, tend in many instances to mask the true changes that are occurring.

SUMMARY

A theory for the mechanism of action of serotonin in brain is proposed. It is suggested that serotonin is probably not a neurohormone but a natural inhibitor of acetylcholinesterase. Through its action on acetylcholinesterase and the acetylcholine receptor protein, serotonin modulates the action of acetylcholine by direct competition with it for the active sites on these important proteins.

REFERENCES

1. Brodie, B. B., and Shore, P. A.: Unified concept of interaction of psychotropic agents with neurohormones, Fed. Proc. 17:353, 1958.

2. Brodie, B. B., Spector, S., and Shore, P. A.: Interaction of drugs with norepinephrine in the brain, Symposium on Catecholamines, Williams & Wilkins Company, Baltimore, 1959, p. 548.

3. Brodie, B. B., Bogdanski, D. F., and Shore, P. A.: The action of psychotropic drugs. A biochemical and physiological interpretation. in Rinkel, M., and Denber, H. C. B., Eds.: Chemical Concepts of Psychosis, McDowell and Obolensky, Inc., New York 1958, p. 190.

4. Shore, P. A., and Brodie, B. B.: Influence of various drugs on serotonin and norepinephrine in the brain. in Garattini, S., and Ghetti, V., Eds.: Psychotropic Drugs, Elsevier, Amsterdam, 1957, p. 423.

5. Brodie, B. B., and Shore, P. A.: On a role for serotonin and norepinephrine as chemical mediators in the central autonomic nervous system. in Hoagland, H., Ed.: Hormones, Brain Function and Behavior, Academic Press, Inc., New York, 1957, pp. 161–176.

6. Kuntzman, R., Costa, E., Gessa, G. L., Hirsch, C., and Brodie, B. B.: Com-

bined use of a-Methyl meta-tyrosine and reserpine to associate norepinephrine with excitation and serotonin with sedation, Fed. Proc. 20:308, 1961.

7. Hess, W. R.: Das Zwischenhirn, Syndrome, Localisationen, Funktionen, 2nd ed., Benno Schwabe, Basle, 1954.

8. Hess, W. R.: Diencephalon, Autonomic and Extrapyramidal Functions, Monog. Biol. Med., Vol. III, Grune & Stratton, Inc., New York, 1954.

9. Aprison, M. H.: Rate of compulsive circling in relation to accumulation of cerebral acetylcholine, J. Neurochem. 2:197, 1958.

10. Nachmansohn, D.: Chemical and Molecular Basis of Nerve Activity, Academic Press, Inc., New York, 1959.

11. Rinaldi, F., and Himwich, H. E.: Alerting responses and actions of atropine and cholinergic drugs, A.M.A. Arch. Neurol. Psychiat. 73:387, 1955.

12. Aprison, M. H., Folkerth, T. L., and Hanson, K. M.: Cholinesterase/monoamine oxidase ratios in the avian central nervous system, Physiologist 3:10, 1960.

13. Davison, A. N.: Physiological role of monoamine oxidase, Physiol. Rev. 38:729, 1958.

14. Twarog, B. M., and Page, I. H.: Serotonin content of some mammalian tissues and urine and a method for its determination, Am. J. Physiol. 175:157, 1953.

15. Crossland, J., Pappius, H. M., and Elliott, K. A. C.: Acetylcholine content of frozen brain, ibid. 183:27, 1955.

16. Aprison, M. H., and Wolf, M. A.: Unpublished data.

17. Gordon, P., Haddy, F. J., and Lipton, M. A.: Serotonin antagonism of noradrenaline in vivo, Science 128:531, 1958.

18. Aprison, M. H., and Folkerth, T. L.: Comparison of Monoamine Oxidase and Cholinesterase Activities in Several Discrete Areas from Pigeon Brain, to be published.

19. Aprison, M. H., and Nathan, P.: Determination of acetylcholine in small samples of fresh brain tissue, Arch. Biochem. Biophys. 66:388, 1957.

20. Dixon, M., and Webb, E. C.: Enzymes, Academic Press, Inc., New York, 1958.

21. Krupka, R. M., and Laidler, K. J.: Molecular mechanisms for hydrolytic enzyme action. I. Apparent noncompetitive inhibition, with special reference to acetylcholinesterase, J. Am. Chem. Soc. 83:1445, 1961.

22. Aprison, M. H., Nathan, P., and Himwich, H. E.: Cholinergic mechanism of brain involved in compulsive circling, Am. J. Physiol. 184:244, 1956.

23. Aprison, M. H., and Nathan, P.: Acetylcholine concentrations in the brain of rabbits exhibiting forced turning movements, ibid. 189:389, 1957.

24. Aprison, M. H. Effect of 5-hydroxytryptamine on cholinesterase activity, Fed. Proc. 19:275, 1960.

25. Woolley, D. W.: A probable mechanism of action of serotonin, Proc. Nat. Acad. Sci. U.S. 44:197, 1958.

26. Wilson, I. B., and Cohen, M.: The essentiality of acetylcholinesterase in conduction, Biochim. Biophys. Acta 11:147, 1953.

27. Costa, E., Gessa, G. L., Hirsch, C., and Kuntzman, R.: On current status of serotonin as brain neurohormone and in action of reserpine-like drugs (Abstr., New York Academy of Science Conference on Some Biological Aspects of Schizophrenic Behavior, New York, April 6-8, 1961.

28. Friess, S. L., and McCarville, W. J.: Nature of the acetyl-cholinesterase surface. I. Some potent competitive inhibitors of the enzyme, J. Am. Chem. Soc. 76:1363, 1954.

29. Malhotra, C. L., and Pundlik, P. G.: The effect of reserpine on the acetyl-

choline content of different areas of the central nervous system of the dog, Brit. J. Pharmacol. 14:46, 1959.

30. Pepeu, G. L., and Giarman, N. J.: The effect of certain neuropharmacologic agents on brain acetylcholine, Fed. Proc. 19:280, 1960.

31. Canal, N., and Maffei-Facciolo, A.: Reversal of the reserpine-induced depletion of brain serotonin by a monoamine oxidase inhibitor, J. Neurochem. 5:99, 1959.

32. Aprison, M. H., Wolf, M. A., Poulos, G. T., and Folkerth, T. L.: Neurochemical correlates of behavior. III. Variation of serotonin levels in several brain parts and other organs during the complete period of maximum behavioral effect after 5-hydroxytryptophan administration, to be published.

33. Aprison, M. H., and Ferster, C. B.: Neurochemical correlates of behavior. I. Quantitative measurements of the behavioral effects of the serotonin precursor, 5-hydroxytryptophan, J. Pharmacol. Exp. Therap. 131:100, 1961.

34. Aprison, M. H., and Ferster, C. B.: Neurochemical correlates of behavior. II. Correlation of brain monoamine oxidase activity with behavioral changes after iproniazid and 5-hydroxytryptophan administration, J. Neurochem. 6:350, 1961.

35. Paasonen, M. K., and Dews, P. B.: Effects of Raunescine and Isoraunescine on behavior and on the 5-hydroxytryptamine and noradrenalin contents of brain, Brit. J. Pharmacol. 13:84, 1958.

36. Brodie, B. B., and Shore, P. A.: A concept for a role of serotonin and norepinephrine as chemical mediators in the brain, Ann. N. Y. Acad. Sci. 66:631, 1957.

37. Shore, P. A., and Brodie, B. B.: LSD-like effects elicited by reserpine in rabbits pretreated with iproniazid, Proc. Soc. Exp. Biol. Med. 94:433, 1957.

38. Besendorf, H., and Pletscher, A.: Beeinflussung Zentrale Wirkungen von Reserpin und 5-Hydroxytryptamin durch Isonicotinsäurehydrazide, Helv. Physiol. Pharmacol. Acta. 14:383, 1956.

39. Stein, L., and Ray, O. S.: Accelerated recovery from reserpine depression by monoamine oxidase inhibitors, Nature 188:1199, 1960.

40. Spector, S., Shore, P. A., and Brodie, B. B.: Biochemical and pharmacological effects of the monoamine oxidase inhibitors, iproniazid, 1-phenyl-2-hydrazinopropane (JB 516) and 1-phenyl-3-hydrazinobutane (JB 835), J. Pharmacol. Exp. Therap. 128:15, 1960.

41. Gertner, S.: The effects of monoamine oxidase inhibitors on ganglionic transmission, ibid. 131:223, 1961.

42. Gertner, S. B., Paasonen, M. K., and Giarman, N. J.: Presence of 5-hydroxytryptamine in perfusate from sympathic ganglia, Fed. Proc. 16:1281, 1957.

43. Gertner, S. B., Paasonen, M. K., and Giarman, N. J.: Studies concerning the presence of 5-hydroxytryptamine (serotonin) in the perfusate from the superior cervical ganglion, J. Pharmacol. Exp. Therap. 127:268, 1959.

CHAPTER 15

The Relationship of Parkinsonism Produced by Drugs to Psychotic Reactions

By DOUGLAS GOLDMAN, M.D.

In Bleuler's classic monograph, in the section on theory [1, p.463], the following statement appears:

...Complete justice to all these factors can only be done by a concept of the disease which assumes the presence of (anatomic or chemical) disturbances of the brain; the course of the cerebral disorder is chronic, for the most part, but there are also phases of acute forward thrusts or of standstill; the disturbance of the brain determines the primary symptoms (disconnection of association, perhaps the disposition to hallucinations and stereotypies, a portion of the manic and the depressive syndromes, and the states of clouded consciousness, etc.). In more severe exacerbations, psychic symptoms, such as certain confusional and stuporous states, are direct consequences of the cerebral process. The rest of the psychic symptoms develop indirectly by way of abnormal mechanisms in the primarily disturbed psyche, inasmuch as the affectivity, in particular, gains pathologic superiority over the weakened logical functions.

This paragraph from Bleuler is indicative of the necessary conclusion to which his studies of the illness to which he gave the name "schizophrenia" led him. It was likewise the opinion of Kraepelin [2] that the illness which he first characterized as "dementia praecox" is fundamentally of organic origin. A number of modern students of this variety of mental illness have in all practical ways turned their backs on the possibility of an organic explanation for the illness and its course and have resorted to theories of psychogenic origin and development to the exclusion of organic factors.

The purpose of this report is to bring to light evidence which is corroborative of the theory of an organic origin of psychotic illnesses. The author has previously reported results of electroencephalographic studies with the use of Pentothal activation which indicate that schizophrenic illness is associated with specific electroencephalographic changes brought to light by Pentothal activation. These studies have been found, in two separate series of subjects (separated individually as well as in time), to have strong statistical validity. The present study represents material of an entirely different sort which may be considered to indicate the strong probability that psychotic functioning is associated with clear evidence of abnormality of brain functioning and therefore with an actual abnormality of the brain under consideration. The evidence consists of three groups of related observations.

EVIDENCE

Schizophrenic Patients Who Develop Parkinsonism

Over a period of more than twenty years a small group of patients admitted to Longview State Hospital, Cincinnati, who were recognizable as classical schizophrenic patients on admission have each developed, after one to ten years, the classical clinical picture of parkinsonism. This began to occur long before the introduction of any of the drugs that have been found to produce this physiological abnormality. Two typical case reports are here summarized:

CASE 1. Patient P. P., white, female, admitted to Longview State Hospital April 19, 1938, at age 17 years. The diagnosis prior to hospitalization in two agencies (University of Chicago clinics and Bureau of Juvenile Research in Columbus, Ohio) was schizophrenia. This diagnosis was reconfirmed after the admission examination, some of the staff members preferring "simple type" and some "hebephrenic type." She received insulin coma therapy with five additional Metrazol treatments from May to August of 1938. She was able to be out of the hospital from December, 1943, to March, 1944. The first recognition of parkinsonism in this sophisticated institution occurred in July of 1947, when the characteristic tremor was recognized in her hands and feet. Parkinsonism persists to the present time but is under fairly adequate control with anti-Parkinson drugs.

CASE 2. Patient A. F. B., white, female, age 22 years, admitted June 8, 1935, to Longview State Hospital. The diagnosis at the time of admission according to the record lay among: (1) early schizophrenia, (2) "mixed" manic-depressive psychosis, and (3) psychoneurotic (situational) depression. The patient was noted to have athetoid movements of the jaw and left arm, but these were not considered significant and were not considered in the diagnosis. In February, 1943, the physician first recognized the patient to have a postencephalitic syndrome. Active parkinsonism has been present until the present time but controlled to a great degree with anti-Parkinson drugs. In 1960 a follow-up mental status examination led an alert resident physician to suggest that the diagnosis be schizophrenia.

Parkinsonism After Phenothiazine Therapy

Recently individuals suffering from minimal residuals of encephalopathic processes were admitted to Longview State Hospital. One had barely perceptible hemiparesis. It was felt that his psychotic manifestations would respond to treatment with one of the newer phenothiazines under study. This phenothiazine, Tindal (acetophenazine), had much less tendency to produce parkinsonism than the well-known group of piperazine and dimethylamino derivatives already in the market. After a relatively short period of time of treatment with marked benefit for his psychologic manifestations, this patient developed an intense tremulous parkinsonism restricted to the side of his hemiparesis.

This observation seemed sufficiently striking by itself, but it also stirred a considerable amount of interpretive activity, particularly with the attempt to develop some harmonizing concept. It presently seemed evident that the parkinsonism that had developed in this patient was a reaction to the stress represented by the pharmacological activity of the drug administered. It is difficult to decide whether the manifestations of pharmacological activity involve a normal group of cells freed from controlling influences and thus indirectly affected by the drug or a group of pathological cells unduly and directly susceptible to the adverse influences of the drug administered.

Survey of Patients Under Drug Therapy

The concept that the parkinsonism reaction represented a reaction to pharmacological stress was very readily carried over to a study of the schizophrenic patients who had been treated with drugs. Motion picture records of a great many of these were available. These were all closely examined, and it was found that practically invariably the parkinsonism produced in the psychotic patients was irregularly distributed. Many examples of monoplegic parkinsonism involving one arm or one leg were evident. Frequent examples of involvement of parts of the mouth, the tongue, or the lips were seen. Even examples of involvement of single digits were available. Several examples of involvement of one arm and the opposite leg were seen. When the parkinsonism became sufficiently intense, the opposite member was frequently involved; and motion picture demonstration illustrated well that as the intensity of the reaction increases, the opposite extremity becomes involved, often in a cyclic fluctuating manner.

To further document this concept, a large number of patients under drug therapy were surveyed to determine the nature of the parkinsonism or its residuals. The survey was made with respect to wards without reference to diagnosis and included all patients on the wards examined, regardless of diagnosis, who were receiving therapy with drugs for psychotic or related illnesses. This represented a kind of instantaneous cross section of the patients on the wards surveyed. Since over two-thirds of the patients in the hospital were receiving drug therapy, it was not too difficult to survey about 700 patients in a relatively short period of time. Table I indicates the chief facts revealed by this survey.

All patients who were receiving the active phenothiazines at the time of the survey, schizophrenic, affective, and other psychotic groups, and many patients who were not suffering from clearly psychotic illness, such as patients suffering from personality pattern disturbances, alcoholism, and organic brain disease, were included. The total group was divided into two groups: (1) patients with psychotic reactions on a functional basis (schizophrenia and manic-depressive psychoses) and (2) nonpsychotic patients and those with organic brain syndromes. The proportion of patients whose parkinsonism was asymmetrical and/or otherwise localized was determined by observation of each individual by the author. It is noteworthy that the functionally psychotic group suffered a much greater proportion of reactions of parkinsonism and that these were preponderantly asymmetrical or restricted to limited portions of the body.

TABLE I

Parkinsonism in Drug Therapy

Drug Therapy for Psychotic States	Number of Patients	Parkinsonism				No Parkinsonism	
		Asymmetrical		Symmetrical			
		no.	%	no.	%	no.	%
Phenothiazines and reserpine							
Schizophrenia	422	190	45	83	19.7	149	35.3
Manic and involutional	51	26	51	8	15.7	17	33.3
Other diagnoses*	216	31	14.4	31	14.4	154	71.2
Other Drugs							
Schizophrenia	10	1	10	1	10	8	80
Manic and involutional	13	1	7.7	0	0	12	92.3
Other diagnoses*	18	2	11.1	2	11.1	14	77.8

*Other diagnoses (234)

    Mental deficiency (45)

    Personality disorders, etc. (30)

    Brain syndromes (134)

    Miscellaneous (25)

DISCUSSION

If the brains of these individuals had normally symmetrically developed cell groups, particularly among the basal ganglia, it is inconceivable that any pharmacological agent distributed via the circulatory system would not affect all cells equally and therefore symmetrically with consequent symmetrical physiological manifestations. It is evident that such a normal symmetrical anatomical and chemical status is significantly often absent in the psychotic group under consideration and that under the stress of pharmacological activity the abnormality of the previously compensated neurological dysfunction is brought to light. In the nonpsychotic group under treatment there was much less parkinsonism as well as much less asymmetrical change. Such an interpretation of physiological or pharmacological stress is certainly not new in clinical medicine. The use of the sugar tolerance test in diabetes mellitus and of the curare tolerance in myasthenia are examples that come readily to mind.

The fact that less than 100% of psychotic individuals develop parkinsonism under drug treatment does not exclude the probability that a much larger proportion would develop parkinsonism if larger doses of drug were to be used. Considering the variegated nature of the psychotic illnesses, particularly those that are usually labeled "schizophrenic," it is hardly to be expected that all patients would react with absolute similarity. The diversity of the psychotic reactions in the "functional" groups (a troublesome fact to Bleuler and to others) is entirely consistent with the pharmacophysiological findings since the parkinsonism of no two patients is exactly similar.

In no sense is it the author's intention to indicate that psychotic reactions are a variety of parkinsonism. Parkinsonism has simply been used as a physiological index of the presence of a stress-susceptible abnormality of neurological function which has been observed as an important concomitant of the psychotic states.

This group of observations must not be considered in itself final but should be considered as a point of departure for further observation of neurological correlates of psychotic processes and possibly as the beginning of a rational understanding and clarification of psychotic illness.

SUMMARY

The strong probability that psychotic illness is accompanied by a localized abnormality of the brain is suggested by: (1) the observation of patients who developed parkinsonism after the recognition of classic psychotic reactions prior to the use of modern drug therapy, (2) the development of localized parkinsonism under drug (phenothiazine) stress in patients with a localized neurological defect, and (3) the demonstration of the localized nature of the drug-parkinsonism reaction in psychotic patients. The observations reported are considered a suitable point of departure for further study of the organic concomitants of psychotic illness.

REFERENCES

1. Bleuler, E.: Dementia Praecox or the Group of Schizophrenias, 2nd ed., International Univ. Press, New York, 1950. (Zinkin, J., Trans.)

2. Kraepelin, E.: Einfuehrung in die psychiatrische Klinik, 2nd ed., Barth, Leipzig, 1905.

CHAPTER 16

Some Acute and Chronic Biochemical Responses to Electroconvulsive Therapy

By BURT COCHRAN, JR., M.D., AND
EDWARD P. MARBACH, PH.D.

INTRODUCTION

Electroconvulsive therapy of neuropsychiatric disorders, widely used for one quarter of a century, is still acknowledged to have an obscure mechanism of action. Considerable theorizing and investigation have produced a number of postulated mechanisms for electroconvulsive therapy (ECT), among the more popular being the suggestion that therapeutic response is reflected and perhaps mediated by the autonomic nervous system [1, 2]. Increased activity in certain areas of the hypothalamic-sympathoadrenal neurohumoral complex after electric shock, particularly after a series of such applications, has been reported [3,4]. Some have claimed that therapeutic response to ECT is associated with increasing reactivity of the sympathetic nervous system [2]. A number of biological phenomena have been cited as reflecting such a response, including the ECT effect of stimulating a plasma rise of adrenal medullary amines [5,6], the well-known glycogenolytic effects of epinephrine and anoxia, and serial changes noted in the pharmacological testing of the autonomic system [7]. A sensitive though nonspecific index of acute sympathetic system stimulation is the liberation of free fatty acids (FFA, NEFA) from what in past years had been considered relatively inert stores of body fat [8, 16, 20, 21].

The technical assistance of Martha Szalay and the actuarial work of Carmonde Grant are acknowledged, as is the cooperation of Drs. Edward Stainbrook, John Ray, Robert Eston, and Leonard Kurland as well as the Psychiatric Unit Staff Physicians.

Supported in part by U. S. Public Health Service, National Institutes of Health Research Grant 79-08-101.

The present study is concerned with defining individual acute and chronic changes as well as any interrelationship in circulating levels of these free fatty acids, glucose, other conventional plasma lipid fractions, and urinary catecholamine excretion in an adult psychiatric hospital population that was unselected except for the receipt of electroconvulsive therapy.

CLINICAL MATERIALS AND METHODS

All 29 subjects were inpatients receiving electroconvulsive therapy (ECT) at the Los Angeles County Hospital Psychiatric Unit. Three times weekly at about 9:30 a.m. ECT was given, with the course of therapy based entirely on local criteria. The acute dynamics of plasma true glucose and lipids were followed serially during 79 individual treatments in a group of 29 patients, 13 male and 16 female, ranging in age from 15 to 67 years. Three rather loosely defined clinical groups were represented: 7 psychotic depressive reactions, 5 psychoneurotic depressive states, and a heterogenous group of 17 schizophrenic reactions usually with varying degrees of depression, catatonia, or paranoia (Table I).

The major areas of interest were certain acute plasma and urine reflections of both a single application of ECT and repeated treatments. In addition, alterations in these basal body chemistries were followed before, during, and after the completion of individual courses of therapy. The study was designed to integrate with the established local ECT protocol (Table II). As indicated there, ECT was modified by pretreatment atropine, thiamylal sodium, succinyl-choline chloride, and oxygen.

Each patient had an initial complete medical examination with the routine hemogram; urinalysis; standard 12-lead electrocardiogram; electroencephalogram; and roentgenograms of the skull, dorsolumbar spine, and chest plus blood chemistry determinations including a serologic test for syphilis. Prior to ECT whenever possible a minimum of three basal lipid batteries were obtained to establish a range of biologic variability for each subject.

Surveillance of the subject's activity, mood, medications, hours of sleep, cigarette practice, and food intake (particularly unauthorized eating) was necessary. Blood and urine samplings were taken as outlined in Fig. 1 with some modifications based on the individual's cooperation. Venous serum at room temperature ob-

TABLE I

Mean Pre-ECT Basal Blood Values in 29 Subjects According to Clinical Groupings by Discharge Diagnoses

Diagnosis	Number of Subjects*	Average			Mean Basal Blood			Response to ECT‡		
		Age	Hospital Days	Number ECTs	Glucose (mg%) 70–100†	Total Cholesterol (m μ%) 160–260†	PBI (m μ%) 4–8†	G	F	P
Psychotic depressive	7 (4M, 3F)	57	61	10	86	235	5.0	4	1	2
Psychoneurotic depressive	5 (2M, 3F)	38	69	8	85	278	4.8	2	1	2
Schizophrenic reaction	17 (7M, 10F)	29	122	17	90	234	5.4	4	6	7
Over-all	29 (13M, 16F)	38	84	12	87	249	5.1	10	8	11

*M–male, F–female
†Normal values.
‡G–good (return to apparently normal extrahospital life)
P–poor (continuing need for further hospital care)
F–fair (all others)

TABLE I
Activity in Open-Field Conditioning
(feet per minute and per cent of time near wall)

Animal Groups	Before Signal Session		During Session		After Session	
	ft	%	ft	%	ft	%
Controls n - 5	4.8	80	8.7	75	0.08	98
Experimentals (bottle-fed) n - 5	18.7	40	11.8	70	3.0	50

Note: A difference between both the amount of movement and percentage of time near the wall exists in the presignal period for the two groups. However, as soon as signals start for the first period, the controls show a rise in amount of activity and the experimentals show a fall, so that the amount now does not significantly differ. Furthermore, the experimentals' percentage of time near the wall rises sharply, whereas the controls' percentage remains about the same, so that in this respect, too, they are now about equal. But as soon as the signal session is over, there is a marked drop in activity for both groups, but the controls' activity drops significantly lower and at the same time the controls spend a higher percentage of time near the wall. All differences mentioned throughout this paper are significant at least at the 5% level, and many as low as 1%. The Kolmogorov-Smirnov two-sample test or Mann-Whitney U test was used in most instances.

TABLE II
Physiological Indices during Conditioning in the Frame
(heart and respiration rates per minute)

Animal Groups	Before Start of Signals (hour session)		During the 2-min Intervals (20 intervals)		During Each 10-sec Signal (20 signals)	
	Heart	Respiration	Heart	Respiration	Heart	Respiration
Controls n - 5	104	48	97	44	99	44
Experimentals (bottle-fed) n - 5	123	87	117	98	114	110

Note: Experimental animals gave higher readings in both indices in all situations. Whereas the onset of signals had little effect on the controls, the respiration rate of the experimentals increased, becoming still faster at each signal, and the heart rate decreased, becoming still slower with the signals. This is true for all the experimental animals, though admittedly the change in each instance is rather slight. The temperature of each animal changed during the session but no correlations were evident.

CLINICAL APPROACH TO ECT STUDY

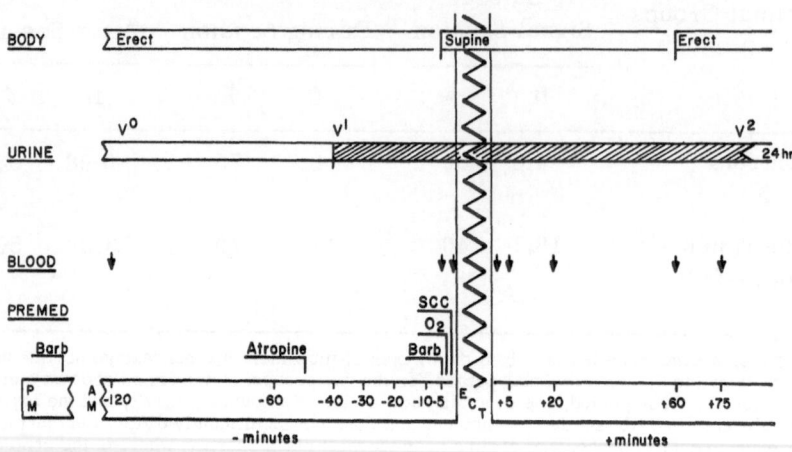

FIG. 1.   Schematic time-line representation of the integration of therapeutic (Table II) and
investigative protocols in the present study.

tained from the fasted, recumbent patient was used for all blood
tests except for the FFA determination. Plasma for the latter
test was collected by venipuncture with minimal stasis and avoiding
physical or psychic trauma.   Blood was received in iced, heparinized tubes and was promptly centrifuged with the plasma drawn
off and stored frozen at -23 C until analysis as a group took
place. Urine collections began with the patient's voiding upon
awakening. Subsequently timed and measured urines were obtained
at the time of atropine premedication, at the initial voiding upon
return from the morning shock treatment, and after twenty-four
hours. Refrigeration and/or acidification to pH 1 were measures
used to stabilize the collecting urines, which were subsequently
frozen until analyzed.   Just prior to thiamylal administration a
15-cc blood specimen was taken from the recumbent patient by
the therapist, after which the syringe was exchanged and the intravenous barbiturate given. With the subject asleep, a previously
heparinized No. 21 needle was used in the opposite arm to collect
venous blood after premedications were given and was kept in-
dwelling via a simple occlusive metal hub and tape for ease in
early post-ECT sampling.

In the convalescent state the subject was kept recumbent until the 60-minute specimen was obtained, after which orthostatic responses of FFA and glucose were checked 10 to 30 minutes after ambulation. Venous blood was obtained under these conditions before premedication, after premedication but before electric shock, and then 1 to 2, 5, 20, 60, and approximately 75 minutes after the seizure. Serial changes of blood glucose, FFA, total cholesterol, and total lipids were followed by this program. Additional basal specimens were checked on non-ECT days.

Chronic responses to an individual course of ECT were sought by checking on changes in the circulating protein-bound iodine (PBI) as well as by the lipid and glucose determinations already mentioned. Intermittent determinations of serum lipid phosphorus and lipoproteins were performed but are not included in this report.

LABORATORY METHODS

All laboratory procedures were performed in the Metabolic Research Laboratory at the Los Angeles County Hospital except for the PBI and catecholamine tests and occasional serum aliquots checked for cholesterol or total lipid and used as a reference value only. Similarly, a standard pooled serum was run as an unknown and repeatedly used as a standard reference value. The following methods were used:

True glucose values were determined by a modified Sunderman-Fuller [12] method, and free fatty acid by a modified Dole [8] method with a one-phase ethanolic titration [13]. Total cholesterol was ascertained by a procedure modified from Pearson and co-workers [14] with temperature control. The total lipid procedure of Kunkel and co-workers [15] was adopted.

The catecholamine tests encompassed some 12 months and unfortunately were performed by three different methods, thereby not allowing very direct comparison. Some such assay was obtained in all but six subjects. One method could provide only a total catecholamine level [16]. The more recent and reliable method was one which utilized differential fluorometry and provided a reasonable estimate of epinephrine. Timed urinary excretion levels seemed a more physiological means of expression. PBI determinations were based on the alkaline ash method of Baker and co-workers [17].

RESULTS AND DISCUSSION

Those subjects followed serially during ECT are grouped clinically and compared in Table I. No great refinements in psychiatric diagnoses were attempted. Thus, the schizophrenic group was not subdivided in spite of its heterogeneity. Certain group differences were evident. The psychotic depressive patients were older, had a relatively short hospital stay, and tended to respond well to an average course of ten shock treatments. The psychoneurotic depressive patients were younger, had a higher pretreatment basal cholesterol level, and did not respond as well to ECT. The schizophrenic patients were still younger and required twice the number of treatments and hospital days while having the greatest number of poor responses. There was generally close agreement in basal PBI and glucose levels among the three groups, all of which levels were within physiological limits. Mean basal cholesterol levels, already noted to be high in the psychoneurotic depressive subjects, very likely should be considered abnormal in the schizophrenic group owing to its share of younger female subjects.

Figure 2 is a line-graph illustration of the acute responses of

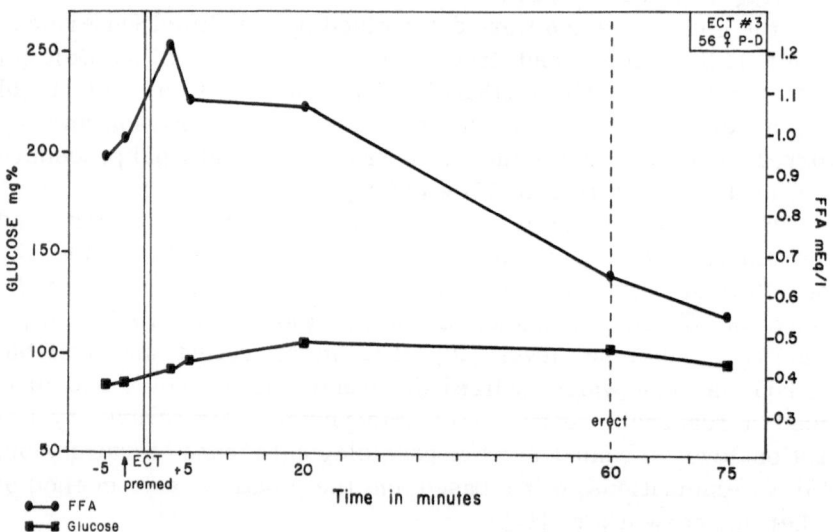

FIG. 2. Line-graph representation of comparative acute changes of blood glucose and FFA in response to single application of electroshock.

blood FFA and glucose to a single electroshock treatment. This 56-year-old woman with involutional psychotic depression had a maximum rise of FFA of 26% above the already elevated basal level at 3 minutes after ECT while the nadir of her blood glucose rise (34%) occurred after 20 minutes. These are representative figures for individual acute responses. After premedications the blood glucose was unchanged, while there was a slight rise (0.03 meq/liter) of FFA (just at the limits of precision for this method). Assuming the upright body position, sitting at her bedside, and ambulating failed to elevate the FFA, which continued to fall off at about the same rate. In spite of some initial improvement the subject had a poor response to a course of eight ECTs.

Table III shows an arbitrary comparison by chronological age of some clinical data from good and poor ECT responders. From 22 subjects followed serially, contrasting groups of eight good and eight poor therapeutic responders were selected. Such an appraisal usually fails to provide any new information.

When biochemical indices are added to such a therapeutic grouping, however, striking differences are seen in maximum acute responses of FFA to ECT (Fig. 3). Further differences are evident when FFA dynamics during early ECT (treatment No. 1 through No. 6) and later ECT (usually beyond No. 10) are compared. The good response group showed an increased rise of FFA and a somewhat increased responsiveness with continued serial ECT. These changes were in contrast to corresponding insignificant glucose shifts. Similarly, the poor responders were distinguished by a low and unchanging FFA response to ECT.

Further analysis of good and poor groups failed to show any close correlation with the abnormal FFA response to orthostatic tolerance. The mean decrease in FFA after the subject's assuming the upright position was 0.05 and 0.03 meq/liter respectively in the two groups. There was, however, a tendency for a return of a normal FFA rise with continued ECT in both groups. The normal orthostatic response of FFA to an upright tilt is often +15 to 75% or more [9,18]. However, the previous intense work during the seizure plays a role in promoting a skeletal muscle uptake of FFA in these subjects [19].

PBI changes were not found to be significantly different (Table IV). Total cholesterol values rose with successive ECTs above 15% of basal value in 19 of 35 subjects during the course of ECT but were returning toward basal levels in 10 of these subjects with continued treatment. Nevertheless, post-ECT levels were

TABLE III

Clinical Responses to Serial ECT in 16 Patients

Patient's Age	Number		Hospital Days	Response	Diagnosis*
	Treatment				
	ECTs	Days			
15	20	44	124	Poor	SR
16	7	24	77	Poor	SR
26	21	48	136	Poor	SR
26	21	41	91	Good	SR
28	8	18	87	Poor	SR
30	8	42	74	Poor	PND
31	20	49	205	Good	SR
33	8	16	80	Good	PND
34	21	55	67	Poor	SR
35	16	38	71	Good	SR
37	21	50	84	Good	PD
40	9	26	70	Good	PND
50	9	19	50	Good	PD
50	12	27	56	Good	PD
56	8	24	77	Poor	PD
65	11	27	60	Poor	PD

*SR — schizophrenic reaction.
PND — psychoneurotic depressive reaction.
PD — psychotic depressive reaction.

BIOCHEMICAL RESPONSE TO SERIAL ECT

MEAN ACUTE MAXIMUM % OF CHANGE

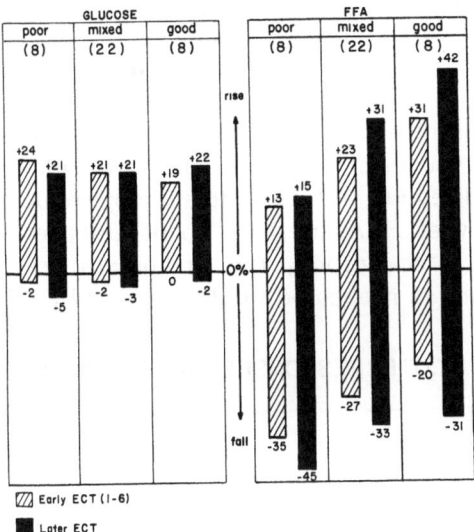

FIG. 3. Bar-graph representation of glucose and FFA changes in early versus later ECT comparing a total of 22 subjects followed serially with 2 selected therapeutic response groups. (All values are group means of percentage maximum deviation from basal — i.e., 0% — values.)

TABLE IV

Unselected Mean Basal PBI and Total Cholesterol
Levels in Different Phases of ECT

ECT Phase	Subjects	PBI (mμ%)	Subjects	Total Cholesterol (mg%)
Prior to ECT	27	5.1	34	238
During ECT	34*	4.6	35	253
Post-ECT			22	262

*Combined pre- and post-ECT PBI reactions.

higher than prior to treatment (Table IV). The average cholesterol rise was 24% above the basal level. A mild (approximately 10%) but frequent decrease in total cholesterol at 60 minutes post-ECT was seen in 47 of 65 individual treatments.

No significant change of serum total lipid was found throughout the study.

Figure 4 illustrates a comparison between the acute FFA and glucose responsiveness at the fourth and sixteenth shock treatment in a 15-year-old female with chronic schizophrenia. Apparent enhanced reactivity of FFA and less so of glucose is seen with the later treatment. In addition, the orthostatic response became normal. The data as presented would be cited by some as showing

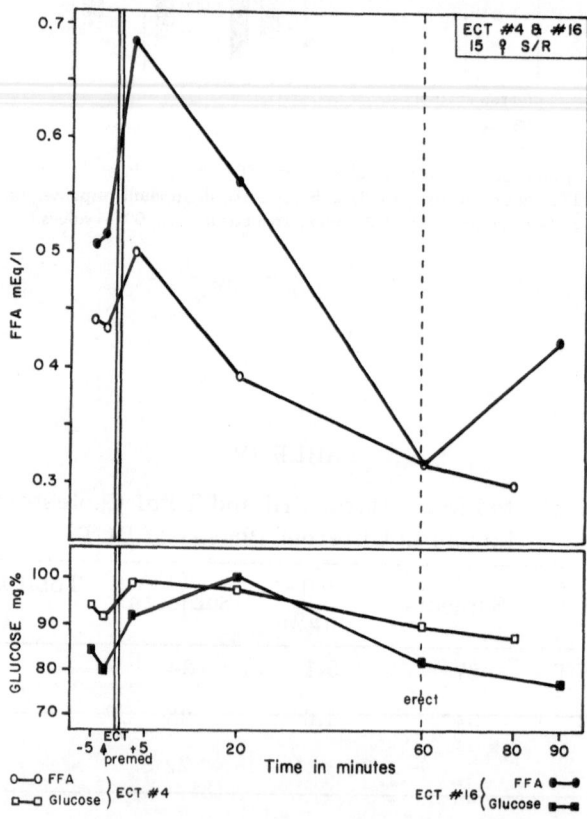

FIG. 4. Line-graph comparison of changes in glucose and FFA acute responses of an individual subject in early versus later ECT. (Note: FFA scale has been expanded.)

TABLE V

Factors Affecting Pre- (Basal) and Postelectroconvulsive Therapy (Reactive) Levels of Plasma-free Fatty Acids under Conditions of This Study. (Only responses of factors shown as major in these subjects are capitalized.)

Factor	FFA Levels	
	Basal	Reactive
Hours fasted [*1]	INCREASE	Increase
Pretreatment anxiety, hostility, and arousal [*2]	INCREASE	Variable
Premedications [*3]	No change	DECREASE
Electrical stimulation [*4] of		
central nervous system	—	INCREASE
adipose tissue	—	INCREASE
skeletal muscle	—	INCREASE then DECREASE
Exercise (muscle work) [*5]	Increase	INCREASE then DECREASE
Anoxemia	—	Increase
Catechol amine liberation [*6]	INCREASE	INCREASE
Body weight loss [*7]	INCREASE	Variable
Body weight gain	DECREASE	Variable
Metabolic acidosis [*8]	Increase	Increase
Hemoconcentration [*8]	None	Increase
Serum calcium rise [*8]	None	Variable
Erect posture [*9]	Increase	Increase

*Uncited studies by Metabolic Research Laboratory: (1) average basal FFA rise of 0.03 meq/liter/hr after 6-hr fast in a mixed psychotic population; (2) FFA mobilization via reticular-activating system and catecholamine response [21, 22]; (3) decreased basal and post-ECT catecholamine excretion reported [4], but no significant basal FFA effect of premedications in this study; (4) electrical stimulation of FFA release from adipose depots in vitro and in vivo [6, 19, 21–24]; (5) exercise promotes initial FFA mobilization [19, 21], with subsequent FFA uptake by striated muscle [24]; (6) epinephrine- and norepinephrine-induced lipolysis of adipose triglycerides [10]; (7) basal FFA rise with hyponutrition and weight loss and converse with weight gain; (8) serial studies in 10 of these subjects showed no significant change in venous bicarbonate, microhematocrit, or pH levels. Similarly, 6 subjects showed no arterial pH change. Average post-ECT rise of ionized serum calcium in 7 subjects was 0.32 mg%; (9) orthostatic rise of FFA [9, 18].

increased sympathetic response with repeated ECTs [3,4]. However, her clinical response was not considered to be more than
fair.

The free fatty acids are a metabolically active but tiny fraction
of transport fat and in the past five years have been accredited an
important role in body caloric homeostasis, being mobilized as the
major body fuel whenever carbohydrate utilization is impaired or
intake is lacking [20]. This very labile fatty acid fraction is responsive to many neurohumoral and nutritional stimuli. For
purposes of orientation in the present ECT study, it should be
noted that plasma venous FFA has been found to rise with skeletal
muscle exercise and to decrease with subsequent rest [19,21]. The
important role of the sympathetic nervous system with norepinephrine (and adrenal epinephrine) bringing about a hydrolysis of
depot fats to liberate FFA must be kept in mind [10]. The close
link among the central nervous system, mood, affect, and the
subject's state of arousal has been emphasized by Bogdonoff and
others [11,22]. Electrical effects on plasma lipids have been reported, including the mobilization of FFA by the stimulation of
rat adipose tissue *in vitro* [23] and the uptake of FFA by the
stimulation of skeletal muscle [24].

Kershbaum [25] reported a short-term (24-hour) study of serum
lipids on patients receiving ECT and concluded that there is no
significant change in the levels of cholesterol, phospholipid, or the
lipoproteins.

Table V lists factors which must be considered as influencing
plasma FFA levels in the present study.

SUMMARY

1. Electric shock, both as a single application and as repeated
   therapy, induced both acute and chronic changes in the levels
   of plasma glucose and lipids of human recipients. Such
   exposure was given as a course of neuropsychiatric therapy
   in 29 subjects with psychiatric disorders.
2. Acute changes as seen in the 72 individual electroshock
   treatments with sufficient data for analysis were expressed
   as percent of maximum deviations from basal levels. Findings were:
   a. a rise of blood glucose: mean +19% usually at 20
      minutes post-ECT.

      b. a rise of FFA: mean +29% usually at 2 to 5 minutes post-ECT.

      c. a fall of blood glucose: mean −2% usually at 60 minutes post-ECT.

      d. a fall of FFA: mean −29% usually at 60 minutes or longer post-ECT.

3. Catecholamine timed urinary excretion was determined by at least one of three methods in 23 subjects. The most frequent change seen was that of slight total elevations in the urine specimen collected during and after ECT. However, only rarely was this value abnormal. Differential fluorometry* showed that epinephrine levels increased in 10 subjects, more often in the pre- than in the post-ECT urines. By all methods abnormal urinary catecholamine excretion was found to be inconstant, being present in only 12 of the 23 subjects tested.

4. ECT in this study was modified by pretreatment with atropine, thiamylal sodium, succinylcholine chloride, and oxygen. Selective plasma samplings failed to show any significant acute effect of these agents on the basal biochemical indices under study. Others have shown such treatment represses catecholamine acute reactivity during ECT [4].

5. The plasma protein-bound iodine (PBI) showed no significant change during ECT treatment in 27 subjects.

6. Serum total cholesterol levels rose more than 15% above basal levels in 19 of 35 subjects during the course of ECT, although 10 of the 19 reverted toward basal levels with continued treatments. No significant change was found in 13 subjects, while 3 subjects exhibited progressive decreases in cholesterol with treatments. Less striking but more consistent (present in 70% of individual treatments) was a mild decrease in the circulating total cholesterol seen 60 to 90 minutes post-ECT.

7. When 22 subjects who were followed serially were selectively grouped on the basis of markedly good or poor therapeutic responses to ECT, some differences in acute biochemical reactivity to electric shock were found. The mean blood glucose maximum rise was about equal in all therapeutic groups. The plasma FFA, however, showed over twice the

---

*Fluorometric catecholamine studies were run through the courtesy of Dr. Shannon Brunjes, Department of Internal Medicine, Loma Linda University School of Medicine.

acute elevation (average 37%) in 8 subjects with good response when contrasted with 8 poor responders (average 14%).

8. Similarly, when a further analysis of the results of early shock treatment (ECT No. 1 to No. 6) was compared with that of later therapy in the same individual, a slight but insignificant increase in glucose rise with successive treatments in all subjects was found. The elevation of plasma FFA was significantly more marked (42%) in later treatments given to the eight subjects with good therapeutic response than in the poor responders (15%).

REFERENCES

1. Funkenstein, D. H., Greenblatt, M., and Solomon, H. C.: Autonomic nervous system changes following electric shock treatment, J. Nerv. Ment. Dis. 108:409, 1948.

2. Gellhorn, E.: Physiological Foundations of Neurology and Psychiatry, Univ. of Minnesota Press, Minneapolis, 1953.

3. Gellhorn, E., and Safford, H.: Influences of repeated anoxia, electroshock, and insulin hypoglycemia on reactivity of sympathetico-adrenal system, Proc. Soc. Exp. Biol. Med. 68:74, 1948.

4. Havens, L. L., Zileli, M. S., Dimascio, A., Boling, L., and Goldfien, A.: Changes in catecholamine response to successive electric convulsive treatment, J. Ment. Sci. 105:821, 1959.

5. Weil-Malherbe, H.: The effect of convulsive therapy on plasma adrenaline and noradrenaline, ibid. 101:156, 1955.

6. Hardy, J. D., Carter, T., and Turner, M. D.: Catecholamine metabolism, Ann. Surg. 150:666, 1959.

7. Funkenstein, D. H., Greenblatt, M., Root, S., and Solomon, H. C.: Psychophysiological study of mentally ill patients. II. Changes in reactions to epinephrine and mecholyl after electric shock treatment, Am. J. Psychiat. 106:116, 1949.

8. Dole, V. P.: A relation between non-esterified fatty acids in plasma and the metabolism of glucose, J. Clin. Invest. 35:150, 1956.

9. Hamlin, J. T. III, Hickler, R. B., and Hoskins, R. G.: Free fatty acid mobilization by neuroadrenergic stimulation in man, ibid. 39:606, 1960.

10. Havel, R. J., and Goldfien, A.: The role of the sympathetic nervous system in the metabolism of free fatty acids, J. Lipid Res. 1:102, 1959.

11. Bogdonoff, M. D., Estes, E. H., Jr., and Weissler, A. M.: Studies on fat mobilization during acute states of arousal, Southern Med. J. 55:680, 1960.

12. Sunderman, F. W., and Fuller, J. B.: A modification of the Benedict method for measuring blood glucose, Am. J. Clin. Path. 21:1077, 1951.

13. Cochran, B., Jr., Marbach, E. P., and Pote, W. W. H., Jr.: Plasma lipid studies in diverse diabetic states, Clin. Res. 8:107, 1960.

14. Pearson, S., Stern, S., and McGavack, T. H.: A rapid, accurate method for the determination of total cholesterol in serum, Anal. Chem. 25:813, 1953.

15. Kunkel, H. G., Ahrens, E. H., and Eisenmenger, W. J.: Application of turbimetric methods for estimation of gamma globulin and total lipid to the study of patients with liver disease, Gastroenterology 11:499, 1948.

16. Sobel, C., and Henry, R. J.: Determination of catecholamines adrenalin and noradrenalin in urine and tissue, Am. J. Clin. Path. 27:240, 1957.

17. Barker, S. B., Humphrey, M. J., and Soley, M. H.: The clinical determination of protein bound iodine, J. Clin. Invest. 30:55, 1951.

18. Euler, U. S. von, Luft, R., and Sundin, T.: The urinary excretion of noradrenaline and adrenaline in healthy subjects during recumbency and standing, Acta Physiol. Scand. 34:169, 1955.

19. Basu, A., Passmore, R., and Strong, J. A.: The effect of exercise on the level of non-esterified fatty acids in the blood, Quart. J. Exp. Physiol. 45:312, 1960.

20. Gordon, R. S., Jr.: Unesterified fatty acid in human blood plasma. II. The transport function of unesterified fatty acid, J. Clin. Invest. 36:810, 1957.

21. Carlson, L. A., and Pernow, B.: Studies on blood lipids during exercise. I. Arterial and venous plasma concentration of unesterified fatty acids, J. Lab. Clin. Med. 53:833, 1959.

22. Bogdonoff, M. D.: The relationship of central nervous system activity to lipid metabolism, A.M.A. Arch. Int. Med. 105:505, 1960.

23. Correll, J. W.: Mobilization of unesterified fatty acids (UFA) from isolated rat adipose tissue by nerve stimulation in vitro, Fed. Proc. 20:275, 1961.

24. Issekutz, B., Jr., and Spitzer, J. J.: Uptake of free fatty acids by skeletal muscle during stimulation, Proc. Soc. Exp. Biol. Med. 105:21, 1960.

25. Kershbaum, A., Bassitt, D. R., and Bellet, S.: The effect of electric convulsive therapy on serum lipids, Am. J. Med. Sci. 237:341, 1959.

Discussion by George N. Thompson, M.D.

The continuing search for the mechanisms of therapeutic response to electroconvulsive therapy has gradually shifted from theories based on purely mechanical and physical changes in the brain to those of biochemical-endocrine changes and their influence on the brain and on the behavior of the individual. A co-winner of the A. E. Bennett Award of this Society in 1958 was the paper by Havens and co-workers entitled, "Catecholamine Responses to Electrically Induced Convulsions in Man." * This paper indicated a shifting emphasis toward a biochemical explanation of how electroconvulsive therapy works.

One of the most frequently asked questions by patients who are to take electroconvulsive therapy (or their relatives) is, "How does it work?" They, too, are interested in knowing what changes are to take place in them to produce a cure or improvement. Most clinicians now find themselves giving some type of biochemical explanation.

The authors of the present paper have done a broad biochemical study on patients taking electroshock therapy and have restudied a number of variables. Of the biochemical studies made, the ones with the most significant changes were the blood glucose rise, the free fatty acid rise, and the free fatty acid fall. The free fatty acid rise was perhaps the most significant change of all since it seems to have some prognostic value (during the early treatment phase) of the probable efficacy of the treatment. The free fatty acid rise is probably related to the catecholamine response to electroshock therapy found by Havens and others. Hence we come back to a basic conclusion that heightened adrenosympathetic reactivity during treatment probably accounts for the other biochemical responses. As yet, we do not have a direct correlation between the capacity of the patient for a degree of adrenosympathetic reactivity and clinical improvement. In fact, to the clinician it often seems that those patients who respond best to treatment are the ones who seem to have the least capacity for adrenal and sympathetic reactivity.

Drs. Cochran and Marbach are to be congratulated for a precise correlative study on biochemical response and clinical change in the patients studied.

*In: Proceedings of the Society of Biological Psychiatry.

CHAPTER 17

Treatment of Autistic Schizophrenic Children with LSD-25 and UML-491

By LAURETTA BENDER, M.D., LOTHAR GOLDSCHMIDT, M.D., AND D. V. SIVA SANKAR, PH.D.

Autistic schizophrenic children present challenging and baffling problems in treatment. Without attempting to deal again with the controversial issues concerning the definitions and etiological factors of either childhood schizophrenia[1] or the autistic reaction pattern [2], we will refer to the various treatment regimes attempted by Bender and co-workers in the past quarter of a century with these children. Many of the children have been followed subsequently into later childhood, adolescence, and adulthood [3]. Meanwhile, a new group of young autistic children are always available for new treatment endeavors as the new modes become available.

THERAPEUTIC MEASURES AND RESULTS

Thus, the following have been tried [4]: Metrazol [5], electric convulsions [6], subshock insulin, many psychopharmaceutical agents [7-10], the milder antihistamines (Benadryl), amphetamines, anticonvulsants, muscle tone stimulants (Tolserol), meprobamates, phenothiazines, reserpines, antidepressants, tranquilizers, etc.

The goal in these therapeutic efforts has been to modify the secondary symptomatology associated with retarded, regressed, and disturbed behavior of the children. There has also been a conviction that the treatment goal was directed at some basic disorders associated with early schizophrenia. It was thought that the treatment not infrequently did succeed in nudging the lagging maturation in all behavior areas, thus enabling the child to carry on with a more normal development. It was also believed that plastic embryonic patterning, characteristically schizophrenic, in visceral-vegetative functions should be overcome and that increased tone and motor patterns should be stimulated in the unstriped muscles of the vascular bed and of the respiratory and gastrointestinal systems as well as in the striped muscles of the motor systems. It was recognized that the perceptual sensitivity of the schizophrenic infant[11] and the perceptual distortion of the older child needed correction, but no direct approach seemed available. Of course, there are other problems: anxiety; stereotyped, rhythmic, and manneristic motility; mutism; inadequate or inappropriate language; psychosomatic or allergic illnesses; negativistic, ambivalent, and erratic attitudes and behavior; and regressive, fixated, and accelerated episodes in maturation. Autism appears to be a defensive reaction in the disorganization resulting from schizophrenic symptoms.

Many of the medical treatment measures, together with new social and educational experiences in a hospital and guidance and therapy for the parents, have been sufficiently successful in some cases and partially successful in an increasing number of cases to justify a search for more potent agents [12]. Furthermore, other significant observations have been made:

1. Prepuberty schizophrenic children react differently from adults to all physiological and pharmacological agents. This different response offers new data for understanding the schizophrenic phenomena, defense mechanisms, and the physiological and pharmacological agents. These areas of investigation justify much more exploration than has so far been done.

2. Children show much less side-effects to drugs so that larger doses can be used.

3. Children also appear to develop tolerance more slowly and do not suffer withdrawal symptoms when the drug is stopped.

4. Childrens' reactions to drugs are often paradoxical; for instance, tranquilizers prove to be maturational stimulants and behavior organizers and amphetamines do not interfere with sleep or appetite and improve interpersonal relations and learning ability.

With these experiences in mind and with awareness of the current interest in LSD-25 as a therapeutic agent[13] because of its psychotomimetic properties, it occurred to us that LSD might be effective in breaking through the autistic defense in chronically regressed, retarded, mute, and withdrawn children.

The theoretical interest in LSD as a serotonin inhibitor, with consideration of the possibility that serotonin is in some way related to schizophrenia, further justified this endeavor. Also, since LSD is an autonomic nervous system stimulant, it could be of particular value in treating schizophrenic children, in whom general tissue tone, especially the tone of the vascular system, and the pattern of the autonomic nervous system functions are impaired.

MATERIALS AND METHODS WITH LSD

A treatment program was planned for 14 schizophrenic children under the age of eleven, who had been under hospital care for a considerable period and previously tried on a variety of treatments with inadequate response. There were 11 boys and 3 girls with an age range of six to ten and a half years of age.

An acute experiment was planned first. In groups of five the children were given 25 μg of LSD-25* intramuscularly while under continous observation. The two oldest boys, over ten years, near or in early puberty, reacted with disturbed anxious behavior. The oldest and most disturbed received Amytal sodium 150 mg intramuscularly and returned to his usual behavior. Neither of these boys was continued on this treatment program at that time.

The twelve other children reacted to the intramuscular injection of 25 μg of LSD with similar behavior in varying degrees. They appeared to be in an elevated or "high" mood. They were gay and playful and accepted contact with an adult in their tentative, teasing, playful activities, which included ball playing, paper tearing, motor play, rhythmic hand clapping, and body swaying. They appeared flushed, bright eyed, and unusually interested in the enviroment. The height of the reaction occurred in 30 to 40 minutes and continued 2 to 3 hours. These acute experiments were repeated several times, and then the LSD was given orally and increased to 100 μg once a week in the early morning. Then it was increased gradually to twice and three times a week as no untoward side-effects were noticed, and it was observed that the reaction to the drug persisted. Finally, it was given daily, and this was continued for six weeks until the time of this report.

As a brief description of these children it may be pointed out that before hospitalization all of these children had been examined by one or several professional workers in the community, and the diagnosis of autism and schizophrenia had been accepted. All these children and their parents had experienced considerable psycho-

* All of the LSD-25 was furnished by Sandoz Pharmaceuticals.

therapy, and all had had some form of physiological and pharmacological therapy in the hospital. The parents of this group of children were all adequate but could not keep the children at home because of the severity of the retarded, regressed, and disturbed behavior. The children were all without any useful language; some were completely mute, some had a few words they used occasionally, and the others had psychotic, noncommunicative language. None of these children were testable with any of the standard psychological tests nor would they perform any paper-pencil tests.

At the outset of the treatment, all were removed from the medication that they then were receiving. Blood, urine, and liver function tests were done. Blood was also drawn for Dr. Sankar's biochemical studies.

A Vineland Maturity Scale determination was made on each child (by Dr. Goldschmidt with ward personnel, teachers, and mothers). On this scale the estimated social maturity score ranged from 2-3 to 5-7 years, while their chronological ages ranged from 6-1 to 10-6 years. The range of the social maturity quotient was 32 to 60.

RESULTS WITH LSD AND CONCLUSIONS

A summary of the re-evaluation of the children in the course of treatment is as follows:

1. All tolerated the drug without side-effects, toxic features, regressive behavior, or other untoward responses.

2. All were able to get along without any further medication, although they had been accustomed to receiving other medication before the LSD was given to them.

3. All have shown some mild degree of favorable response with slow and steady progression. The amount has varied from child to child. There have been no regressions although some children have had episodic recurrence of behavior familiar to them, such as feces smearing and aggressive contact with other children.

4. In general, they were happier; their mood was "high" in the hours following the ingestion of the drug, and this tended progressively to carry over through the whole day.

5. They have become more spontaneously playful with balls and balloons. They participate with increasing eagerness in motility play with adults and other children if directed by adults.

6. They no longer push other children away or show hostile agression to them as much as they formerly did.

7. They seek positive contacts with adults, approaching them

with face uplifted and bright eyes, and respond to fondling, affection, etc.

8. Habit patterning is improved. They handle food better and eat better. Two became toilet trained.

9. Their physical condition has improved. Their color is rosy rather than blue or pale, and they have gained weight.

10. There is less stereotyped whirling and rhythmic behavior.

11. Ordinary environmental stimuli and situations are better understood and are reacted to appropriately. Thus, they respond to their own name and react appropriately to "yes" and "no." They fall into routine more spontaneously, and several carry out small commands. One anticipates routine and assists in holding a door open and directing other children to the dining room.

12. The Vineland Maturity Scale rating was qualitatively higher in all children. A quantitative gain of 1 point was shown by one child and 2 points by another child.

13. No children showed a recordable gain in the use of language.

Dr. Sankar's biochemical findings were as follows: the administration of LSD-25 to children seems to increase the inorganic phosphate of both plasma and erythrocytes. Thus, out of 26 laboratory analyses of 14 children, 18 samples showed an increase in the plasma inorganic phosphate within an hour after the drug was given parenterally. This increase amounted to approximately 26% on the average. Similar results (unpublished) have also been obtained in animals in our laboratories. However, as the therapeutic effects of LSD-25 given orally seem to become noticeable, this phosphate effect of LSD-25 either decreases or, on the other hand, there is a decrease in the plasma inorganic phosphate with an equal number of subjects showing an increase in the inorganic phosphate content of the erythrocytes. On repeated administration, out of 14 cases only 7 showed an increase in plasma inorganic phosphate while only 4 showed an increase in erythrocyte inorganic phosphate.

Our conclusions were that LSD-25 given daily in oral doses of 100 μg to prepuberty autistic schizophrenic children appears to be an effective autonomic and central nervous system stimulant. It appears to have some effect on the tone of the vascular system, on the level of mood, and on the phosphorous level of the blood serum and erythrocytes as well as in the organizing of perceptual experiences. These changes appear to be chronic with continuous administration of the drug and to have a favorable influence on the clinical course.

EXPERIENCES WITH UML-491

Meanwhile, UML-491 (Sandoz) has become available. This is L-methyl-D-lysergic acid butanolamide, a methylated derivative of LSD. It is considered to be (like BOL) nonpsychotomimetic but a more powerful serotonin-inhibiting agent and more effective in relation to the autonomic nervous system. It has been promoted as a prophylactic against migraine headaches.* It is in this connection that one of us (Dr. Bender) became acquainted with this pharmaceutical agent, in the search for relief from life-long classical migraine or vascular headaches.

During the years when schizophrenic children have been observed and migraine symptoms experienced, intriguing similarities of the two conditions have been noted. This includes the various autonomic nervous system disorders, distorted and hypersensitive reactions to perceptual experiences, the disorder in the tone of the vascular bed, the tendency to autistic withdrawal, and the familial histories. Serotonin has been under consideration as a factor in both conditions [14, 15]. It may be suggested also that the two conditions are self-exclusive.

The principle in the use of UML-491 for migraine headaches is based on its serotonin-inhibiting and autonomic nervous system effective properties. It is given prophylactically in sufficient dosage to maintain a chronic blood level (beginning with 8 mg daily in four divided doses and maintained with 4-mg Spacetabs twice daily).

After the first dose of UML, a reaction was observed similar to that of the children after their first dose of LSD. Subsequently, other similarities were noted between the response of schizophrenic children to LSD and that of the migraine symptoms to UML. The following were experienced: a lift in mood; motor restlessness; irritability; localized muscle tensions or spasms; mild "crawling" skin sensations; more clearly defined and satisfying visual (color) and auditory (music) experiences; a smoothing out of the autonomic nervous system functions; relief of episodic headaches; relief in perceptual hypersensitivity in visual, auditory, olfactory, and skin sensations and in allergic reactions; and a general sense of well-being with an improved sleep pattern.

Needless to say, this experience has encouraged us in the plan to pursue the study of LSD and its derivatives, especially UML, as therapeutic and investigative agents in childhood schizophrenia.

*Sandoz Pharmaceuticals, especially Rudolph P. Bircher, M.D., has made available to us the information about this compound as well as the UML-491 itself for this study.

We immediately placed eight autistic schizophrenic children on UML-491, 8 mg in four divided doses orally. During the three initial weeks the children have tolerated the drug well. There have been some brief (20-minute) episodes of reactions to changing muscle tensions and kinesthetic sensations with clowning, staggering gait, and twisting of the neck, back, and arms. One child had a brief episode when his extremities were pale and cold and the superficial veins were conspicuous. He shivered and crawled into bed as though cold, but he soon recovered. In general, they reacted as the children receiving LSD, with a lift in mood and increased activity. They appear brighter, more outgoing, and less stereotyped in behavior.

CONCLUSION

The use of these two drugs with the possible use of other derivatives, such as BOL, in autistic schizophrenic children with combined clinical and biochemical investigations will give us more knowledge about both the basic schizophrenic process and the defensive autism in children and also about the reaction of these dilysergic acid derivatives as central and autonomic nervous system stimulants and serotonin antagonists. Hopefully these drugs will also contribute to our efforts to find better therapeutic agents for early childhood schizophrenia.

REFERENCES

1. Bender, L.: Diagnostic and therapeutic aspects of childhood schizophrenia, in Bowman, P. W., Ed.: Mental Retardation, Proceed. First Internat. M. Conf. Grune & Stratton, Inc., New York, 1960, p. 453.

2. Bender, L: Autism in children with mental deficiency, Am. J. Ment. Defic. 64:81, 1959.

3. Bender, L: Clinical research from in-patient services for children, 1920–1957, Psychiat. Quart. 35:531.

4. Bender, L., and Faretra, G.: Organic therapy in pediatric psychiatry, Dis. Nerv. Syst. (Monog. Suppl.) 22:110, 1961.

5. Cottington, F.: The treatment of childhood schizophrenia with Metrazol shock, Am. J. Psychiat. 98:397, 1941.

6. Bender, L.: One hundred cases of childhood schizophrenia treated with electric shock, Trans. Am. Neurol. Assoc. 72:165, 1947.

7. Freedman, A. M., Effron, A. S., and Bender, L.: Pharmacotherapy in children with psychiatric illnesses, J. Nerv. Ment. Dis. 122:479, 1955.

8. Bender, L., and Nichtern, S.: Chemotherapy in child psychiatry, New York J. Med. 56:2791, 1956.

9. Nichtern, S.: Chemotherapy in child psychiatry, in Child Psychiatry and the General Practitioner, Charles C. Thomas, Springfield, 1961.

10. Bender, L., and Cottington, F.: The use of amphetamine sulphate (Benzedrine) in child psychiatry, Am. J. Psychiat. 99:116, 1942.

11. Bergman, P., and Escalona, S.: Unusual sensitivities in very young children, Psychoanal. Study Child 3/4:333, 1949.

12. Bender, L.: Twenty years of research on schizophrenic children, with special reference to those under six years of age. in Caplan, G., Ed.: Emotional Problems of Early Childhood, Basic Books, New York, 1955.

13. Abramson, H. A., Ed.: The Use of LSD in Psychotherapy, Trans. Conf. on d-Lysergic Acid Diethylamide (LSD-25), New York, Josiah Macy, Jr. Foundation, 1960.

14. Kety, S. S.: Biochemical theories of schizophrenia, Science 29:1528, 1959; ibid 29:1590, 1959.

15. Ostfeld, A. M.: Migraine headache, its physiology and biochemistry, J.A.M.A. 174:110, 1960.

16. Dalessio, D. J., Camp, W. J., Goodall, H., and Wolff, H. A.: Studies on headache, A.M.A. Arch. Neurol. 4:235, 1961.

Discussion by Alfred M. Freedman, M.D.

It is a pleasure for me to have the opportunity of commenting on Dr. Bender's paper. For many years I have been convinced of the necessity for new and experimental approaches to the treatment of childhood schizophrenia. My former teacher, Dr. Bender, has long been a pioneer in this regard, and her willingness, even eagerness, to attempt and to evaluate new treatment methods in this field has been demonstrated once again.

I have been particularly interested in the experience described by Dr. Bender today since two years ago I undertook an acute experiment in the use of LSD with a group of twelve autistic schizophrenic children. Our experiment was a brief one and differed from Dr. Bender's in that it involved only a single administration of LSD to most of the children. Two of the group of twelve were given the drug on two occasions, but there was no attempt to continue its use on a therapeutic basis.

Before our experiment in the use of LSD was undertaken in the spring of 1959 [A], there had been no indication in the literature that the drug had been used with children elsewhere. Since that time, there have appeared a few scattered references [B-E] to its use with children, but the number of children involved has been very small and the results for the most part inconclusive. The few patients I have come across in whom the treatment was considered a success were not classified clearly as schizophrenic children.

Actually, the use of LSD even with adults has been primarily in the area of the neuroses, and most investigators have agreed for some years that it is of very questionable value in the treatment of schizophrenic individuals. Such patients have been found to be markedly resistant to the drug and required relatively higher doses than did normal or neurotic subjects for it to produce any effects. However, we were particularly interested in a paper by Cholden, Kurland, and Savage [F], who studied the reactions of a group of chronic, regressed schizophrenic subjects to LSD. They reported that some catatonic individuals who had been mute for years burst into speech or laughter under the influence of the drug. It was this report particularly that led us to our own experiment.

Our patients were a group of twelve autistic schizophrenic children, ten boys and two girls ranging in age from five years and eleven months to eleven years and ten months, who attended a day school for schizophrenic children. Seven of the children were mute and the remaining five used words or phrases occasionally, most often for no apparent reason. Each had a characteristic compulsive motor behavior. Six of the twelve received tranquilizers regularly. These were discontinued twenty-four hours before the LSD was administered.

The experiment was conducted over a period of several weeks so that only one child received LSD on any one day, although two were given the drug on two separate occasions. The drug was administered orally in a vehicle to which the children were accustomed—cocoa, milk, orange juice, etc. The dosage was set at 100 μg for each child except for one smaller girl who received 50 μg and one boy who received 200 μg on a second administration, 100 μg initially and another 100 about two hours later. Each child received the drug immediately after arriving at the school in the morning and was under the constant observation of a pediatric psychiatrist with whom he was familiar until the obvious effects had worn off.

The onset of the effect of the drug was apparent in from 15 to 30 minutes, and the obvious symptoms continued for a minimum of 4 hours and a maximum—in one case—of over 5 hours. The somatic reactions of the children to the drug included the commonly observed facial flush and pupillary dilatation, which appeared at varying times for from 5 minutes to over 2 hours. There was no change in pulse rate or blood pressure other than that normally associated with a general state of anxiety. In three children there were evidences of catatonia. These included strange fixed positions of the hands, maintenance of various bizarre positions, and true waxy flexibility of the left arm in one child who received 200 μg of LSD. Appetite was markedly affected, none of the children accepting the food that was offered at the usual time and place. Muscle tone varied from relaxed to tense, depending on mood. Increased body awareness was evidenced by the repeated stroking or touching of parts of the body, most often the lips or mouth; and many of the children showed a desire for increased physical contact and cuddling. The usual physical mannerisms of the children disappeared, but they reappeared as the effects of the drug wore off.

The most striking of the observable psychic effects were the mood swings, which were sharp and rapid from extreme elation to extreme depression or anxiety varying in duration and degree among the children. In five there seemed to be a flattening of affect rather than depression. Behavior suggestive of auditory and visual hallucinations, never seen before in these children, was observed on seven occasions. This included standing quietly, apparently listening to something and smiling, clapping the hands over the ears frequently as though hearing something unusual, following something on the ceiling with the eyes, and so on. Half the children seemed to demonstrate decreased alertness, while several showed an increase in this quality. Remoteness was increased in most of the children; eye contact was increased in two but was decreased in four. Verbalization and vocalization were increased in quantity but not in quality. There was some experimentation with new sounds, but the hoped-for change from muteness to speech did not occur.

In contrast with our experience, the children Dr. Bender has been treating showed an elevation of mood, better contact with both adults and children, and a generally improved object relationship. Dr. Bender also indicates no interference with appetite; none of the children in our group had any appetite for food while under the influence of LSD.

I consider it entirely possible that most of the differences between her group of children and ours in their reactions to LSD may be due to the development of tolerance in Dr. Bender's patients who had been receiving the drug regularly. This development has been reported by a number of investigators including Cholden, Kurland, and Savage [F], who found that by the third day their schizophrenic patients were practically unaffected by LSD.

In any event, this experimental approach is certainly praiseworthy and to be encouraged.

REFERENCES

A. Freedman, A. M., Ebin, E. V., and Wilson, E. A.: An experiment in the use of LSD-25 with autistic schizophrenic children, to be published.

B. Abramson, H. A., Ed.: The Use of LSD in Psychotherapy; Transactions of a Conference on d-Lysergic Acid Diethylamine (LSD-25), Josiah Macy, Jr., Foundation, New York, 1960.

C. Murphy, R: Personal communication.

D. Peck, T. T.: Personal communication.

E. Hoffer, A.: Personal communication.

F. Cholden, L. S., Kurland, A., and Savage, C.: Clinical reactions and tolerance to LSD in chronic schizophrenics, J. Nerv. Ment. Dis. 122:211, 1955.

CHAPTER 18

Children Born to Mothers Maintained on Pharmacotherapy During Pregnancy and Postpartum

By ELSE B. KRIS, M.D.

Reports on hospital admissions reveal that between 2 and 10% of women entering mental hospitals suffer from a psychosis appearing at the time of pregnancy or during or after childbirth. Generally, the literature on psychiatric complications arising during pregnancy or the postpartum period indicates that almost all authors agree that the rapid and dramatic changes in the course of normal life processes frequently are accompanied by emotional reverberations. Many authors feel that a latent schizophrenia can become manifest or be exacerbated during these periods and consider pregnancy and childbirth to be immediate precipitants of schizophrenic reactions. There seems to be general agreement that persons with a history of earlier emotional and personality disorders are liable to become overtly psychotic in reaction to the stress of childbearing and childbirth.

The risk of a recurrence of the psychosis in subsequent pregnancy or parturition has been generally acknowledged, and various authors agree that women who have already had mental disorders are particularly predisposed to the development of a psychotic reaction at such times. This realization has made it necessary to search for some type of prophylaxis. As a result, insight type of psychotherapy, supportive psychotherapy, and prophylactic electric shock therapy have been recommended to prevent such breakdowns.

While chlorpromazine has been widely used in the treatment of nausea and vomiting in pregnancy, very little so far has been recorded on the use of this drug for the prevention of psychiatric complications during pregnancy and childbirth. However, some authors have expressed their concern over the effect the administration of ataractic drugs might have on the mother, the fetus, and the infant.

REVIEW OF SIX-YEAR EXPERIENCE

While closely following groups of patients returned to the community after hospitalization because of a psychotic breakdown, several women who became pregnant were kept under continuous observation. In the past six years, 31 children were born to mothers maintained throughout pregnancy, confinement, and postpartum on psycho-pharmacotherapy. A previous report by this author [10] dealt with the observations made on the first few children and their mothers, and it was stated that apparently maintenance therapy can be safely carried on during pregnancy and postpartum as a preventive measure in those cases where the danger of renewed psychotic breakdown exists. It was then reported that these mothers went through pregnancy without any undue side-effects caused by such pharmacotherapy and that the children at the time of their birth seemed to be normal. Today's report concerns itself mainly with these children, the oldest of which now have reached the ages of between four and five years. Moreover, several of the mothers have given birth to a second child while again being kept for reasons of prevention on one or the other phenothiazine derivative. Thus, to 14 mothers admitted to this study about six years ago, 17 babies have been born up to the present.

One woman, who had not been on maintenance pharmacotherapy, during the fourth month of her pregnancy became very disturbed and had to be rehospitalized. A second woman, who after the institution of maintenance therapy failed to take the medication, relapsed two weeks before term. Another woman, entering the maternity hospital for delivery, was advised by a resident physician that she did not need and therefore should not continue to take chlorpromazine. A few days after her return home, the Research Unit was notified by the family that she had become vividly hallucinated. Several home visits were made and intensive pharmacotherapy reinstituted. Two weeks later she was again symptom-free.

The children were born at term except in one case in which two children born to a mother maintained on pharmacotherapy were born prematurely. But the five children this woman gave birth to before her psychotic breakdown were all born prematurely. Birth weights of all these children were within normal range, and so was their general development. Five of the mothers nursed their infants up to three months; one, up to the end of the fourth month. All the other children were bottle fed. The average maintenance dose of these mothers consisted of 50 to 150 mg chlorpromazine daily taken at bedtime only. One of the mothers complained after the child was born that when taking her medication at nighttime she could not hear the baby crying. When the hour of medication was changed to daytime for a few weeks, she had no difficulty in caring for the infant.

The following case histories tend to illustrate better the role of pharmacotherapy in the prevention of a psychiatric breakdown in individuals with histories of previous psychosis than any statistical evaluation could do.

CASE REPORTS

CASE 1. Terry, who was born in September, 1956, is an alert friendly, good-natured child. His maternal grandparents were separated on and off, and the grandfather, diagnosed as a psychospathic personality, is reported as having died in a state hospital. His mother's childhood is described as uneventful. She married at the age of nineteen but was separated a few months later. At the age of twenty-two she became irritable and tense, gradually developed auditory hallucinations, and was finally hospitalized in 1954 and diagnosed as having catatonic-type schizophrenia. She responded well to chlorpromazine therapy and was placed on convalescent care in 1955, when she was admitted for aftercare to the Research Unit; the maintenance therapy of chlorpromazine 150 mg daily recommended by the hospital was supervised.

Shortly after her release from the hospital she married a man whom she had known for some time, and in January, 1956, she was found to be pregnant. The maintenance therapy was continued at a reduced level of 50 mg daily. The family doctor and the maternity hospital to which she planned to go for delivery were advised of this maintenance pharmacotherapy, as was done in all cases in this study. The entire pregnancy, during which time Mrs. A. J. was seen regularly, was uneventful.

She gave birth to Terry, the baby weighing 7 lb $4\frac{1}{2}$ oz at term. His early development is described as normal. He was bottle fed and started to walk at the age of one year and to talk at eighteen months, and toilet training is said to have been completed at the age of two. He is described as obedient and easy to manage. At Sunday school, which he attended for the past year, he is said to learn quickly and to get along well with the other children.

The psychological test report indicates that Terry, who will be five in September, was found to be a bright, alert, assertive child who was responsive to the demands of the testing situation. On the Stanford-Binet Form L test he attained an MA of 4—5 with an IQ of 98. He scored basally at year III-6 and passed four tests at year IV, two at year IV-6, two at the year V, and one at year VI with no successes at year VII. There is no clear-cut pattern of successes or of failures in any particular area. His performance seemed normal. His speech and comprehension are reasonably clear for his age, and he displays precarious shrewdness and ability to manipulate situations. He displayed characteristic restlessness toward the end of the session, but with some prodding was able to respond to limits. The over-all impression from the examination is that Terry is an essentially normal boy of at least average intelligence.

CASE 2. Mrs. R. L. was born in 1935. She completed high school at the age of eighteen and a half and worked in a factory until she married at the age of twenty. Her first child, Sheila, was delivered by Cesarean section in June 1956. She became depressed, described auditory and visual hallucinations, and was hospitalized two weeks postpartum. The infant was taken into the care of the maternal grandparents.

After three months of hospitalization the patient was released on convalescent care with a recommendation for a 150 mg chlorpromazine daily maintenance dose. She became pregnant shortly after her return home and was maintained on 100 mg of chlorpromazine throughout pregnancy and the postpartum period. Danny, who was also delivered by cesarean section in August 1957, showed significantly the same developmental history as the first child. The birth weight of both children differed only by 4 oz. Both children started to walk and to talk at about the age of one year and were toilet trained at the age of two. Both children attend Sunday school, where they are described as alert, easily learning youngsters who get along well with the other children and who present no problems of any kind. Neither the Sunday school teacher nor the parents are able to describe any particular difference in these two children except that the mother states that, being less nervous herself, she feels more comfortable in handling the younger child. Maintenance pharmacotherapy of the mother was discontinued a year ago and up to date she has maintained her good level of adjustment.

Psychological tests on both these children (one born before and the other after the mother's psychotic breakdown) indicate the following:

Sheila, the first child, is shy and somewhat fearful. On the

Stanford-Binet Form L test she attained an IQ of 94. Her speech and comprehension are clear for her age. At times she was slow in answering and showed considerable apprehension, but there was no area of failure. The over-all impression is that of an essentially normal but somewhat apprehensive child of about normal intelligence. It is felt that her shyness might possibly be due to the fact that she had been separated from her mother for nearly the full first year of her life.

Danny, who will be four in August, is described as alert and responsive and showed normal performance during testing, displaying some shrewdness. Speech and comprehension were found to be in accordance with his age level. He gave the over-all impression of a normal child of somewhat above-average intelligence. He appeared to be more at ease than his older sister, showing none of her apprehension throughout the testing.

CASE 3. Mrs. M. T's childhood is described as uneventful. She married at the age of twenty, and one year later gave birth to her first child. Ten days postpartum she became very disturbed and confused, talked about people being against her and wanting to harm her, and described vivid auditory hallucinations. She was hospitalized in September 1954 and received 35 electric shock treatments with little improvement resulting, but when later placed on chlorpromazine (300 mg daily) she responded well. She was released on convalescent care in September 1955, after maintenance therapy had been discontinued for about two months.

In July 1957, she became pregnant again and, because of her previous history of a postpartum psychosis, was placed prophylactically on 75 mg Thorazine. On March 7, 1958, she gave birth to a 7-lb 5-oz boy, Charles. He showed normal development, and the mother got along well. In June 1958 the medication was discontinued gradually, and the patient maintained her good level of adjustment. In 1960 she became pregnant again but objected to a reinstitution of pharmacotherapy, insisting that she felt very well and did not need any medication.

On February 27, 1961, she gave birth to her third child, a 6-lb 5-oz boy; two weeks later—on March 14, 1961—the Research Unit was notified that the patient had become increasingly disturbed, tense, and hallucinated. An immediate attempt was made to institute chlorpromazine medication. However, the patient was disturbed, failed to take the medication, and finally had to be rehospitalized. This case is particularly noteworthy (presenting a control in itself), for twice when the patient was not on pharmacotherapy she became actively psychotic after childbirth while remaining free of post-partum psychosis when on drug therapy.

DISCUSSION

Findings on all the other children in this group are essentially similar. There was in none of the cases any indication of the presence of any problems of behavior, or of any emotional or mental disturbance. It will be interesting to follow these children for the next few years and to observe their future developments. In particular, it will be interesting to see how other siblings compare in learning ability, drive, aspirations, interpersonal relationships, and general life adjustment. Special attention will be paid with regard to the incidence of schizophrenia in those children whose mothers had undergone pharmacotherapy during pregnancy. There are in addition, a number of questions which still require answering. For instance, does a mother maintained on pharmacotherapy provide a better environment for the development of her children?

SUMMARY

As is apparent from what has been described here, pharmacotherapy for the prevention of recurrent psychotic breakdown during pregnancy and the postpartum period seems to have no adverse effect on either the mother, the fetus, or the early years of the child's development. These children showed no unusual restlessness, were not unusually quiet, and, in general, showed no particular differences when compared with their siblings or peers of the same social class and cultural background. Several of the mothers stated that they themselves were less nervous while under pharmacotherapy during pregnancy and the postpartum period and that this reflected on the children, who, they felt, were much easier to manage than their previously born children.

In cases where pharmacotherapy on a maintenance basis was either not instituted or was interrupted for some reason, a recurrence of overt psychotic symptoms was observed. On the other hand, mothers maintained on pharmacotherapy throughout pregnancy and the postpartum period remained symptom-free and were able to take care of their homes and families in a relaxed manner, beneficially influencing the development of these young children.

REFERENCES

1. Bleuler, E: Textbook of Psychiatry, Macmillan, New York. 1939, 210.

2. Henderson, D. K., and Gillespie, R. D.: Textbook of Psychiatry. Oxford Univ. Press, New York. 1947.

3. Hallvard, V.: Puerperal mental disorders, Acta Psychiat. Neurol. Scand. Suppl. III, 1956.

4. Klein, Henriette: Anxiety in Pregnancy, Paul B. Hoeber, Inc., New York, 1954.

5. Yonmans, J. B.: The prevention of psychiatric complications of pregnancy and puerperium, Am. Pract. Dig. Treat. 6:1315, Sept. 1955.

6. Stevenson, G. H., and Geoghegan, J. J.: Prophylatic electroshock therapy, Am. J. Psychiat. 107:743, Feb. 1951.

7. Linn, L., and Polatin, P.: Psychiatric problems of the puerperium from the standpoint of prophylaxis, Psychiat. Quart. 24:2, 375, Apr. 1950.

8. Dickel, H. A., and Dixon, H. H.: Inherent dangers in the use of tranquilizing drugs in anxiety states, J.A.M.A. 163:422, Feb. 9, 1957.

9. Gellis, S. S.: Personal communication.

10. Kris, E. B., and Carmichael, D. M.: Chlorpromazine maintenance therapy during pregnancy and confinement, Psychiat. Quart. p. 685. Oct. 1957.

Discussion by Martin Gross, M.D.

Dr. Kris reported that of 17 babies born to 14 mothers under ataractic medication, none were born prematurely (except 1 where 5 other children of the same mother were also born prematurely). None of the children had an abnormal birth (except for 1 boy who was delivered by cesarian section, as had his sister been fourteen months earlier). None of the children showed particular difficulties compared to their siblings, and none showed any problems of behavior or any emotional or mental disturbance. Sobel* reported that in 52 pregnant women treated with chlorpromazine the incidence of fetal morbidity was not raised as compared to a control group. Only one baby in this group, who had convulsions, "was developmentally retarded."

After reading Dr. Kris' report, I searched the files of our outpatient department in Baltimore and found records of six mothers who had given birth to eight children while under medication with ataractic drugs. One woman had twins; another had a boy and a girl in succession, both while she was taking Thorazine. All deliveries were at full term and normal, except in one case in which the birth was one month premature. All patients were under Thorazine medication during their confinement and one, in addition, under Frenquel. Some patients had been previously under Compazine or Sparine. The children, now from three months to four years old, are well developed and on a level at least equal to that of their siblings, as judged by parents and pediatricians.

The experienced social worker who visited the homes of these eight children reported—startled—that the behavior of the children as she observed them in the home confirmed the parents' descriptions of them as: physically attractive, normal, healthy, and socially well adjusted. Five of the mothers function adequately, taking care of their homes and their children. One is experiencing difficulties in performing her duties as a housewife, but she has a set of twins and a third child all under

*Sobel, D. E.: A.M.A. Arch. Gen. Psychiat. 2:606, 1960.

six years of age. Also, she is in the terminal stage of another pregnancy. Thus, our own experience coincides with that of Dr. Kris.

Her second and third case, reported in detail, are especially interesting. Both of these mothers had their previous bout of psychotic illness shortly after the birth of a child, and both did not relapse during a confinement under Thorazine treatment. It is true that no binding conclusions can be drawn from two cases, but the good result obtained here plus the absence of side reactions during confinement represent a definite indication for this kind of treatment in pregnant convalescent psychotic women. We therefore recommend routine continuation of drug treatment in convalescent schizophrenic women during and after confinement. It stands to reason to include women with the diagnosis of postpartum psychosis. Not only that, but also those women who have experienced an acute psychotic breakdown during a former pregnancy and are off medication should be started on ataractic drugs before confinement and continued on these drugs for a few months thereafter.

Two women of our group are pregnant again and that brings us to a question of considerable interest: Is the often withdrawn and frigid schizophrenic woman sexually more relaxed through ataractic medication, so much so that conception is facilitated? I do not think that this question can be answered at present, but it should be kept in mind for further investigation.

IV CLINICAL STUDIES

The Differentiation of Psychiatric Patients by EEG Changes After Sodium Pentothal

By BASRI SILA, M.D., MARIE MOWRER, M.D.,
GEORGE ULETT, M.D., AND MARGARET JOHNSON, B.S., R.N.

INTRODUCTION

Goldman [1, 2] has reported that the Pentothal-activated EEGs of schizophrenic patients differ from those of patients with other psychiatric diagnoses. In his reports a technique is described which is based upon a subjective assessment of EEG changes, primarily in the beta range, that occur within a 5-minute period after the intravenous injection of 300 mg of Sodium Pentothal.

There have been several studies of the effect of barbiturates on the EEG. Characteristically, these agents initially provoke an increase in activity with later slowing as the depth of the anesthesia increases. Shagass [3] developed the concept of the sedation threshold, for which he measured the quantity of Amytal necessary to produce a given EEG and behavioral effect. More drug was required in patients with symptoms of anxiety and neurosis than was the case in patients with depression and psychotic reactions. According to the concept of Shagass, with a high threshold there is a production of less beta activity for a given amount of barbiturate, and, conversely, a low threshold would correspond to a high beta index by the Pentothal-EEG test of Goldman. In his own studies, Shagass reports a lower sedation threshold for psychotic depressions than in the case of a mixed group of acute and chronic schizophrenic subjects. This finding is opposite to that claimed by Goldman. Although one must consider that Pentothal and Amytal are different drugs, their over-all reaction upon the EEG should be quite similar.

Supported in part by U. S. Public Health Service Grant MY 2756 and the Neuromedical Foundation of St. Louis.
Sodium Pentothal furnished through the courtesy of Abbott Laboratories.

This report is of the attempts of our laboratory to replicate the work of Goldman using an electronic EEG analyzer to obtain an objective quantification of the Pentothal-induced changes in the brain-wave spectrum.

A preliminary report of our work seemed to indicate the success of this technique in discriminating between a group of hospitalized schizophrenic patients and patients with depression [4, 5]. These studies relied upon clinical diagnosis in the selection of patients and our efforts to exclude questionable or compound diagnosis resulted in the admission to the research study of only 39 schizophrenic and 19 depressed patients from a population of 1600 psychiatric admissions in a twelve-month period. In an attempt to learn more about the types of patients seemingly differentiated by the Pentothal-EEG activation test, this sample was more closely scrutinized and refined on the basis of the symptom picture shown by the individual patient.

MATERIALS AND METHODS

This study included 58 patients from the admissions to the Malcolm Bliss Mental Health Center, St. Louis. Patients were selected by using the American Psychiatric Association's description for (1) schizophrenic reaction and (2) psychotic depressions, including psychotic depressive reaction, involutional psychotic reaction depressed type; and manic-depressive reaction, depressed type.

Patients were admitted to the study only if they had received no electroshock therapy (ECT) or continuous drug administration within a period of two months prior to hospital admission and had not received even a single dose of any drug active on the central nervous system (i.e., alcohol, tranquilizers, psychic energizers, or barbiturates) within forty-eight hours of testing.

All patients with serious complicating organic illnesses were eliminated. There were 39 schizophrenic subjects, 24 female and 15 male, with an average age of 34.2 years (range 17 to 54 years). Nineteen patients were diagnosed as having a psychotic depression. Of these, ten were male and nine female with an average age of 50.4 years (range 26 to 62 years). All patients were independently seen by at least two of the project psychiatrists, who agreed upon the diagnosis before admitting the patient to the study.

All patients were tested in the EEG laboratory at least 2 hours postprandially. The studies were conducted in a soundproof, air-conditioned laboratory. Recording was done with Gilson ten-channel EEG equipment and with conventional lead placement. After 5 minutes of resting EEG recording, 100 mg of Sodium Pentothal was injected intravenously in 5 to 7 seconds. This drug was injected on two more occasions at 2-minute intervals, thus giving a total of 300 mg in a 4-minute period. The patients were observed until the EEG tracings had returned to their premedication levels. All records were analyzed by means of a modified Walter-type electronic EEG analyzer [6].

RESULTS

Examination of the electronic analysis of resting EEG patterns is shown in Fig. 1. It can be clearly seen that the 39 schizophrenic patients and the 19 patients with psychotic depression have, on the average, similar basic resting EEGs. Figure 2 demonstrates the electronically analyzed EEG profile taken during the first minute after the injection of 300 mg of Sodium Pentothal. The difference in the plotted mean value of the EEG frequencies between the schizophrenic and the depressed group is significant beyond the 0.0001 level of probability (using nonparametric analysis). Although this difference in the means is seen to exist at all frequencies, the greatest difference appears in the range of beta activity (13.5 to 24.5 cps) as described by Goldman [1].

In a search for correlations between this increase in beta activity and specific symptoms, we carefully reviewed the charts of all patients previously admitted to the study. On the basis of this symptom analysis we found that a number of patients with symptoms common both to schizophrenia and to depressive illness had been included. Eliminating these patients from the study left us with a group of 24 patients (Fig. 3), 12 schizophrenic patients (mean age 41.8 years, range 35 to 50 years) and 12 patients with psychotic depressions (mean age 54.5 years, range 38 to 62 years) with relatively little overlapping symptomatology. Figure 4 illustrates the basic resting EEG, and Figures 5, 6, and 7 illustrate the profile plots of electronically analyzed EEG activity as seen 1, 3, and 5 minutes repectively after the intravenous injection of 300 mg of Sodium Pentothal. Because of the small number of patients remaining in this carefully selected sample, the medians of EEG frequency values were used in plotting these curves.

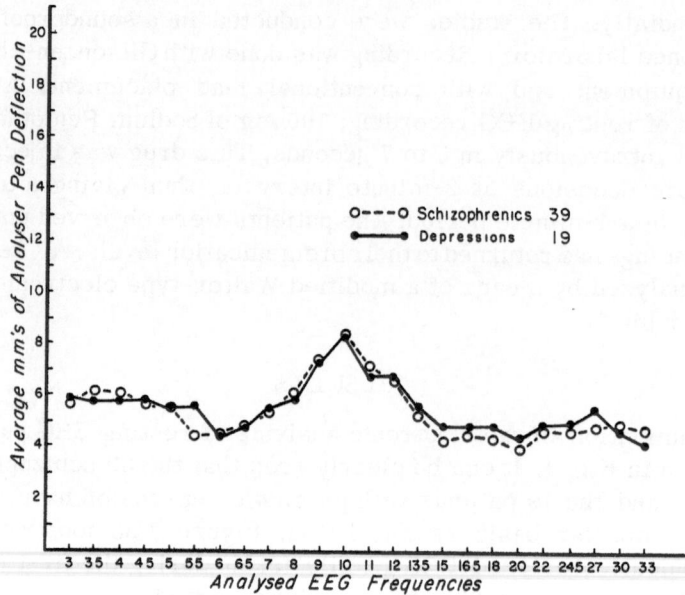

FIG. 1. EEG activity before Sodium Pentothal administration in 39 schizophrenic and 19 psychotic depressive patients.

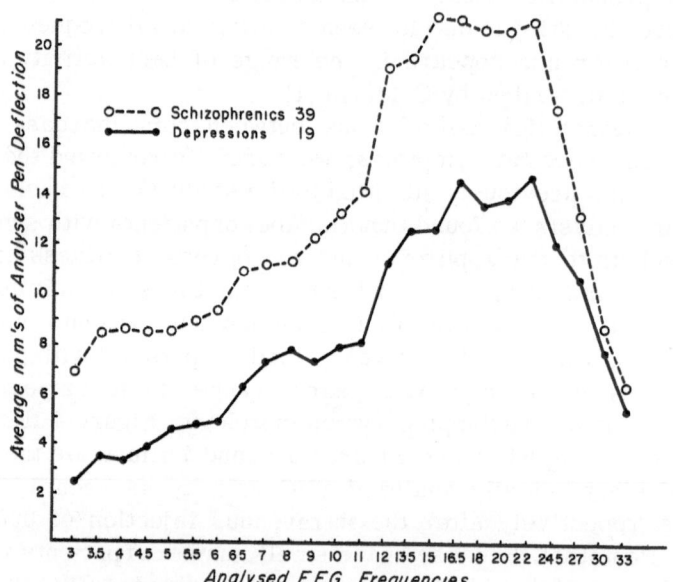

FIG. 2. EEG activity during first minute after Sodium Pentothal administration in 39 schizophrenic and 19 psychotic depressive patients.

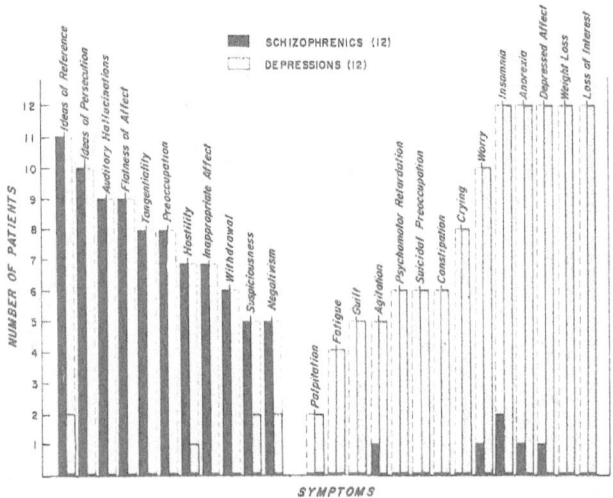

FIG. 3. Graph illustrating distribution of symptoms among 24 psychotic patients with clinical diagnoses of schizophrenia (12) and depression (12).

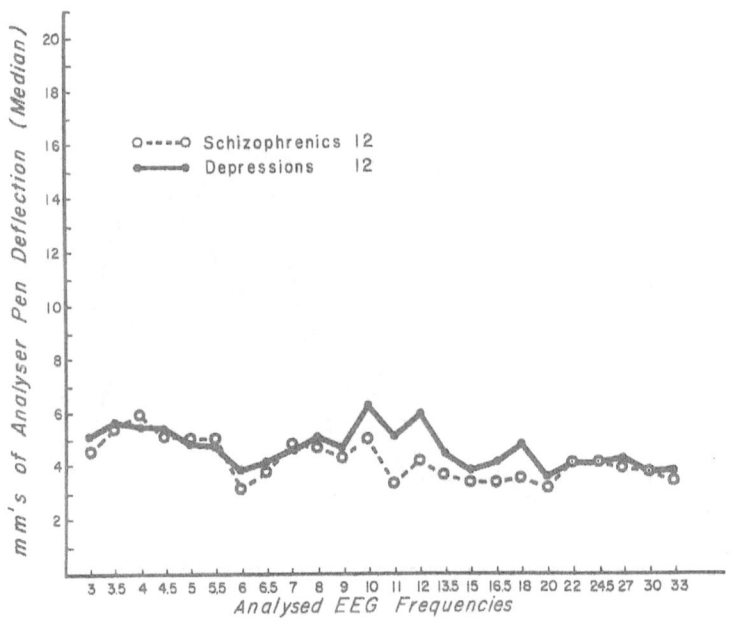

FIG. 4. EEG activity before Sodium Pentothal administration in 24 psychotic patients.

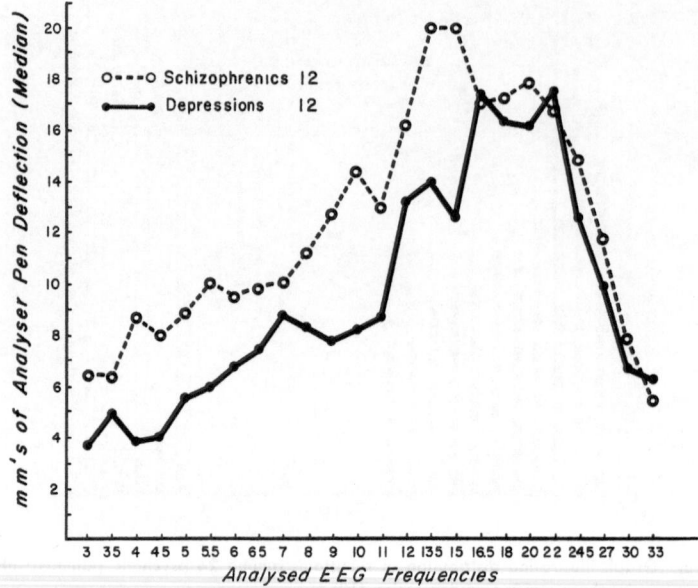

FIG. 5.   EEG activity first minute after Sodium Pentothal administration in 24 psychotic patients.

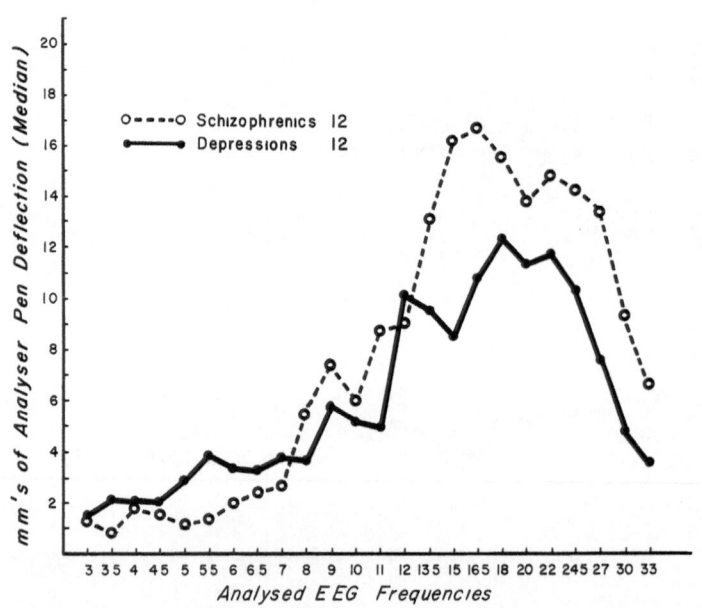

FIG. 6.   EEG activity third minute after Sodium Pentothal administration in 24 psychotic patients.

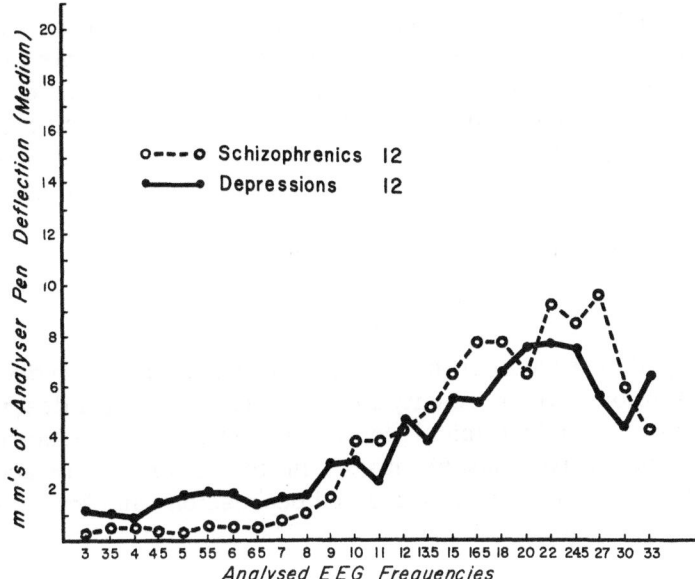

FIG. 7.   EEG activity fifth minute after Sodium Pentothal administration in 24 psychotic patients.

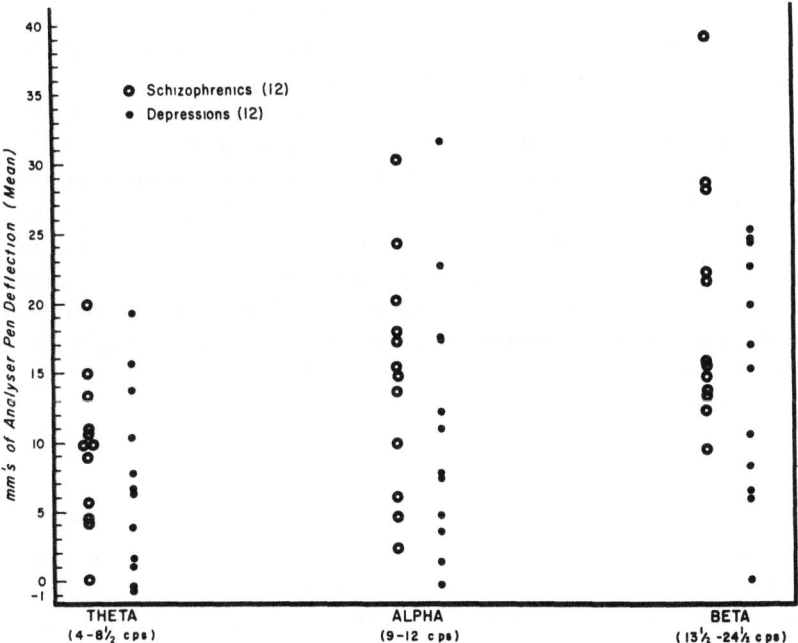

FIG. 8.   Individual mean theta, alpha, and beta indices of EEG activity during first minute after Sodium Pentothal administration.

As can be seen from the data, the Pentothal test did not differentiate significantly between the two groups of patients selected in this manner. Figure 8 shows the distribution of mean values for theta (4 to 8.5 cps), alpha (9 to 12 cps), and beta (13.5 to 24.5 cps) activity of the 12 schizophrenic and 12 depressed patients. The amount of overlapping in the two groups would appear to render the test useless for discriminating between groups of schizophrenic and depressed subjects as diagnosed by these criteria.

DISCUSSION

The greatest value of this study would appear to be a very clear demonstration of the necessity for a careful behavioral description of patients used in clinical research studies. The reliance upon "agreement of two psychiatrists" in terms of widely accepted clinical labels for schizophrenia and depression can obviously lead to different results from those achieved by the careful differentiation of patients on the basis of their presenting symptoms. It is our belief that much confusion in the field of psychiatry could be avoided if experimenters would describe their patient populations in greater detail. It now appears from this study that even the same clinical labels given by the same psychiatrist in the same institution can imply quite different population samples.

The size of the sample reported upon here is obviously too small for a definitive opinion of the usefulness of the Pentothal-EEG index as a valid instrument for detecting neurophysiological differences between certain types of patients called "schizophrenic" or "depressed." We plan to continue our work in this area and to enlarge on the sample here presented while continuing to describe as objectively as possible, on the basis of behavior and symptoms, the patients admitted to the experimental groups. It is our hope that others working in this field will similarly objectify their own observations.

SUMMARY

Sodium Pentothal was injected intravenously in a group of 58 patients diagnosed as having either schizophrenia or depression. EEGs were taken before and for 5 minutes following the injection. These data were electronically analyzed, and the post-Pentothal records were compared with the pre-Pentothal records.

Pentothal produced an increase in EEG activity at all frequencies, but particularly in the beta range. In the group of 58 patients selected on the basis of clinical diagnosis, there was a significant difference in the reaction of the patients diagnosed as having depression or schizophrenia, with a quantitatively greater EEG response in the schizophrenic subjects. When a group of 24 patients was carefully selected from the larger group and dichotomized on the basis of symptoms typical for schizophrenia or depression and with little or no overlapping, there was found to be no significant difference in response between the two groups of patients.

REFERENCES

1. Goldman, D.: Differential response to drugs useful in treatment of psychoses revealed by Pentothal-activated EEG. In Wortis, J.,: Ed: Recent Advances in Biological Psychiatry, vol. III, Grune & Stratton, Inc., 1960, p.250.

2. Goldman, D., Balzhizer, J., and Rosenberg, B.: Specific electroencephalographic changes with Pentothal activation in psychotic states., EEG Clin. Neurophysiol. 11:657, 1959.

3. Shagass, C.: A measurable neurophysiological factor of psychiatric significance, ibid. 9:101, 1957.

4. Ulett, G. A.: Discussion of Goldman, D.: Differential response to drugs useful in treatment of psychoses revealed by Pentothal-activated EEG. In Wortis, J., Ed.: Recent Advances in Biological Psychiatry, vol. III, Grune & Stratton, Inc., 1960, p. 265.

5. Mowrer, M., Sila, B., Ulett, G. A., and Johnson, M.: The differentiation of schizophrenics from non-schizophrenics by the Pentothal index., Soc. Proc., Central Assoc. EEG'ers, EEG Clin. Neurophysiol., 13:145, 1961.

6. Ulett, G. A., and Loeffel, R. G.: A new resonator-integrator unit for the automatic brain wave analyser, ibid. 5:113, 1953.

Discussion by Douglas Goldman, M.D

I have appreciated very much the opportunity to read and study the paper of this group of authors, particularly since it involves a special area of my interest.

Since the technique was originally described from my laboratory, I am very happy that the larger groups of patients were clearly distinguishable by the analyzer technique, with significance in the fourth decimal place for probability against the difference being of accidental or random occurrence. This finding in patients removed both in time and space from our own subjects is in agreement with our own findings.

However, this study represents a replication of our work only in a relatively narrow segment. Our work has involved Pentothal-activation studies in about 2000 patients with collection in two separate intervals of carefully screened, previously untreated patients for statistical study. A relatively large number of patients with several kinds of psychotic illness were followed with Pentothal-activated EEGs prior to treatment, during treatment, the period after recovery or failure to achieve recovery, and in a number of patients through several cycles of relapse and recovery. Some of this work was presented before this society two years ago and is published in our volume for that year [A].

In our initial report [B] a group of patients in the schizophrenic categories, on the one hand, and in the nonschizophrenic categories plus a number of normal non-patient subjects, on the other hand, all untreated for at least one year, were compared statistically (Fig. I). The comparison resulted in discrimination by the chi-square technique at the 0.01 level of significance. Since the original report, we have gathered another group of individuals divided into (1) schizophrenic and (2) nonschizophrenic psychiatric categories which discriminate by the chi-square technique at the 0.001 level of significance (Fig. II) by the use of the scoring scheme which these authors have considered "a subjective assessment."

This scoring scheme (Fig. III) I would like to defend as being objective in the sense that a millimeter ruler is objective and that the time lines in an EEG tracing are objective. The only valid criticism of this technique is that it is laborious and time consuming.

It is not quite fair to Dr. Shagass' sedation threshold to compare it with the Pentothal activation, since Pentothal and Amytal, when used in sharply analogous techniques, hardly produce similar changes in the EEG. This was pointed out in the

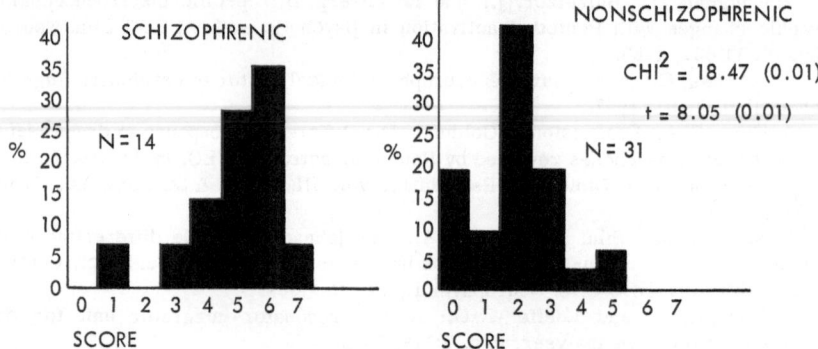

FIG. I.   Statistical comparison of schizophrenic and nonschizophrenic patients (first series).

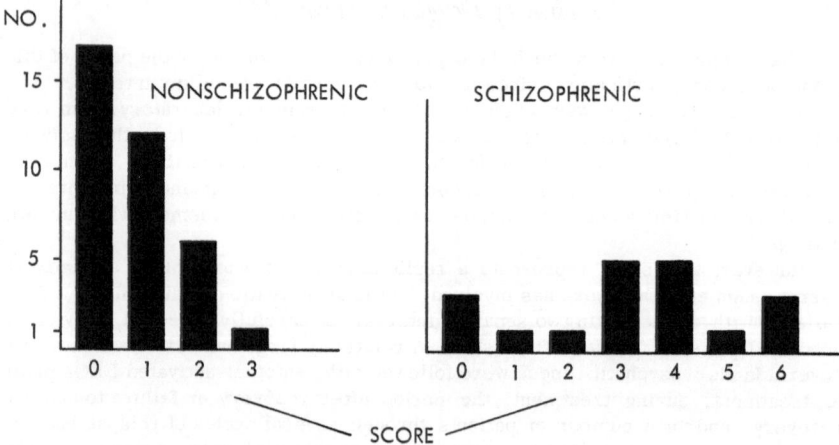

FIG. II.   Schizophrenic and nonschizophrenic patients (second series).

		SCORE
I	"BETA ACTIVITY" 20 PER SECOND FREQUENCY OR OVER, MORE THAN 50% OF TIME IN ANY ONE LEAD, DURING 30 SECOND EPISODES.	
	1. OCCURRING WITHIN 2 MINUTES FROM TIME OF INJECTION.	1
	2. OCCURRING BETWEEN 2 AND 4 MINUTES FROM TIME OF INJECTION.	2
	3. OCCURRING OVER 4 MINUTES AFTER THE TIME OF INJECTION.	3
	SCORE IN ONLY ONE CATEGORY (1, 2, OR 3).	
II	"BURSTS" OVER 0.25 SECOND DURATION, 15 PER SECOND OR MORE FREQUENCY, VOLTAGE OVER 25 MICROVOLTS PEAK TO PEAK, MORE THAN SIX PER MINUTE, PRESENT AFTER 1 MINUTE FOLLOWING INJECTION.	
	A. DURATION	
	1. 0.25 TO 0.6 SECOND	1
	2. 0.6 SECOND OR OVER, TWO OR MORE PER MINUTE	2
	SCORE IN ONLY ONE CATEGORY (1 OR 2)	
	B. OVER 50 MICROVOLTS, PEAK TO PEAK; ADDITIONAL SCORE	1
	C. 15 BURSTS PER MINUTE OR MORE	1
	D. EXTRA CREDIT BEFORE 1 MINUTE AFTER INJECTION ONLY IF ABOVE QUALIFICATIONS ARE PRESENT; MORE THAN 5 BURSTS PER MINUTE, ALL OVER 0.5 SEC. DURATION, AND ALL OVER 50 MICRO- VOLTS PEAK TO PEAK.	2
III	THETA ACTIVITY — 4 TO 7 PER SECOND FREQUENCY, VERY REGULAR, OVER 1 SECOND DURATION, SYNCHRONOUS IN MORE THAN 1 LEAD. VOLTAGE PEAK TO PEAK, MICROVOLTS:	
	1. 100 TO 200	1
	2. OVER 200	2
	SCORE IN ONLY 1 CATEGORY (1 OR 2)	

FIG. III. Scoring scheme.

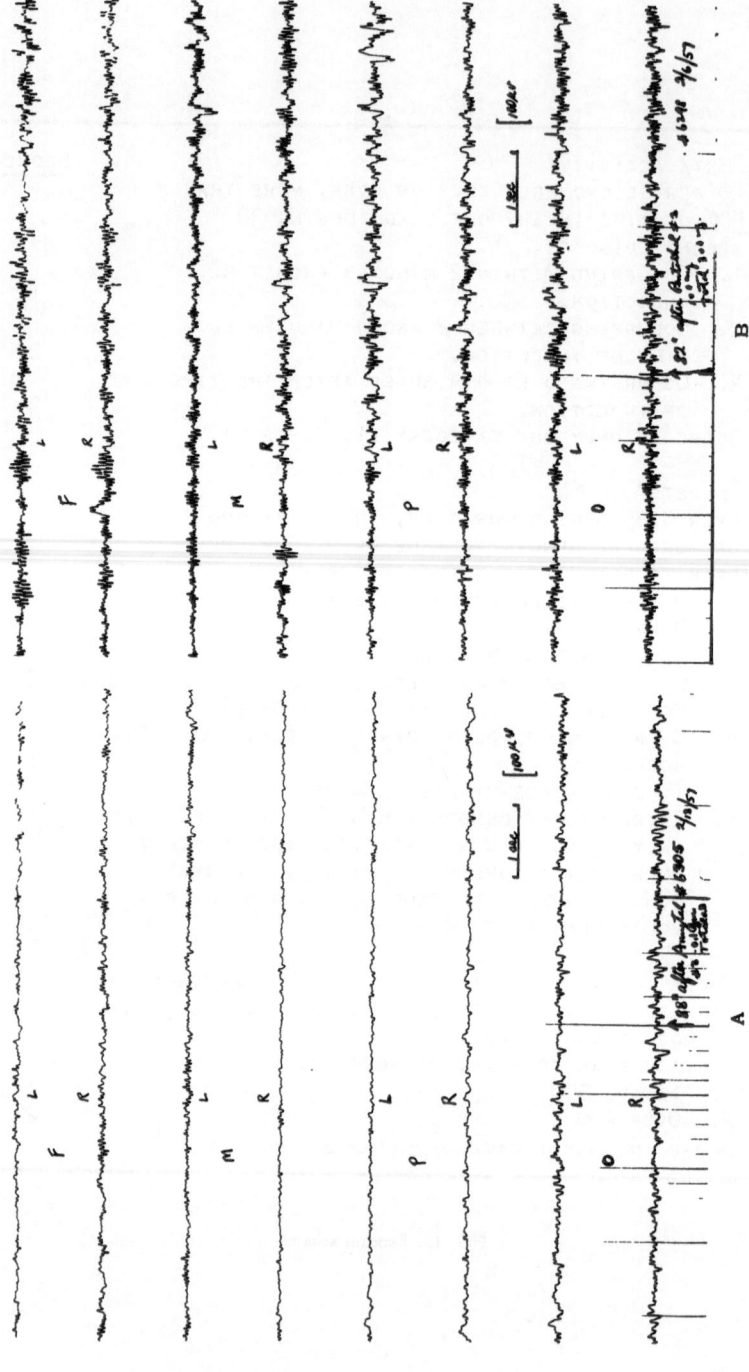

FIG. IV. Comparison of EEG changes with Pentothal and Amytal.

initial description of Pentothal activation and was appropriately illustrated (Fig. IV). It is therefore not to be expected that the sedation-threshold technique should result in findings similar to those of Pentothal activation. There are fundamental differences between the drugs chemically and pharmacologically and in the application of the two techniques, so there is really no reason why "their over-all reaction upon the EEG should be quite similar," as indeed they are not.

Certain inadequacies in the technique applied by Drs. Sila, Mowrer, and Ulett and Miss Johnson are of some importance. Two months without treatment prior to application of the Pentothal activation is probably not long enough in a study in which statistical validity is being tested. Forty-eight hours without any drug may also not be sufficient for clearing of the EEG, particularly with some drugs that are metabolized or excreted slowly. The method of injection of Pentothal, both for dose and for timing is too rigid for the production of maximum effect in all patients. Actually in some, the interval of 2 minutes is sufficiently short so that cumulative anesthetic effects rather than the stimulating cycle may be produced.

In the particularly chosen subgroups of 12 schizophrenic and 12 depressive individuals in whom the EEG differentiation was clearly less distinct than in the larger group, the authors considered that it was indicated that this finding reflected upon the value and significance of the Pentothal-EEG activation; yet it is a matter of simple arithmetic to conclude that the discrimination must have been even more significant between the remaining 27 schizophrenic and 7 depressive patients than in the total group, since the nonsignificant elements had been subtracted. These could have been involved in the criteria for separation as well as the patients. It should be obvious that any method which can discriminate between large groups of psychotic individuals must have meaning.

It is the preoccupation with behavioral and apparent psychological reactions that should be the object of criticism. It is evident to many serious workers at this time that the kinds and intensities of behavioral manifestations producible by human beings are limited. It may be considered that disturbances in neurological function which may affect behavior can take only a limited number of "final common paths." We have therefore come to the time when the discrimination between behavioral differences alone cannot be acceptable as a foundation for a psychiatric nosology.

It is evident in the authors' larger series of patients that diagnoses were better differentiated by the global clinical picture in which component factors and their interrelation were considered than by simply extracting and listing in two columns of descriptive elements while leaving the total clinical picture and its complexity out of consideration. I am in considerable agreement with the authors' appeal for describing as objectively as possible differences among the patients, and I perhaps disagree with them by believing that the deflection of an oscillograph is more objective than the recognizing and naming of behavioral and psychopathological manifestations.

REFERENCES

A. Goldman, D.: Differential response to drugs useful in treatment of psychoses revealed by Pentothal-activated EEG. In Wortis, J., Ed.: Recent Advances in Biological Psychiatry, Vol. III, Grune & Stratton, Inc., New York, p. 250, 1960.

B. Goldman, D.: Specific electro-encephalographic changes with Pentothal activation in psychotic states, EEG J. 11:657, 1959.

CHAPTER 20

Porphyric Psychosis and Chelation Therapy

By HENRY A. PETERS, M.D.

Since 1954 we have reported frequently on the seeming effectiveness of chelation treatment with ethylenediaminetetraacetate (EDTA) and dimercaptopropanol (BAL) in over two-thirds of the patients suffering from acute, chronic, and mixed porphyria, even when many of these patients were in extremis prior to chelation therapy [1-7], while negative results in isolated cases have also been noted [13]. Intensive screening of neurological and psychiatric patients at University Hospital, Madison, as well as increased awareness of physicians referring patients to this institution has resulted in the identification of almost 100 cases of abnormal porphyrin metabolism since 1953.

SCREENING METHODS

Twenty-four hour urine collections in deleaded containers were conducted, and the urine was analyzed by colorimetric means for copper, zinc, and lead and also for coproporphyrin and uroporphyrin. Fresh urine samples were also obtained and analyzed by the method of Mauzerall and Granick [14] for porphobilinogen and delta-amino levulinic acid. Wherever possible, and especially when the clinical inventory was suggestive, repetitive tests were run to pick up those patients who were excreting these metabolites intermittently.

Fecal specimens were analyzed according to Dean's method [15] for the presence of increased amounts of protoporphyrin (consisting of coproporphyrin and protoporphyrin); an abnormality in any one of these categories caused us to repeat frequently our screening

We are especially indebted to Dr. F.L. Kozelka, David Stuiber, Barbara McCann, and Lyra Hekmatpanah for their assistance in the toxicological work. Dr. H.H. Reese, Dr. P.L. Eichman, and Dr. S.A.M. Johnson likewise collaborated in the clinical study. This work has been aided by National Institutes of Health Grant B-1943(C1).

efforts. Cases of chronic and mixed porphyria showing predominantly photosensitive dermatological lesions generally showed positive uroporphyrin values in their urine and positive protoporphyrin values in their feces. Porphobilinogen and delta-amino levulinic acid were seldom elevated in this category but were found in the acute hepatic porphyric patients.

We have also called attention to an increased urinary excretion of zinc and/or copper in the acute and mixed porphyric patients who are in the process of developing neurological and psychiatric symptomatology, these increased excretion values often paralleling the severity of the disease more so than the excretion of abnormal porphyrin metabolites [3-7]. Patients in the remission stage and those with primarily abdominal colic excrete more normal amounts. Patients with chiefly light-sensitive dermatological disturbance (chronic porphyria) tended to show increased urinary excretion of copper. Patients showing an elevation of delta-amino levulinic acid plus an increase in urinary zinc and/or copper or a positive fecal protoporphyrin value as well as a history suggestive of porphyria we have labeled as paraporphyric (to the extent that we excluded in therapy all barbiturate and sulfa drugs). Further study on some of these patients has enabled us to reclassify them as porphyric.

SIGNS AND SYMPTOMS

We have previously summarized and given detailed case reports on the symptomatology presented by our porphyric patients and the effects of chelation therapy [1-7]. The medical literature in recent years has been rich in descriptions of the gastrointestinal, dermatological, psychiatric, and neurological symptomatology observed in these patients; we would especially direct your attention to the descriptions of Dean and Barnes [15], Goldberg [16], Waldenstrom [17], Watson and Larson [18], and Brunsting and co-workers [19].

The symptomatology that we have observed may be summarized as follows, recognizing that symptoms vary from patient to patient and in the same patient to the extent that a patient with abdominal colic or back pain may, after using sulfa or barbiturate drugs or as a result of some other stress, develop profound neurological and psychiatric symptoms in the form of seizures, psychosis, peripheral neuropathy, bulbar signs, and so forth. It should be emphasized, however, that neurological and psychiatric symptoms may exist entirely alone or apart from gastrointestinal symptomatology.

Psychiatric

Psychiatric symptoms were present in over half of our patients. Symptoms varied from toxic psychoses with bizarre, catatonic-like excitement, misidentification, déjà vu, auditory and sometimes visual hallucinosis resembling acute delirium tremens to a chronic brain syndrome, sometimes with Korsakoff psychotic features. Aphasic disturbance was also noted. Levels of consciousness ranged from torpor to coma, and a marked delay in response to questioning or in the following of directions suggested cerebral abscess. Over a dozen patients have manifested a schizophrenic-like psychosis, often as the only symptom present, which could not be differentiated from classical schizophrenic symptomatology by Rorschach test or independent psychiatric evaluation. It is our feeling that a definite schizophrenic porphyric syndrome exists. Often the erroneous diagnosis of hysteria had been attached to patients prior to the development of more severe and obvious neuropsychiatric symptomatology. Other patients gave a history of classical phobic neurosis, while depressive and schizoaffective symptomatology likewise was noted.

Neurological

Neurological signs and symptoms included bulbar involvement, such as dysphagia, diplopia, anisocoria, dysarthria, facial paralysis, and laryngeal palsy. Tracheotomy is often indicated in patients showing early evidence of respiratory insufficiency. Grand mal seizures were frequently observed, while Jacksonian and psychomotor seizure activity was seen accompanied by focal EEG localization of a shifting nature. Migrainous-type headaches have been noted. Several patients manifested homonymous hemianopsia, which in one patient alternated from one side to the other and normalized on recovery. Status epilepticus of severe degree was often recorded, and intolerance to diphenylhydantoin medication has been noted in some of the patients treated for seizure activity. Occasionally cerebellar ataxia and extrapyramidal symptoms have occurred.

The peripheral nervous system was involved in the form of tetraparesis in eight patients, paraplegia in five, and monoplegia in one. These more severe neurological symptoms were often precipitated by sulfonamide or barbiturate medication, especially the quick-acting barbiturates such as thiopental (Pentothal). The paresis was as often distal in onset as proximal and frequently accompanied by recurrent myoclonic jerks and asynchronous muscle contractions, especially against resistance. A spreading excitation of the muscles was seen when a single extremity was moved against resistance, an effect not unlike that seen in strychnine intoxication. This heightened motor irritability existed despite complete tetraplegia and muscle atrophy. Deep-tendon reflexes were at times retained in paralyzed limbs. Sensory alterations were surprisingly absent despite severe motor weakness. Fatigability of the muscles sometimes resembled myasthenia gravis though not responding in characteristic manner to the administration of Prostigmin. Muscle and joint pain was recorded during the onset and sometimes in the recovery phase of the neuropathy. These pains were so fleeting and vague or poorly localized as to suggest hysteria reflecting most probably an altered level of consciousness.

We have previously reported one patient who sustained a fracture dislocation of the shoulder and did not complain of her pain until after her level of consciousness was improved following BAL treatment. Another patient sustained a severe dorsal spine fracture in a fall from bed with resultant paraparesis and a sensory level. The altered level of consciousness obscured this clinical feature until a more careful neurological examination and x-ray films were obtained. Laminectomy was performed in two patients because of symptoms suggesting a cord tumor.

Other symptoms that may exist alone or along with neurological and psychiatric syndromes must be considered.

Gastrointestinal

Gastrointestinal symptoms include recurrent abdominal, back, and at times chest pain, often without muscle guarding, sometimes of burning or atypical description, and usually accompanied by nausea, emesis, intermittent diarrhea (at times blood), or severe constipation. During acute attacks fecal impactions occur, and the pain may mimic gallbladder disease, pancreatitis, lower chest pathology, or a pelvic disturbance.

A history of polysurgery should always be a cause for considering the diagnosis of acute, intermittent porphyria. One woman had a series of 12 major abdominal operations. The differentiation between porphyric pains, which can be extremely severe, and other organic causes of acute abdominal distress may be very difficult.

Urinary incontinence or retention may occur, and oliguria or anuria, especially after the administration of sulfonamide drugs including sulfisoxazole (Gantrisin), has been observed. Several patients had multiple cystoscopic examinations, and nephrectomy was performed in several patients because of suspected primary kidney disturbance. Urinary complaints at times have been thought secondary to conversion hysteria or a schizophrenic psychosis until the metabolic alterations indicative of porphyria were noted. Contrary to popular belief, the burgundy-wine or brownish urine described as typical in textbooks may never be mentioned by the acute porphyric patient, and many urine specimens have been observed to be normal in color even after exposure to sunlight and acidification and despite the presence of increased porphobilinogen in the urine. Nurses observe that the urinary odor is often offensive during exacerbations.

Dermatological

A malar flush over the "butterfly" area resembling lupus was frequently observed during the acute phase in acute and mixed hepatic porphyria. Other patients showed a dusky, metallic complexion and increased melanosis resembling a mask of pregnancy. The chronic and mixed porphyric patients often showed violaceous hues over light-exposed areas, and some of the acute porphyric patients also showed this feature. The chronic and some mixed porphyric patients manifested skin which abraded easily, often showing actinic and photosensitive bullae, dryness of the skin, and absence of normal sweating. One chronic porphyric patient was suffering from mongolism.

Intolerance to Chemicals and Sun Bathing Precipitating Symptoms

A history of intolerance to oil base paints and chemical solvents was seen in approximately one-third of the patients. In several of these patients the use of oil-base paints and in another patient the exposure to gasoline products in his work seemed to play a part in precipitating acute neurological and psychiatric symptoms. Particularly the quick-acting barbiturates used for sedation or Pentothal used in operative procedures seemed to produce acute neuropsychiatric symptoms. Frequently, periods of prolonged somnolence postoperatively accompanied by gastrointestinal and frankly psychotic symptoms were ascribed by the patients and relatives to the surgery itself rather than to the use of barbiturates. Where intolerance to one barbiturate was recorded, it was noted that almost all drugs of this family produced symptomatology, although the slow-acting barbiturates such as phenobarbital were by far the best tolerated. Occasionally one would get a history of previous tolerance, sometimes for several years, to these agents with most probably a loss of tolerance prior to the development of more overt porphyric symptoms.

The sulfonamide drugs frequently induced either skin rashes, abdominal pain, or in some instances psychosis. In the last year we have treated two patients in whom the acute episode of severe porphyria seemed to have been precipitated by the use of chlorothiazide (Diuril). A marked weakening effect on prolonged sun bathing has also been noted, and in one patient her first attack was precipitated after she fell asleep in the sun and developed a severe case of sunburn.

THERAPEUTIC APPROACH

Once the diagnosis is made or suspected, complete avoidance of drugs, especially barbiturate and sulfa derivatives, was insisted upon. Occasional cases seemed to have been aggravated by use of Dexedrine-like compounds. We have seen porphyric symptoms of psychosis or seizures aggravated by diphenylhydantoin (Dilantin), and we generally avoid its use. When seizures were present, we attempted to treat the patients primarily with chelating agents although on occasion phenobarbital and Mysoline were required; administration of these drugs was generally not necessary after or during chelation. When status epilepticus was present, rectal Avertin seemed helpful in breaking up the cycle when chelation alone seemed ineffectual. Symptoms of abdominal colic were sometimes controlled by the use of phenothiazine derivatives, especially Chlorpromazine or Compazine. (However, we have noted marked intolerance to low doses of phenothiazine compounds in several instances, and one patient developed severe trismus and asthenia on Compazine medication.)

Once a base line of control with the phenothiazine derivatives, as advocated by Monaco et al. [20] and Melby, Street, and Watson [21], was established in the patients showing only abdominal colic, the comparative influence of a chelation regimen was then determined. Some of our porphyric schizophrenic patients in the past had tolerated electric shock treatment with good results therapeutically. (One patient previously reported developed status epilepticus after her first two electric shock treatments.) Parenteral chelation was utilized in cases which failed to respond to supportive measures and the withdrawal of barbiturates and sulfa drugs. Patients considered critical, often after previous failure of steroid therapy attempted elsewhere, were subjected to an immediate course of chelation.

The current EDTA dosage averaged from $1\frac{1}{2}$ to $2\frac{1}{2}$ g of the disodium or disodium calcium salt daily, administered in 1000 cc 5% glucose in water for courses of from five to seven days with a repeat course at lower dosage if necessary. In all instances fluids were pushed to a daily intake of at least 3000 cc with careful attention to electrolyte balance. Dimercaptopropanol (BAL) was used as a 10% solution in 20% benzyl benzoate in peanut oil, and the dosage ranged from 50 to 1200 mg per twenty-four hours although generally our dosage ranged from $\frac{1}{2}$ to 1 cc four to five times daily with reduction in dosage as the patients improved. When there was a question of lead exposure or increased urinary lead excretion, BAL was never used initially, and in more recent years we have usually initiated a chelation regimen using EDTA alone, at least for the first three to five days.

During the convalescent stages in the more severe cases and in those showing recurrent abdominal colic, oral regimens were prescribed after a trial of parenteral chelation when the use of phenothiazine derivatives either had sufficient side-effects or failed to give adequate control. Disodium calcium versenate (EDTA) in $\frac{1}{2}$-g tablets was used in a dosage ranging from two to four tablets per day with reduction of dosage as symptoms improved. More recently, we have added powdered glycine during maintenance regimens because of its precursor role in the formation of porphyrin substances. Vitamin B_{12} likewise was added once the clinical response to chelation alone had been evaluated. Chlorpormazine, meperidine (Demerol), paraldehyde, azacyclonal (Frenquel), chloral hydrate, and intravenous procaine were also used occasionally. Frenquel at times seemed helpful in acute toxic psychosis due to porphyria. In most instances steroids were studiously avoided, and in many of our most severe cases steroid therapy had been ineffectual in halting a downhill course prior to the use of chelation treatment. In two cases oliguria and edema of the extremities developed and failed to abort during the initial stages of chelation. Brief courses of hydrocortisone were then utilized with benefit.

To be emphasized in the management of these patients is the fact that exceptional nursing care, tracheotomy, occasionally gastrostomy, and careful attention to fluid and electrolyte balance must be maintained in order to bring about clinical recovery in the most severe cases.

RESULTS

A total of 65 patients have now been treated with chelating agents, including 48 patients with acute intermittent porphyria, 5 with mixed hepatic porphyria, 3 with chronic porphyria, and 9 with paraporphyria. Thirty-six of the 48 acute intermittent cases, 5 of the mixed porphyric cases, 9 of the paraporphyric cases, and 3 of the chronic porphyric cases seemed to benefit from chelation schedules. Of the acute porphyrics not showing a favorable response, one died with periarteritis nodosa that had been diagnosed by biopsy prior to chelating efforts, and this patient died despite prior steroid medication that was continued concomitantly with a final attempt to improve his status with chelation.

Another severe acute intermittent porphyric patient who developed complete tetraplegic and bulbar paralysis died of a staphylococcal bacteremia despite what seemed to be an initial favorable response to chelation. Two acute hepatic porphyric patients with predominantly abdominal symptoms and with associated opiate addiction commited suicide some time after their discharge from the hospital. Twenty of the acute hepatic porphyric patients and two of the mixed porphyric patients were in very critical condition from advanced neuropsychiatric symptomatology prior to chelation efforts despite prior ineffectual use of ACTH in six cases. All but four of this group seem to have benefited from chelation efforts, with complete recovery from tetraparesis having been noted in eight patients. We had previously reported one tetraparetic patient who derived benefit from ACTH after BAL treatment alone seemed inadequate. All the patients with chronic porphyria (manifesting predominantly photosensitive dermatitis with easily abraded skin, loss of sweating, and pigmentary changes) responded to chelation efforts, and a follow-up on one of these patients after a five year period has demonstrated complete clinical remission despite his frequent exposure to the sun and his use of alcoholic beverages.

In judging the effectiveness of chelation therapy in the severely involved patients, we wish to point out that recovery from peripheral neuropathy may be dependent in part upon the degree to which axon cylinders have been altered in addition to the known demyelinization that takes place. We have, however, noted immediate gains in strength in some of these patients after the addition of BAL or EDTA compounds to their regimen when their recovery from peripheral neuropathy prior to chelation treatment had remained static. In some instances chelation efforts alone stopped the occurrence of recurrent epileptic seizures, and rapid improvement in schizophrenic and other psychiatric symptoms was frequently noted after the initiation of chelation efforts. Eight porphyric schizophrenic patients have shown reversals of psychotic symptoms on chelation therapy alone, while a number of other patients with combined neurological and psychiatric symptomatology also recovered on chelating treatment.

When symptoms included mainly abdominal colic, we attempted to compare the effect of phenothiazine derivatives on the recurring colic with the effect of chelation schedules. Those in whom addiction to opiates had taken place were especially difficult to evaluate. Often oral maintenance regimes with disodium calcium EDTA, sometimes supplemented with B_{12} and glycine, seemed capable of aborting later attacks or reducing their severity, although additional courses of intravenous EDTA have at times been necessary. During the onset of peripheral neuropathy as well as during the recovery phase pain has at times been a problem requiring the use of intravenous procaine, although generally these efforts have not been necessary especially since we have utilized EDTA. In addition, we have a series of four patients who were severely involved with peripheral neuropathy and psychiatric symptoms and who were not treated with a chelation schedule; one died shortly after dismissal from the hospital after having been placed on cortisone because of arthralgic symptoms, and the other three have shown a prolonged period of hospitalization and poor clinical recovery.

On occasion we have combined the use of BAL and EDTA toward the end of the treatment period, but we now use EDTA alone during the initial stages of therapy. Many of the patients who showed melanotic discoloration of the skin, in addition to those suffering from chronic porphyria with skin changes, experienced an improvement in their dermatological status in the form of a toughening of the skin, loss of photosensitivity, and a marked decrease in melanotic coloring.

DISCUSSION

The variability of the clinical course in acute porphyria is notorious and naturally makes evaluation of therapeutic regimens difficult. Nevertheless, the frequent prompt response to the use of chelating agents in the more severely involved patients plus the observable improvement in skin lesions seen in the chronic porphyric patients, despite the use of ethanol and continued sun exposure in one patient over a five-year period, make us feel that we are observing a true therapeutic influence. In attempting to explain the seeming effectiveness of chelation therapy, we have focused our attention on the increased urinary zinc and at times copper excretion seen in porphyric subjects who were developing neurological and psychiatric symptomatology; the excretion often seemed to parallel the clinical severity of the condition better than did the excretion of abnormal porphyrin metabolites [3-5].

We have also noted an increase in urinary copper excretion, especially in the chronic and mixed porphyric patients during periods of clinical activity. Those patients showing predominantly abdominal symptomatology revealed generally less abnormal or at times normal values. The values for elevated copper excretion before chelation ranged from two to five times the norm, and for zinc from two to thirty-six times the norm. These values became grossly augmented during chelation therapy but tended to approach normal values during the recovery phase, despite the continued administration of chelating agents and the frequently continued elevation of abnormal porphyrin excretion. Where these cations or some other still unidentified cations may be derived from during periods of exacerbation would seem to be debatable, although a probable shift from the usual fecal to the urinary route of excretion, perhaps owing to some intrahepatic block, seems possible. An increased alimentary absorption, as in Wilson's disease, likewise cannot be excluded. Since some cases of alcoholism, particularly those showing delirium tremens and Wernicke's encephalopathy or neuropathy, and patients with collagen disease, such as periarteritis nodosa and other chronic brain syndromes, reveal increases in urinary zinc and copper and sometimes lead prior to chelation efforts, the elevation of urinary excretion of these cations is not in itself diagnostic of porphyria, but does suggest some common metabolic alteration.

Cases of heavy metal intoxication due to mercury, lead, and arsenic also tend to show a zinc and/or copper diuresis during periods when the patients are developing neuropsychiatric symptomatology. We have seldom encountered patients showing copper and/or zinc diuresis who were clinically asymptomatic. It should be emphasized that it is the concentration of these cations rather than their 24-hour urinary excretion that bears this relationship, since a normal person drinking sufficient amounts of fluid can diurese sufficient amounts of urine to put out lead, zinc, and copper in an elevated range. Moreover, the urinary concentration of these cations seems to be remarkably constant in aliquot samples taken during a 24-hour period and as measured from day to day.

Gunther [22] recognized that urinary porphyrins were often combined with a metal, and Watson and Schwartz [23] noted the zinc metal complexing of uroporphyrin and coproporphyrin. Watson and Larson [18] called attention to the zinc complex being relatively larger in amount in a case of porphyria showing relapse. We have previously postulated that the metabolic block in acute intermittent porphyria, which presumably lies beyond the porphobilinogen stage, might be due to an excess retention of zinc, copper, or perhaps some other cation. We noted that an excess of zinc is said to inhibit the enzymatic activity of lactic and alcohol dehydrogenase and also delta-amino levulinic dehydrase and insulin, ACTH, and equine gonadotropin activity are also retarded on the addition of zinc. Edman [24] has demonstrated the zinc-induced relaxation of muscle fibers that is relieved by the complexing of the zinc with ATP, thus suggesting that some of the motor weakness in porphyria may be related to muscular inhibition due to excess zinc. The zincuria and cupruria observed in the porphyric subjects could represent nature's attempts to rid the body of toxic cations by means of increased excretions of porphyrin metabolites in combination with zinc or some other cations as a last desperate effort to mobilize these porphyrin substances for the needed purposes of chelation.

Solomon and Figge [25] noted that coproporphyrin-III and protoporphyrin are present in the peripheral nerves, and the authors postulate that the porphyrin substances may actually be involved in the process of conduction of nerve impulses. Klüver [26] also noted the presence of these porphyrin substances in the central nervous system. The increased excretion of coproporphyrin-III in porphyria as well as in polio and lead intoxication lead one to question whether the urinary porphyrins could be derived at least in part from the central nervous system. Granick and Gilder [27] feel that coproporphyrin may serve as a regulator of oxygen consumption by living cells, and Watson and Larson [18] have added that nervous tissue might produce and liberate porphyrins more rapidly under certain circumstances. Keilin [28] suggests that cytochrome may be the parent substance of coproporphyrin.

It seems possible that the withdrawal of these porphyrin compounds or a failure for these porphyrins in the central nervous system to be replenished, owing to a metabolic block either in the nervous system or at a hepatic level, could account for some of the symptomatology. Price, Brown, and Peters [29] have noted an elevation of kynurenic acid or kynurenine or both after a loading dose of tryptophan during the acute stages of some cases of acute, chronic, and mixed porphyria, a finding resembling the tryptophan metabolic pattern seen in patients with scleroderma by Rukavina et al. [30]. Price et al. [29] have noted that some of these tryptophan metabolites are in themselves excellent metal-binding agents.

Finally, one might postulate that the withdrawal of cations might be responsible for the symptoms of porphyria and that the tremendous zinc and copper diuresis observed during chelation is undesirable. The effectiveness of chelation might be related only to a redistribution of the cations within the body owing to these chelating agents rather than to their urinary elimination. The ready availability, however, of zinc and copper in the diet plus the observation that these cations are no longer diuresed after recovery sets in despite the continued administration of chelating agents suggests that during exacerbations these cations are toxic in their metabolic effect and capable of producing various enzymatic blocks.

Recently a massive epidemic of chronic porphyria in Turkey as the result of the ingestion of grain that had been treated for seed purposes with hexachlorbenzene and mercury compounds has been reported. This would suggest that at least the chronic porphyric syndrome may be induced by chemical means in patients who do not have a predisposing genetic factor [31].

SUMMARY

Disturbances of porphyrin metabolism are not rare findings when screening tests are conducted on psychiatric and neurological patients. The signs and symptoms of this type of disturbance cover the entire spectrum of neurological and psychiatric disorders. Over two-thirds of the patients seemed to have been helped by chelation therapy. Increased urinary zinc and/or copper excretion is seen when neurological and psychiatric symptoms are developing in porphyric patients as well as in alcoholic syndromes, collagen disorders, and heavy metal intoxication.

REFERENCES

1. Peters, H. A.: BAL therapy of acute porphyrinuria, Neurology 4:477, 1954.

2. Peters, H. A.: Therapy of acute porphyria with BAL and other agents, Dis. Nerv. Syst. 17:177, 1956.

3. Peters, H. A., Woods, S. M., Eichman, P. L., and Reese, H. H.: The treatment of acute porphyria with chelating agents: A report of 21 cases, Ann. Int. Med. 47:889, 1957.

4. Peters, H. A., Eichman, P. L., and Reese, H. H.: Therapy of acute, chronic and mixed hepatic porphyria patients with chelating agents, Neurology 8:621, 1958.

5. Peters, H. A.: Chelation therapy in acute, chronic and mixed porphyria. in Seven, M. J., and Johnson, L. A., Eds.: Metal-Binding in Medicine, J. B. Lippincott Co., Philadelphia, 1960, p. 190.

6. Woods, S. M., Peters, H. A., and Johnson, S. A. M.: Cutaneous porphyria with porphobilinogenuria: A review and report of a case treated by chelation, A.M.A. Arch. Dermat. 77:559, 1958.

7. Peters, H. A.: Trace minerals, chelating agents, and the porphyrias, Fed. Proc., Vol. 20, No. 3, Sept. 1961, Supplement 10.

8. Treanor, W. J., and Rupe, C. E.: Porphyra—An "enzyme lesion": Review of basic and clinical aspects, Henry Ford Hosp. Bull. 3:162, 1957.

9. Painter, J. T., and Morrow, E. J.: Porphyria: Its manifestations and treatment with chelating agents, Texas J. Med. 55:811, 1959.

10. Galambos, J. T., and Peacock, L. B.: The use of chelating agents in the treatment of acute porphyria, Ann. Int. Med. 50:1056, 1959.

11. Paul, K. G., and Thyresson, N.: The effect of BAL on a case of cutaneous porphyria, Acta Dermatol.-venereol. 34:403, 1954.

12. Schrumpf, A.: Porphyria improved after treatment with BAL, Acta. Med. Scand. 145:338, 1953.

13. Wirtschafter, J. D., Turner, F. W., and Dow, R. S.: Case report: Convulsive seizures as the presenting manifestation of intermittent porphyria, Neurology 10:787, 1960.

14. Mauzerall, D., and Granick, S.: The occurrence and determination of delta-amino levulinic acid and porphobilinogen in urine, J. Biol. Chem. 219:435, 1956.

15. Dean, G., and Barnes, H.: Porphyria, Brit. M. J. 5066:298, 1958.

16. Goldberg, A.: Acute intermittent porphyria, Quart. J. Med. 28:183, 1959.

17. Waldenstrom, J.: The porphyrias as inborn errors of metabolism, Am. J. Med. 22:758, 1957.

18. Watson, C. J., and Larson, E. A.: The urinary coproporphyrins in health and disease, Physiol. Rev. 27:478, 1947.

19. Brunsting, L. A., Mason, H. L., and Aldrich, R. A.: Adult form of chronic porphyria with cutaneous manifestations: Report of seventeen additional cases, J.A.M.A. 146:1207, 1951.

20. Monaco, R. N., Leeper, R. D., Robbins, J. J., and Calvy, G. L.: Intermittent acute porphyria treated with chlorpromazine, New England J. Med. 256:309, 1957.

21. Melby, J. C., Street, J. P., and Watson, C. J.: Chlorpromazine in treatment of porphyria, J.A.M.A. 162:174, 1956.

22. Gunther, H.: Ergebn, Allg. Path. 20:608, 1922.

23. Watson, C. J., and Schwartz, S.: The excretion of zinc uroporphyrin in idiopathic porphyrin, J. Clin. Invest. 20:440, 1941.

24. Edman, K. A. P.: Zinc-induced relaxation of muscle fibres, Acta Physiol. Scand. 49:330, 1960.

25. Solomon, H. M., and Figge, F. H.: Occurrence of porphyrins in peripheral nerves, Proc. Soc. Exp. Biol. Med. 97:329, 1958.

26. Klüver, H.: Porphyrins in relation to the development of the nervous system, Proc. 1st Internat. Neurochem. Symp., Academic Press, Inc., New York, 1954.

27. Granick, S., and Gilder, H.: The structure, function and inhibitory action of porphyrins, Science 101:540, 1945.

28. Keilin, D.: On cytochrome, respiratory pigment, common to animals, yeasts, and higher plants, Proc. Roy. Soc. London 98(B):312, 1925.

29. Price, J. M., Brown, R. R., and Peters, H. A.: Tryptophan metabolism in porphyria, schizophrenia and a variety of neurologic and psychiatric diseases, Neurology 9:456, 1959.

30. Rukavina, J. G., Mendelson, C., Price, J. M., Brown, R. R., and Johnson, S. A. M.: Scleroderma, J. Invest. Dermat. 29:273, 1957.

31. Schmid, R.: Cutaneous porphyria in Turkey, New England J. Med. 263:397, 1960.

Discussion by Carl C. Pfeiffer, M.D.

Dr. Peters should be commended for this careful and continued study on the incidence, diagnosis, and treatment of porphyric psychosis. As I listened to the array of possible symptoms, I recalled distinctly several patients seen many years ago who were diagnostic problems because of their socalled "abdominal epilepsy," epilepsy with lupus erythematosus, or periodic schizophrenia. If we had had the knowledge to test thoroughly for possible abnormalities in their trace metal and porphyrin metabolism, we might have instituted better care. This leads to my first question for Dr. Peters. He states that he has treated 65 patients with chelating agents. What percentage of these patients came from state hospitals in Wisconsin? In other words, if a simple test were available, what would be the estimated incidence of this syndrome in patients institutionalized for mental disease?

Dr. Peters and his colleagues apply many complicated tests on stool specimens and 24-hour urine specimens collected in chemically clean bottles. None of these procedures is easy to accomplish on the untidy or uncooperative patient. We might, therefore, ask Dr. Peters about the possibility of the future development of blood tests for porphyric and paraporphyric patients.

Dr. Peters appears to be unnecessarily on the defensive in regard to the efficacy of chelating agents in the amelioration of the symptoms of the patients. Case histories detailing the effects of treatment have appeared in his previous published reports, and these certainly suggest that the removal of excess copper and zinc from the tissues is a factor in the remission of many of the patients. The exact biochemical details of this effect may elude us for many years, but this should not now delay either diagnosis or treatment. Finally, do complications of chelating therapy, such as unmasking of lead poisoning and vitamin B_6 deficiency, occur?

CHAPTER 21

Psychophysiological Patterns in Chronic Schizophrenia

By ALBERT F. AX, Ph.D., P. G. S. BECKETT, M.D.,
B. D. COHEN, Ph.D., C. E. FROHMAN, Ph.D.,
G. TOURNEY, M.D., and J. S. GOTTLIEB, M.D.

This study was done at the Lafayette Clinic, Detroit, where the chief research activity is the interdisciplinary study of schizophrenia. There have been reports of previous studies on carbohydrate metabolism in schizophrenia [1] and on the use of a psychiatric coding system to correlate clinical and biological data [2]. Now our psychophysiology laboratory is completing a series of studies of which this is the second to be reported [3]. As with the previous studies mentioned, there have been many measurements made on the same subjects (often simultaneously) by techniques of biochemistry, physiology, psychology, and psychiatry. In this report we shall deal exclusively with the autonomic responses to three experimental stressors—pain apprehension, the psychodynamic stress interview, and insulin injection.

MATERIALS AND METHODS

Half the subjects were ten chronic schizophrenic males with symptoms of four years or more, 26 to 38 years of age with a mean age of 32. Their diagnoses were: one paranoid, five chronic undifferentiated, two hebrephrenic, and two catatonic. The other group was composed of ten male nonpsychotic patients having an age range of 19 to 49 years with a mean age of 27, not significantly different from the schizophrenic group. The diagnoses for the nonpsychotic group were: two passive-aggressive personality, two conversion reaction, one inadequate personality, three sociopathic personality, and two anxiety reaction.

This investigation was supported in part by Research Grant MY 2950 from the National Institute of Mental Health, U. S. Public Health Service.

All subjects were hospitalized at the Lafayette Clinic for three months or more, were off all drugs for at least three weeks, and had similar diets. The physiological variables recorded simultaneously during the various experimental conditions were: ballistocardiogram, frontalis muscle tension, face and finger skin temperatures, palmar conductance, finger pulse pressure, systolic and diastolic blood pressure, respiration rate, and heart rate. Several aspects of some variables were computed. For example, palmar conductance was scored for level, as an incremenet to produce the well-known GSR and also to ascertain the number of GSRs per minute. By scoring separately both the maximum rises and maximum falls of a variable during a stress epoch, a more faithful representation of the changes is obtained since usually the variable both rises to higher values and falls to lower values than its preceding resting level. This scoring of increments and decrements separately prevents change scores from canceling out when members of a group are averaged. The maximum response of some individuals may be an increment in heart rate, but for other individuals the maximum change in heart rate may be a decrement.

For frontalis muscle tension both the tonus level between contractions and the number of contractions per minute were scored. The heart rate was recorded as a heart period by a cardiotachometer and superimposed on the respiration record obtained from chest and abdomen circumference strain gauges. This superimposition of the heart rate on the respiration record enabled easy scoring of the sinus arrhythmia and other longer-wave activity in heart rate not related to respiration.

Palmar conductance was measured between two $ZnSO_4$-saturated sponges in $1/4$-in. plastic cups with zinc electrodes applied without electrode paste to the washed finger pads of the second and third fingers of the left hand. The polarity of the battery to the skin conductance bridge was reversed every second, thereby eliminating base-line drift due to electrode polarization. The finger pulse pressure transducer was made from a tiny piezoelectric crystal applied with elastic tape to the left thumb pad. The amplitude of this pulse pressure in the finger tip is a good index of the degree of vasodilatation of the digital blood vessels and thus is a fair index of blood flow in the finger tip. The muscle-potential electrodes were silver disks applied to the forehead over each eye with saline electrode paste and held in place by a rubber head band. The potentials were fed into a preamplifier, rectified, and integrated by a leaky storage condenser with a time constant of approximately 1 second.

The blood pressures were obtained by the auscultatory method with the cuff on the right arm and the microphone under the cuff over the artery. The Korotkoff sounds were superimposed on the rising pressure curve. Inflation was automatic once per minute. The ballistocardiograph is a standard Starr-type high-frequency bed. Both the HI and IJ wave amplitudes of the ballistocardiogram were scored. We believe that these amplitudes are indices of the heart stroke force, which appears to be as interesting as stroke volume for our purposes.

The room temperature was kept at 25 C ± 0.2 C. A pain stimulus was produced by a direct current applied via $\frac{1}{4}$-in. saline-soaked sponges to the left great toe pad, an application which produces a sensation of heat. A large saline sponge encircling the left ankle served as the general subject ground.

All four experimental sessions were begun at 8:00 a.m. The subjects came down from the wards without breakfast and without having indulged in any strenuous physical activity on the preceding day. The first session served for orientation to familiarize the subjects with the polygraph procedure and to help allay anxiety. No distressing stimuli were given. The second session (hereafter referred to as the "pain stress") consisted of 15 minutes for attaching the transducers, 15 minutes of rest, 5 minutes for the first blood sample, 5 minutes of instructions, 10 minutes of pain stress, 5 minutes for a second blood sample, and finally 10 minutes of rest— a total period of 65 minutes of which 50 minutes was used for recordings.

The subject was instructed that a painful stimulus to his toe would occur and a beeping tone would sound at frequent intervals and that he could turn both off simply by calling "help" in a loud voice. The exact instructions were: "We want to find out how much stimulation your nervous system can take. The stimulation will be sound and pain. You will hear the beeping noise and feel the heat in your foot. These sensations will become increasingly more painful as time goes on. Now, if you feel at any time that it is getting to a level that might be harmful to you, call 'Help! ' into this microphone. Your call will turn off the sound and the pain for a rest period. Let's try it to ·see how it works." (The experimenter then turned up the sound and pain to the test amplitude at a moderately rapid rate and instructed the subject to yell "Help." This was repeated until the subject was able to respond appropriately.)

"The stimulation will return after a rest period whenever you call 'Help.' Feel free to call 'Help' again as much as you want. Now remember, we want you to stand as much as you can—but when you suspect that it is getting to a harmful level, call 'Help.' Don't be a hero about it, as this could do damage to your nervous system. Remember, when you feel it is getting to a harmful intensity, call 'Help!'"

Several practice trials were given to make. sure the subject understood and could cooperate. The pitch of the 2/sec beeping tones was started at 500 cps and incremented by 100 cps each minute. Ten seconds after the beginning of each tone stimulus, the pain current was turned on, starting for the first minute at 2.20 ma— just above the sensory threshold—and increased by 0.2 ma each minute, reaching a maximum of 4 ma—a quite painful stimulus if allowed to remain on continuously for the 50 seconds of each minute trial. The voice microphone control was set so that whenever the subject called "help" loudly the pain and tone would be turned off and remain off for 5 seconds. If the subject would call "help" immediately upon hearing the tones he could avoid all pain. The number of help calls was scored as a behavioral index of stress response.

During the third session, after 15 minutes of rest and the first blood sample, there was a 20-minute interview by one of the psychiatrists designed to probe the areas of known conflict for this patient. The interview was followed by the second blood sample and a final rest period. The patient's emotional arousal was observed during this interview by a second psychiatrist and rated on the emotional arousal scale independently immediately after by both psychiatrists. The emotional arousal was rated on a nine-point scale for the following variables: facial expression (immobile to animated), gestures and bodily movements, freedom of speech, formality of language, modulation of voice, sociability, anger, anxiety, amount of affect, and mood (depressed to exhilarated). Reliability intercorrelations between the two psychiatrists were 0.76 for sociability, 0.60 for anger, 0.55 for anxiety, 0.80 for mood, and 0.78 for total emotional arousal.

In the fourth session, after the usual rest period and the first blood sample, an intravenous injection of 5 units of insulin was given. Exactly 15 minutes later the second blood sample was taken followed by 10 minutes of rest.

The physiological recording was continuous throughout all four sessions. The experimental epochs of these sessions selected for analysis for this report consist of: for the first pain session (1) the last 5 minutes of the rest period just prior to the first blood sample and (2) the pain stress period starting just after the first blood sample and ending just before the second blood sample. This pain stress session was also scored a second way so as to include the response to the two blood samples. It was noted that a few subjects made larger responses of GSR and muscle tension to the venous puncture than to the experimental pain stimulus. Either scoring produced essentially the same over-all results. For the third session the scoring epochs were (1) the rest period prior to the interview and (2) the last 10 minutes of the interview. For the fourth session the periods scored were (1) the last 5 minutes of the rest period prior to the blood sample and injection of insulin and finally (2) the last 5 minutes of the insulin period prior to the second blood sample. Maximum and minimum values were found for each stress period. Increments and decrements were computed as deviations from the preceding resting levels.

Prior to the analysis of the data, we constructed a formula of eight physiological scores which on our previous studies had been descriptive of two emotional states we called "fear" and "anger" and which we had suggested were possibly related to blood levels of epinephrine and norepinephrine respectively [4,5]. Subsequent studies of infusions of these two hormones have supported these polygraph patterns.

RESULTS AND DISCUSSION

As was apparent in our 1951 study (Fig. 1), the injection of epinephrine caused a greater rise in systolic blood pressure, heart rate, ballistocardiogram values, and respiration rate, whereas the injection of norepinephrine produced a greater rise in muscle tension and number of GSRs and a greater fall in heart rate. Basing ourselves on these prior results and on reports by Funkenstein et al. [6] that patients of poor prognosis tended to be in norepinephrine-like states, we predicted that our polygraph patterns in response to pain apprehension stress would resemble the norepinephrine pattern for chronic schizophrenic subjects (poor prognosis), whereas the response pattern would be more like the epinephrine pattern for the nonpsychotic group. We were aware that Schachter [7] had found essentially pure norepinephrine-like patterns in response to the

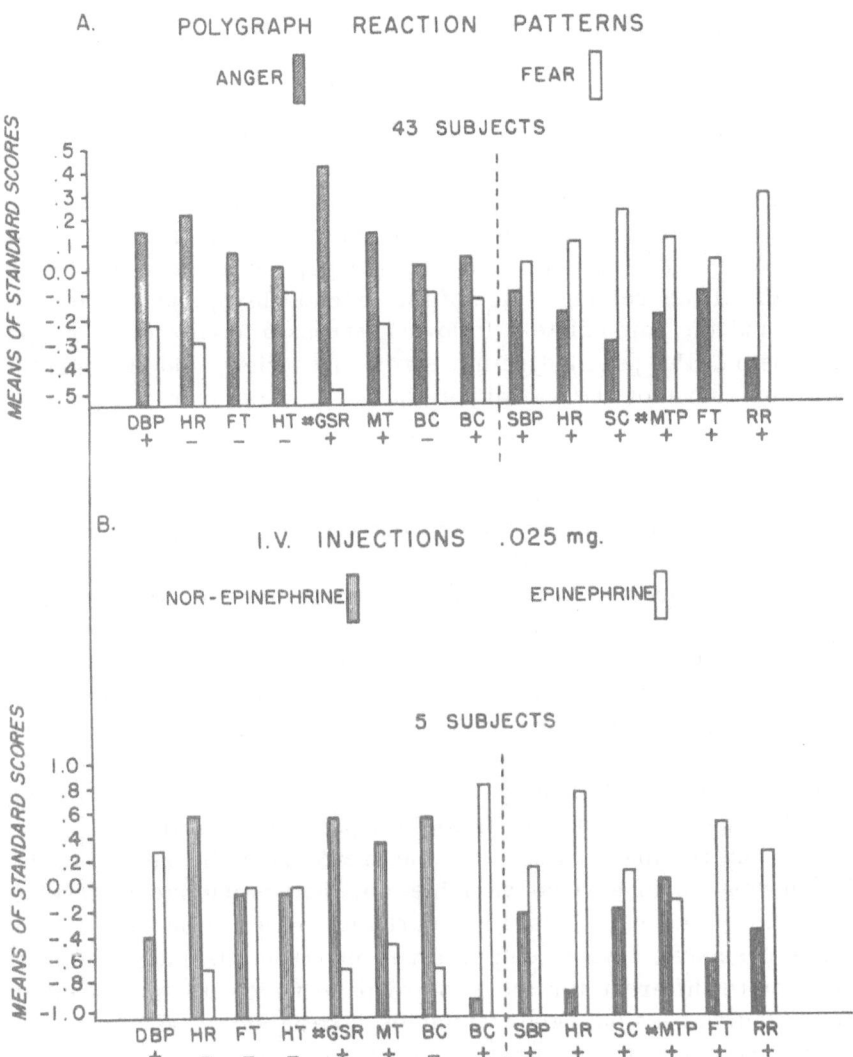

FIG. 1.   The top section of this figure* shows the mean differences in physiological response pattern between experimentally induced "fear" and "anger" for 43 subjects. The lower section shows the mean response pattern for five of the same subjects to injections (0.025 mg) of epinephrine and norepinephrine. (*Published in Psychiat. Res. Rep. #12, Jan. 60.)

pain stress of the cold-pressor test. In our present pain-apprehension stress test, the stress was largely apprehension for most subjects because they were able to avoid the pain stimulus due to the 10-second prior onset of the tone stimulus. The chief stress was the psychological conflict between being a baby by calling "help" and being a hero by suffering pain.

Before discussing the results of applying this predictive formula for epinephrine and norepinephrine-like response patterns, some characteristics of the present data should be inspected.

All possible group and experimental condition differences were explored by doing a 2-by-6 analysis of variance. The two groups were, of course, our two criteria groups, and the six conditions were the three resting states of the second, third, and fourth sessions and the immediately following stressor states of pain-apprehension, the psychodynamic stress interview, and the insulin injection. Most of the variables showed a significant change with respect to the six experimental conditions.

For both groups the pain stress produced the largest changes in all variables except for the diastolic blood pressure, face temperature, ballistocardiogram, and muscle tension. Psychodynamic interview stress produced the largest changes for both groups for face temperature and muscle tension. Insulin stress produced larger changes in the pulse volume increment, ballistocardiographic increment, heart rate decrements, and diastolic blood pressure decrements. The diastolic blood pressure increased more for schizophrenic subjects during pain, but for nonpsychotic subjects it increased more during the interview. Since these various differences are not individually statistically significant, it is not very useful to speculate very far as to their possible meanings.

An interesting finding was the trend from the second to the fourth session in several variables for the resting periods (Table I). Some of the variables, like heart rate, respiration rate, finger pulse pressure, finger temperature, and frontalis muscle tonus, were quite different for the two groups at first but came together by the fourth session. Other variables, like palmar conductance and ballistocardiogram, remained significantly different throughout the sessions. This suggests systems of flexibility that may be more readily modified by environmental circumstances and other systems which are inflexible and may be more fundamentally characteristic of the group differences. Certainly the ballistocardiogram was one of the most unresponsive variables to our stressors but at the same time one of the most diagnostic. Palmar conductance was highly diagnostic during the resting states and also by its stress levels to both pain and psychodynamic stress.

All these group differences in trends for resting levels from the second to the fourth session suggest higher sympathetic arousal for the schizophrenic group for the earlier session. It appears that schizophrenics are more disturbed by the testing situation and are slower to adapt to it. The ballistocardiograph index of heart stroke force, on the contrary, was consistently lower for the schizophrenic group during all rest and stress conditions. Since the ballistocardi-

TABLE I

Resting Level Trends

Physiological Variable	Pain Stress		Psychodynamic Stress		Insulin Stress	
	Schiz.	Non-Schiz.	Schiz.	Non-Schiz.	Schiz.	Non-Schiz.
Heart rate	80.0	72.1	79.7	74.8	73.9	73.0
Respiration rate	16.2	13.9	17.5	17.2	17.7	16.6
Diastolic blood pressure	70.1	69.1	74.1	69.3	71.1	70.5
Systolic blood pressure	116.4	117.8	118.0	118.6	118.2	119.0
Finger pulse pressure	14.9	18.8	13.9	14.1	15.3	15.6
Palmar conductance	5.7	4.0	6.2	3.5	5.2	3.8
Humber GSR/minute	0.20	0.14	0.55	0.20	0.38	0.26
Maximum GSR	0.45	0.09	0.57	0.20	0.55	0.30
Finger temperature	30.56	31.90	30.82	31.00	30.49	30.29
Face temperature	33.77	33.58	33.65	33.77	33.69	33.79
Muscle tonus	8.12	6.00	8.86	5.23	6.22	5.86
Ballistocardiogram	16.0	21.5	16.9	20.4	16.6	21.4

ogram is normally an index of sympathetic arousal of the epineph-rine type, this finding appears to be in direct conflict with the other emotional arousal indices. If, however, as we have already sug-gested, the schizophrenic subjects tend to respond to stress with a norepinephrine-like response, their tension state during rest would not necessarily be associated with a raised ballistocardiograph index. The fact that the consistently smaller ballistocardiograph index for schizophrenic subjects during rest is not associated with other cardiovascular changes, and is usually associated with a pure norepinephrine state, such as lowered heart rate and raised diastolic blood pressure, may be due to an adjustment or "tuning" of the autonomic nervous system in the chronic tension state of schizo-phrenia. Such a tuning may, of course, involve certain parasym-pathetic readjustments, which could readily account for the higher heart rates, unraised blood pressure, and lowered ballistocardi-ogram. Poor physical condition in the athletic sense would also pretty well fit this picture.

As seen in Table II, 11 scores for three physiological variables (palmar conductance, muscle tension, and ballistocardiogram) have statistically significant group mean differences for one or more experimental conditions. Due to the small number of subjects and large variability, the group mean differences had to be quite large to establish statistical significance. Resting levels for palmar conductance and ballistocardiogram discriminated the two groups significantly, but muscle tension reached significance only during the insulin epoch. In all six conditions the schizophrenic group produced the higher stress levels for palmar conductance and muscle tension but the heart stroke force index (ballistocardiogram) for the schizophrenic group was always lower. The striking difference in muscle tension was due to a marked lowering of tension during insulin for the nonpsychotic group, whereas the schizophrenic group showed little change.

With these results in mind it may now be helpful to examine the application to this data of the "epinephrine minus norepinephrine" formula previously mentioned. The epinephrine-like score is the sum of the standard scores of increments for systolic blood pressure, heart rate, ballistocardiogram, and respiration rate. The norepi-nephrine-like score is the sum of the standard scores for increments of diastolic blood pressure, muscle tension, and number of GSRs plus the decrements for heart rate. These seven increment and one decrement scores were in response to the pain-apprehension stress (including the intravenous punctures) as maximum deviations from the just prior resting level for these variables. Each subject's epinephrine-norepinephrine difference score is computed from the sum of the first four scores minus that of the second four scores.

TABLE II

Group Differences of Physiological Variables

Physiological Variable	Mean		Difference	Significance
	Schiz.	Non-psychot.	Schiz.-Non-psychot.	
Resting heart rate (P*)	80.0	72.1	7.9	NS†
Palmar conductance				
Maximum (P)	11.6	8.5	3.1	0.05
Resting (Pd‡)	6.2	3.5	2.7	0.05
Maximum (Pd)	9.6	6.1	3.5	0.05
GSR				
Maximum number (P)	1.7	0.6	1.1	0.05
Maximum (P)	3.1	1.8	1.3	0.05
Maximum (Pd)	1.5	0.5	1.0	0.05
Muscle tonus				
Resting (Pd)	8.9	5.2	3.7	NS
Maximum (P)	23.8	15.3	8.5	NS
Minimum (Ins.§)	16.1	2.9	-3.2	0.05
Maximum finger pulse pressure (Ins.)	18.3	24.6	-6.3	NS
Ballistocardiogram				
Resting (IJ) (P)	16.0	21.5	-5.5	0.02
Maximum (IJ) (P)	16.1	22.5	-6.4	0.05
Resting (IJ) (Pd)	16.9	20.4	-3.5	NS
Resting (IJ) (Ins.)	16.6	21.4	-4.8	0.02
Maximum (IJ) (Ins.)	19.9	23.9	-4.0	NS
Maximum (HI) (P)	8.0	11.1	-3.1	0.05

*Pain.
†No significance.
‡Psychodynamic interview.
§Insulin.

The result of applying this a priori scoring formula to the data of this study is seen in Fig. 2. The white bars are the mean of the standard scores for the nonpsychotic group and the black-and-white-striped bars are the mean of the standard scores for the schizophrenic group. Clearly, the white bars of the nonpsychotic control group are all higher on the left side where the epinephrine-like variables are tabulated (increments in respiration rate, ballisto-cardiogram, heart rate, and systolic blood pressure); and, conversely, the black bars of the schizophrenic group are all higher on the right side of the figure where the norepinephrine-like variables are located (increments in diastolic blood pressure, number of GSRs, muscle tonus, and decrements in heart rate).

In Fig. 3 the tabulation of each individual's epi-norepi score reveals that nine of the ten nonschizophrenic control subjects fall above the mean zero line whereas seven of the ten schizophrenic subjects fall below the critical line. This 9:1-3:7 contingency table has a significant chi square. In other words, all but one of the non-psychotic control subjects responded to the pain-apprehension stressor situation with an epinephrine-like physiological response

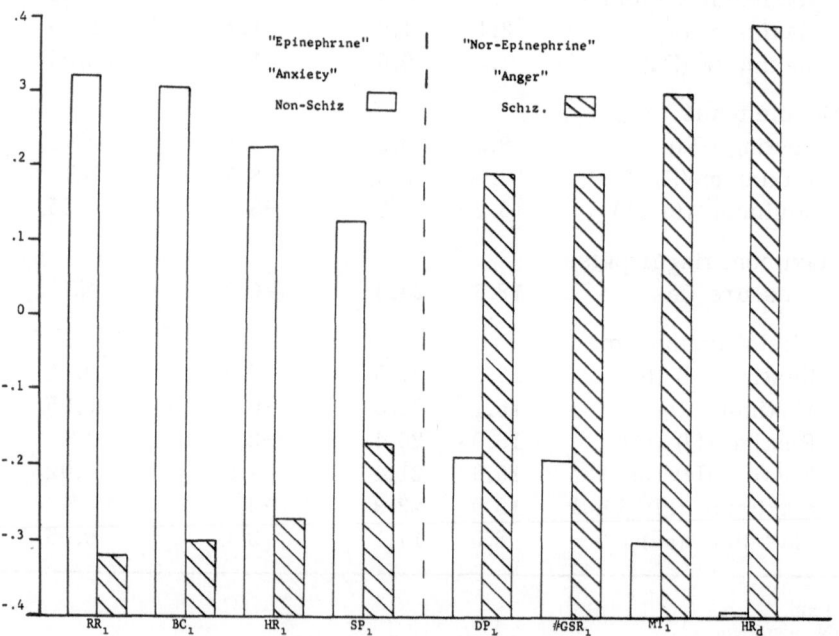

FIG. 2.   Standard score means.

pattern. Seven of ten chronic schizophrenic subjects responded with a more strongly norepinephrine-like physiological response pattern.

It is clear that two of the three schizophrenic subjects who responded with a more epinephrine-like response pattern are not merely border-line cases but are well up into the epinephrine-like region. The one nonschizophrenic subject who responded with a norepinephrine-like pattern is also not a strict border-line case.

Such a finding suggests that chronic schizophrenia as diagnosed at the Lafayette Clinic may very well consist of two types: (1) the larger proportion having a norepinephrine-like physiological response pattern and (2) a smaller proportion with an epinephrine-like response pattern. Similarly, among the non-psychotic group there is the one norepinephrine-like responder. More data can be brought to bear on this point.

There was a very wide range among these 20 subjects as to the number of "help" calls made during the 10 minutes of the pain-apprehension stress. Two subjects made no help calls at all. One was a mute catatonic schizophrenic patient, and the other was a very hostile psychopath. The two making the highest number of help

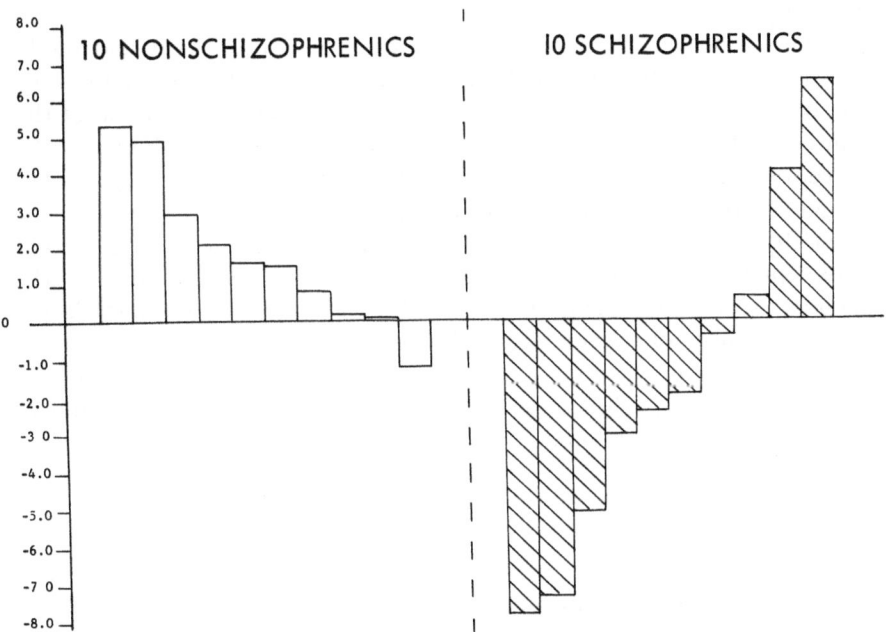

FIG. 3. "Epi-norepi" scores for pain stress.

calls (122 and 107) were pathetically frightened schizophrenic subjects who were also the same two of the three schizophrenics who
had a predominantly epinephrine-like response pattern. The actual
correlation between "help" calls and the epi minus-norepi score is
0.56. This correlation of 0.56 is spuriously low because of an incidental correlation of 0.80 between "help" calls and the number of
frontalis muscle contractions, which of course occurred with each
"help" call and which elevates the norepi score. With muscle
tension contractions removed by partial correlation, this correlation
between "help" calls and the epi-norepi factor is raised to 0.62.
The number of "help" calls also correlates 0.75 with resting finger
temperature just prior to the stress. Thus, cold hands (and I'm sure,
"cold feet") also contribute to the description of a fearful, dependent emotional state.

    This strong association between the high epinephrine-like
physiological response pattern and the dependent, fearful behavioral
response pattern, on the one hand, and the converse strong association between the aggressive refusal to call "help" and the norepinephrine-like physiological response pattern emphasizes the power
of these physiological patterns to discriminate between anxiety and
hostility.

    The association is unambiguous with regard to the dangerously
hostile aggressive criminal sexual psychopath who refused to call
"help" even once at the cost of severe suffering. The case of the
mute catatonic subject and the association in general between the
norepinephrine-like physiological pattern and schizophrenic patients
suggests that most schizophrenic individuals possibly have more
hostility than anxiety. Another suggestion from this finding is that
this epinephrine-norepinephrine-like variable running through the
schizophrenic syndrome may well be related to the emotional lability frequently observed clinically and thought to be important for
treatability and prognosis, as Funkenstein proposed long ago. We
are investigating this aspect by our follow-up studies and also by
correlations with the coded clinical case history variables.

SUMMARY

    Ten physiological variables were simultaneously recorded
during four stress conditions (rest, pain-apprehension, stress interview, insulin injection) on groups of chronic schizophrenic and nonpsychotic patients. Previous studies of epinephrine and norepineph-

rine injections had revealed physiological response characteristic of these two agents. When these a priori patterns were tested on the response data for these subjects, it was found that 90% of the non-psychotic patients responded to the pain-apprehension stress with the pattern characteristics of epinephrine whereas 70% of the schizo-phrenic patients responded with the pattern characteristic of norepinephrine. A behavioral response of calling "help" to avoid the pain was highly correlated with the epinephrine response pattern. Results suggest that a majority of chronic schizophrenic patients react to pain-apprehension stress with a norepinephrine type of response but that a subgroup responds with the epinephrine-like response.

REFERENCES

1. Gottlieb, J. J., Frohman, C. E., Beckett, P. G. S., Tourney, G., and Senf, R.: Production of high-energy phosphate bonds in schizophrenia, A.M.A. Arch. Gen. Psychiat. 1:243, 1959.

2. Beckett, P. G. S., Senf, R., Frohman, C. E., and Tourney, G.: Relations between energy transfer systems and the symptoms of schizophrenia, presented at the Am. Psychiat. Assoc. Meeting, May 1961.

3. Ax, A. F., and Luby, E. D.: Autonomic responses to sleep deprivation, A.M.A. Arch. Gen. Psychiat. 4:55, 1961.

4. Ax, A. F.: The physiological differentiation between fear and anger in humans, Psychosom. Med. 15:433, 1953.

5. Ax, A. F.: Psychophysiology of fear and anger, Psychiat. Res. Rep. no. 12, p. 167, 1960.

6. Funkenstein, D. H., Greenblatt, M., and Solomon, H. C.: Autonomic changes paralleling psychologic changes in mentally ill patients, J. Nerv. Ment. Dis. 114:1, 1951.

7. Schachter, J.: Pain, fear and anger in hypertensive and normotensives, Psychosomat. Med. 19:17, 1957.

Discussion by John I. Nurnberger, M.D.

The pursuit of biological correlates of schizophrenic reaction types, qua noso-logical entities, has been a singularly unproductive one over the past seventy or more years. It is refreshing, as well as reassuring, to note that the investigations in progress at the Lafayette Clinic, of which the present is one, do not add silt to this stagnant pool. The biochemical studies of systemic and erythrocyte-nucleotide activities, reported within the past several years from this research group, were correlated with meaningful behavioral parameters in patients who (quite incidentally, to this discussant's point of view) had been clinically identified as schizophrenic.

The present study goes even further in creating virtually ideal conditions for noting and manipulating functional correlates. The fact that the observations under discussion were made on a limited population of patients identified as schizophrenic is of limited importance. More important is the fact that the observations were made on clinically familiar subjects and under specified and controlled clinical conditions and that responses were not to incidental circumstances but to reproducible contingencies in most, though not all, phases of the study. These facts, plus the now well-established judgment that Dr. Ax is himself an exquisitely careful psychophysiologist whose data are collected with great care under excellent instrumental conditions, make the present work a solidly meaningful contribution.

However, it is most likely that the real value of this careful study will be revealed not by analyses based on oversimplified categorizations of responders as "epinephrine- or norepinephrine-like" but, rather, by meticulous individual analyses of response variations and stereotypes for each individual subject. When such individual analyses are supplemented by studies of expanded populations of subjects, more discrete and less stylized information should be forthcoming. One of the implicit assumptions of the investigators is that they were studying an experimental population of subjects meaningfully homogeneous with respect to the diagnostic category, chronic schizophrenia. The control population was considered homogeneous with regard to the category, nonschizophrenia. My contention, supported by a rich literature, is that they have been studying an experimental population as categorically discrete as apples plus oranges. There is good evidence that predominantly paranoid schizophrenic individuals are a class unto themselves, that catatonic schizophrenic patients cannot be grouped usefully with hebephrenic patients, that chronic undifferentiated schizophrenic individuals run a wide gamut, and finally that, with time, intergroup drifts occur within the same subject. There is a wealth of information supporting a fundamental discrimination of process or nuclear from symptomatic or reactive "schizophrenia."

It is true that the psychophysiological response patterns observed seemed to discriminate, with some confidence, between the so-called experimental and control groups. What does this mean? The control population selected is an unusually provocative one. Six of the ten controls were thought to have a "personality disorder." The line which separates so-called "acting out" schizophrenic individuals from environmentally controlled (hospitalized and restricted) patients with personality disorders, especially sociopathic disorders (three of the controls), is a fine line indeed. I would wonder whether the reactions which discriminated the control from the experimental groups might have been substantially altered had the control population been maintained under conditions that make environmental manipulation and acting out unlikely. Such patients within a veterans' installation, where reasonably good control of manipulative acting out was maintained, showed adaptive changes difficult to differentiate, psychologically and clinically, from frankly paranoid and regressive psychotic behavior.

One problem which every investigator within this important field must face is the following: How fixed, durable, and typical are the elicited response patterns? Dr. Ax and his associates provide no data to answer this problem, nor can one assume either analogy or identity between any of the stressor situations used. I should mention that the simple pain-apprehension-postponement situation developed is a first-rate testing tool. If the authors had repeated this particular stressor situation on three or four occasions in the same subjects, the inferences to be drawn might have been quite different. One of our associates, Dr. Hanus J. Grosz, studied a larger population of hospitalized schizophrenic patients several years ago. These were, in general, symptomatically disturbed for not more than six months prior to the study. He administered intramuscular Mecholyl to the entire population on three separate occasions over a one-week period under identical experimental conditions. A substantial percentage of that population showed clear shifts in reaction pattern, drifting from one major response category to another. Even more perplexing, he noted that vasomotor response patterns (blood pressure changes) recorded from the left and right arms in the same subjects were unequivocally different in a considerable number of subjects. These are very sobering observations. The excellent experimental condition created by Dr. Ax and his associates in their pain-apprehension situation could, if repeated, provide a highly sensitive and meaningful measure of constancy and lability with the familiarization factor involved itself being a probably individuating element in the study.

I would question the condensation and homogenization of complex psychophysiological response sequences composed of 12 partially independent variables as "epinephrine- and norepinephrine-like." Such categories may simplify the presentation of data, but one is forced to ask: "What of the transitional forms, their frequency and their heterogeneity, and how pure are the extremes?" In this regard, the interesting studies of Bridger and Reiser on normal human neonates should be mentioned. They recorded heart rate changes following gentle air blasts to the abdomen. When the resting heart rate was at the high extreme of the individual response distribution, the pulse rate tended to decrease with air blast. When the initial rate was relatively low, stimulation was followed by a heart rate increase. Now, insofar as heart rate changes provide one measure of the epinephrine or norepinephrine reaction type, would one conclude that the fall from high levels reflects the "norepi" type of response while the rise from low levels is more like the "epi" type? If this be so and if this variation occurs in the same organism under different resting conditions, what does this augur for the interpretation of Dr. Ax's patterns unless they be analyzed, response by response?

Now, finally, a question addressed to the significance of the discriminations based on response pattern "types." In an experimental population of ten subjects, the authors note seven with a norepinephrine-type pattern. How likely is it that this particular distribution will be borne out when the experimental population, similarly diversified, is expanded to 50 or 100 subjects? If the final distribution of reactors comes out more nearly 50-50, what will be the interpretable aspects of such a distribution? Frankly, I do not believe they will be able to interpret such results in a meaningful way if their stressor situations are not carefully and controllably repeated over a period of time in each subject. If they do the latter and if they can demonstrate, as is likely, stable and variable responders and if, finally, they continue to compare such pattern variations with the wealth of psychological, descriptive and other data they are collecting, then I am certain they will have amassed information of very great importance for clarifying the biological substrates of behavior in their subjects.

CHAPTER 22

Affective Change in Thyrotoxicosis and Experimental Hypermetabolism

By W. P. WILSON, M.D., J. E. JOHNSON, M.D.,
AND R. B. SMITH, B.A.

Since the hyperthyroid patient may present himself with psychiatric symptomatology, many investigators have concerned themselves with the psychiatric findings in these patients. A review of the literature [1-15] allows one to construct the natural history of the psychiatric symptoms. Typically, the disease may be precipitated by an emotionally significant event. This is frequently followed by a period in which only symptoms of a psychiatric order may occur. After weeks, months, or even one to two years, the physical signs of the disease will become overt. With the onset of these physical findings, the emotional instability may be intensified, according to some investigations. This instability is apparently manifest by symptoms which are related to disturbances in affect since frequent mention is made in the literature of the high incidence of melancholia and mania. After treatment, although the psychiatric symptoms may be reduced in intensity, the patient may continue to show personality disturbances.

Since none of the studies reviewed were complete in their description of the affective changes, we have attempted to: (1) describe in detail the natural history of the affective symptoms, (2) to test the validity of the concept that catastrophic emotional events are invariably present as has been stated by some investigators, (3) to test or reject the observation that psychiatric symptomatology persists after specific antithyroid treatment (in our series radioactive iodine), and (4) to determine whether thyroid hormone *per se* will produce psychiatric symptomatology.

This work was supported by a grant from the Hogg Foundation for Mental Health, University of Texas.

MATERIALS AND METHODS

The 26 patients examined here were 1 adult male and 25 adult females who had presented themselves to the outpatient clinics of the University of Texas Medical Branch Hospitals in Galveston, Texas. In a few instances the private patients of one of us (JEJ) were also included. These patients were for the most part of social classes IV and V. The Hollingshead two-factor index was used to determine social class. The mean age of the thyrotoxic patients was 37 years, with a range of 22 to 57 years. Eighteen patients were white and eight were Negro. All patients included were examined physically for evidence of hyperthyroidism, and in all instances the activity of the thyroid gland was determined. The radioactive iodine uptake and protein-bound iodine were used as indices of this increased activity.

To obtain an anamnesis of the psychiatric symptomatology each patient was interviewed by one of us (WPW). In these structured interviews, attempts were made to obtain as much specific information related to changes in affect and the associated biological concomitants (sleep, appetite, sexual function, and psychomotor activity) as was possible. In all cases, except one, at least one reliable informant was interviewed to verify the information obtained from the patient. In many cases additional informative material was obtained.

In an effort to further document the affective changes in this group of patients, the Clyde Mood Scale[16] was applied to 16 of the 26 patients. Correlations were then made between some of the clinical findings and the mean scores on the mood scale.

The experimental subjects used to determine the effects of triiodothyronine on affect were nine male medical students and two female technicians. The eleven subjects were known to be endocrinologically and emotionally stable. Each of these subjects was administered the Clyde Mood Scale test immediately prior to beginning the ingestion of triiodothyronine. Each then received 300 μg of the hormone a day for three days. After seventy-two hours and while still receiving triiodothyronine, the Clyde Mood Scale test was again administered.

RESULTS

"Precipitating factors" were elicited in 14 patients. Ten patients had their illness precipitated by the loss or threatened loss of a significant person in the enviroment. In seven instances this person was a male, in two a female, and one was a stillborn child of undetermined sex. The four other patients had their illness precipitated by pregnancy (two cases), an infectious disease, or an operative procedure.

The relationship of the onset of the first hyperthyroid symptoms to the onset of mood change, or the affective biological concomitants (sex, appetite, sleep, and psychomotor activity), was established in 24 patients. In 11 patients symptoms, interpretable as being affectively determined, preceded the first symptoms of hyperthyroidism. The mean duration here was 9.2 months with a range of one month to three years. In 13 patients the symptoms developed at the same time. None of the patients reported the development of changes in affect after the onset of the hyperthyroid signs. Seventeen patients reported a change in affect as determined by their mood statement. Fifteen patients described their mood as depressed, two described elation, and seven denied a change.

Anxiety, characterized by a feeling of impending doom or disaster or nameless dread, associated with tachycardia and other autonomic symptoms, was observed in six patients. Fourteen patients reported only bouts of tachycardia or an absence of symptoms suggesting anxiety. No information was available in six patients.

Sixteen patients reported insomnia; however, no typical pattern of sleep disturbance was seen. One patient was hypersomnic. Nine reported no change.

Libido and potentia were changed in nine patients. Three reported an increase in both, six reported a decrease, and nine reported no change. Eight patients were either sexually inactive or were reluctant to discuss their sexual life.

Appetite was disturbed in 23 of the 26 patients. Eleven patients reported an increase, in both desire for food and intake of food. Twelve patients reported a decreased desire for food; however, it was determined that in spite of the anorexia, many of the patients had an increased intake. Only three reported no change.

The data related to changes in psychomotor activity were interesting. Eight of the patients were observed to have rapid movements, rapid speech, and restlessness associated with a stated increase in speed of thinking. Fourteen patients were retarded in both the speed of their movements and their thinking. Four patients demonstrated and reported no change. In three patients an abrupt change from decreased to increased psychomotor activity occurred with the development of the physical symptoms of hyperthyroidism. As a concomitant of the psychomotor retardation, nine patients reported affective confusion with subjective memory loss. Five patients reported no such confusion. The eight patients with increased psychomotor activity denied this symptom.

Increased irritability was one of the most commonly observed symptoms. Nineteen patients reported this symptom; seven patients reported no increase or decrease. Diurnal variation was present in 16 patients, where mood, as well as energy levels were changed. Eleven patients were worse in the evening. Five were worse in the morning, and seven reported no change. No reliable information could be obtained in three patients.

Delusions, incidental to affect, were observed in only four patients. These were of guilt and sinfulness. In spite of their obvious somatic change, none of the patients admitted to hypochondriacal imaginations.

Suicidal ideation was observed in six patients, although only one patient had planned this action.

Formed hallucinations were observed in two patients. One saw Jesus, the other her dead grandmother. No auditory component was present in either instance. The hallucinations occurred only on one occasion and did not recur.

Sensorium disturbances were not observed in any of the patients examined. Memory, orientation, calculation, and retention and immediate recall were always intact on clinical examination.

Two patients were found to have depersonalization and derealization.

When the data for each patient were analyzed to determine the occurrence of a complete picture of an affective disorder, it was noted that nine patients' anamneses and mental status examinations were indistinguishable from manic-depressive psychoses. All but two of these patients had an illness precipitated by an emotionally significant event, and five of the nine had suicidal ideation. One patient with elation was considered typically manic.

The mean data for the correlations of the Clyde Mood Scale results with individual symptoms are summarized in Table I. Here it may be observed that the mean scores on the individual scales correlated well with the presence or absence of the symptom. Patients who were depressed had a higher score than did patients who denied this symptom. Those with psychomotor retardation had decreased energetic scores. Those with anxiety were more jittery, and those with affective confusion less clear thinking. Patients with irritability, however, were no more or less friendly than those who were not. It was interesting that the patients with irritability did present themselves as more aggressive, even though their scores were still low. The mean score for all patients did not show a deviation from the normal mean on the depressive, energetic, and friendly scores. However, the jittery score was increased and

TABLE I

Mean Clyde Mood Scale Results Correlated with Clinical Symptoms

Clinical Symptom	Clyde Mood Score
Predominant affect	Depression
Depressed	58
No change	33
All patients	50
Psychomotor activity	Energetic
Decreased	31
Increased	53
All patients	42
Anxiety	Jittery
Present	79
Absent	58
All patients	68
Affective confusion	Clear thinking
Present	29
Absent	46
All patients	39
Irritability	Friendly
Present	58
Absent	49
All patients	55
Irritability	Aggressive
Present	39
Absent	21
All patients	24

TABLE II

Mean Clyde Mood Scores in 11 Normal Subjects
Before and After Triiodothyronine

Entity Scored	Clyde Mood Score		P
	Control	Experiment	
Friendly	65	41	0.02
Energetic	65	55	NS*
Clear thinking	63	52	NS
Aggressive	58	49	NS
Jittery	33	59	0.01
Depressed	26	31	0.05

*No significance.

the clear-thinking and aggressive scores were decreased from the mean.

The results of the use of the Clyde Mood Scale as a measure of affective change in the normal subjects receiving triiodothyronine (Table II) indicated an effect of this substance on feeling tone, although there was gross individual variation in the subjective reports obtained by the experimenter. There was a significant increase in the depressive score (P-0.05), a significant increase in the jittery score (P-0.01), and a significant decrease in the friendly score (P-0.02). The aggressive, energetic, and clear-thinking scores were not significantly changed.

DISCUSSION

The data presented here corroborate the findings of others that affective symptomatology is a frequent concomitant of thyrotoxicosis and that in many instances the presentation of this symptomatology is indistinguishable from severe depressions [1,4,15]. Certain of our findings do, however, seem contradictory to previous reports. The generalization that many patients are seriously disturbed long before developing hyperthyroidism [15] is in part substantiated and in part refuted by this study. If one means by "long" a period of several months to three years, this statement is true. However, inspection of the data reveals that most of the patients who had psychiatric symptoms for a long period preceding the development of the physical symptoms had illnesses precipitated by emotionally significant events and were considered normal prior to that time. Once the illness was physically manifest, the only dramatic change in symptomatology that was observed was the change in psychomotor activity. It was indeed rare to discover a patient whose basic mood disturbance had appreciably and dramatically changed concurrent with the appearance of the physical signs of hyperthyroidism. This finding is in part contradictory to the statement of Cleghorn [15] that "once the gland becomes overactive, the emotional instability is heightened." On the other hand, an intensification of irritability was frequently associated with the development of the physical symptoms of the disease. It is conceivable that this latter finding could be interpreted as emotional instability.

Although the patients in this series were not all re-examined after specific antithyroid therapy, enough follow-ups [15] were obtained to form some conclusions as to the persistence of symptomatology. Not one of the patients in this series required psychiatric treatment because of persistent symptoms. This observation is in contrast to the observation of Moschowitz [5], who felt that the patient continued to have symptoms after treatment. Our clinical observation is documented by observations on another group of patients who were treated and were euthyroid at the time of examination. These patients were indistinguishable from a group of normal controls when examined with the Clyde Mood Scale [17]. The changes observed in the experimental studies reported here lend some credence to the hypothesis that increased secretion of thyroid hormone produces alterations in feeling tone. Although the changes observed are small, they are consistently in the same direction and are not related to chance variation since many of these subjects had shown remarkable stability in their test scores on previous occasions.

Finally, the social classes and intellectual abilities of the patients and subjects included here must be considered. Since the patient material was of class IV and V, whose intellectual abilities are presumed to be normal or below normal, it is conceivable that the Clyde Mood Scale was not as good a measure of the affective state as it was for the experimental subjects who were an intellectually superior group. This may then account for the small deviation from normal on all scales except the "jittery" one. On the other hand, the scattering of symptoms in the patients seems the most probable factor responsible for the lack of correlation.

SUMMARY

Complete medical and psychiatric examinations were performed on 26 hyperthyroid patients. The Clyde Mood Scale test was administered to 16 of these patients. Large doses of triiodothyronine were administered to eleven normal subjects, and changes in affect were determined according to the Clyde Mood Scale. It was observed that the predominant symptomatology of thyrotoxic patients is affectively determinated and that the presence or absence of symptoms correlates well with scores obtained on the Clyde Mood Scale. The administration of thyroid hormone produces depression, decreases friendliness, and increases jitteriness in normal subjects.

REFERENCES

1. Robertson, A.: On Graves' disease with insanity, J. Ment. Sci. 20:573, 1875.

2. Lewis, N.D.C.: A psychoanalytic study of hyperthyroidism, Psychoanal. Rev. 10:140, 1923.

3. Mayo, C.H., and Plummer, H.W.: The Thyroid Gland, The Beaumont Foundation Lectures, C.V. Mosby Co., St. Louis, 1926, pp. 45–83.

4. Bram, I.: Psychic trauma in pathogenesis of exophthalmic goiter, Endocrinol. 11:106, 1927.

5. Moschowitz, E.: The nature of Graves' disease, A.M.A. Arch. Int. Med. 46:610, 1930.

6. Mittelmann, B.: Psychogenic factors and psychotherapy in hyperthyreosis and rapid heart imbalance, J. Nerv. Ment. Dis. 77:465, 1933.

7. Goodall, J.S., and Rogers, L.: The effects of the emotions in the production of thyrotoxicosis, M. J. Rec. 138:411, 1933.

8. Conrad, A.: Psychiatric study of hyperthyroid patients, J. Nerv. Ment. Dis. 79:505, 1934.

9. Lidz, T.: Emotional factors in the etiology of hyperthyroidism, Psychosom. Med. 11:2, 1949.

10. Lidz, T., and Whitehorn, J.C.: Psychiatric problems in a thyroid clinic, J.A.M.A. 139:698, 1949.

11. Ham, G., Alexander, F., and Carmichael, H.F.: Dynamic aspects of the personality features and reactions characteristic of patients with Graves' disease, life situations and bodily diseases, Res. Publ. Ass. Nerv. Ment. Dis. 29:451, 1950.

12. Ham, G., Alexander, F., and Carmichael, H.F.: A psychosomatic theory of thyrotoxicosis, Psychosom. Med. 13:18, 1951.

13. Porta, V., and Palozzoli-Selvini, M.: Indagini sulla personalita degli ipertiroidei, Arch. Psicol. Neurol. Psichiat. 14:315, 1953.

14. Lidz, T.: Emotional factors in the etiology of hyperthyroidism. J. Mt. Sinai Hosp. 20:27, 1953.

15. Wittkower, E. D., and Cleghorn, R. A., Eds.: Recent Developments in Psychosomatic Medicine, J. B. Lippincott Co., Philadelphia, ch. 10, p. 190.

16. Clyde, D. J.: Construction and validation of an emotional association test, Unpublished Ph.D. Thesis, Pennsylvania State College, 1950.

17. Smith, R. B., Wilson, W. P., and Goolishian, H. A.: Affect and hyperthyroidism, a psychological study, to be published.

18. Longier, M., Wittkower, E. D., Stephens-Newsham, L., and Hoffman, M. M.: Psychophysiological studies in thyroid function, Psychosom. Med. 18:310, 1956.

Discussion by Roland P. Mackay, M.D.

The interesting work reported by Dr. Wilson and his associates appears to have been addressed mainly to answering two basic questions: (1) what are the affective concomitants of hyperthyroidism, and (2) do the affective disturbances cause or result from the toxic state?

Their finding that the emotional features of thyrotoxicosis are in many cases indistinguishable from those of depression is surprising if one defines "depression" in the usual way. For example, in the depressive phase of the manic-depressive psychosis (which might be called a "pure" depression), one commonly sees emotional gloom and intellectual and psychomotor retardation in varying proportions. On the other hand, patients with so-called agitated or psychoneurotic depression usually show affective gloom but some (admittedly misdirected) acceleration of intellectual and psychomotor activity, i.e., the clinical picture of the well-known "alarm reaction." Now, it would appear that thyrotoxic patients exhibit—in the majority of cases—this combination of gloom and intellectual and psychomotor acceleration, just as in the "alarm reaction." The affective portion of this state is, indeed, "depressive," insofar as it is sad, anxious, or discouraged, but the patients do not exhibit the cognitive and conative retardation of the primary depressions. Thus, thyrotoxic patients appear to present a good imitation of the typical anxiety neurosis rather than of the true depression. This feature, of course, is the reason why the clinical distinction of thyrotoxicosis from anxiety neurosis is so often difficult and so dependent upon recourse to such physical signs as a large pulse pressure, elevated production of heat (e.g., hot, wet hands, rather than cold, damp hands), and an elevated basal metabolic rate.

Dr. Wilson and his associates find that 14 of 26 patients had a history of emotional precipitating factors implying stress. Again, in 11 of 24, affective symptoms preceded somatic signs by a mean period of 9.2 months; while in the remaining 13 of the 24, affective and somatic features appeared together. To be pragmatic here, one must ask, "What does 'precede' mean?" Obviously, the affective symptoms are dated by the patients' statements, while the somatic signs are dated by objective proof of thyrotoxicosis. In short, of the two dates, the one subjective, the other objective, the subjective may well be the better for estimating the actual onset of thyrotoxicosis. What I am saying is that the onset of "nervousness" as reported by the patient may be the true indication of the onset of hyperthyroidism; the objective proof is more apt to be achieved after the event. Indeed, it is usually the subjective "nervousness" that leads to the search for objective evidence of thyrotoxicosis. Thus, the "earlier" onset of affective disturbances is in no sense an evidence that these affective features in reality preceded or exercised a causative role in producing the thyroid intoxication.

Finally, the authors' report that none of the patients required psychiatric therapy after resolution of the thyrotoxicosis seems to suggest that the intoxication was, in fact, the cause of the affective disorders. The control cases, in which the administration of triiodothyronine produced the same affective states as were observed in the hyperthyroid patients, lead to the same conclusion.

Thanks are due the authors for an imaginative and instructive contribution.

V PSYCHOPHARMACOLOGIC RESEARCH

Metabolic Effects of Psychoactive Drugs

By D. V. SIVA SANKAR, PH.D., ELEANOR GOLD, B.A.,
AND D. BARBARA SANKAR, B.A.

The advent and widespread use of psychotomimetic and psychotherapeutic drugs, while of indisputable value, pose certain questions as to their effects on several somatic and metabolic functions—growth in children, resistance to infection, production of antibodies, etc. Furthermore, there is a great need for investigations aimed toward an elucidation of the action of these drugs at the biochemical, cellular, and molecular levels. With this in view, we have attempted to study the metabolic effects of some psychoactive drugs. We have previously reported [1] the metabolic effects of lysergic acid diethylamide (LSD). In the present study, results of the administration of 2-bromolysergic acid analogue (BOL), phenylisopropyl hydrazine (JB 516 or Catron), and chlorpromazine are presented.

MATERIALS AND METHODS

For purposes of convenience and reproducibility of results, the albino rat was chosen as the experimental animal. Adult rats of our stock colony, which were originally of the Wistar strain, were used. A total of 16 rats were used for the studies on LSD, while 12 were used for each of the other drugs. The values for each group were averaged (Table I, II, and III). The rats were placed in metabolism cages in advance of the actual experiment to acclimatize them to the cage.

The amount of food consumed was estimated by carefully weighing the food placed in the food cups and the residue at the end of every 24-hour period. The technique of paired feeding was not used because of (1) possible metabolic changes in the control animals and (2) the difference between the experimental

TABLE I

Metabolic Effects of LSD and BOL in Rats
(mean values)

Metabolic Entity	LSD			BOL		
	Control	Experimental	% Change	Control	Experimental	% Change
Food intake (g)	19.26	16.26	-15.6	14.8	15.8	6.7
Water intake (ml)	34.4	33.2	- 3.5	—	—	—
Weight of feces (% food intake)	22.0	22.8	3.6	20.0	20.0	0.0
Urinary N (mg/day)	422	348	-17.5	443	453	2.2
Urea N (% urinary N)	72.4	61.2	-15.5	75.4	79.7	5.7
Urinary inorganic phosphate (μM/day)	535	487	- 9.0	544	530	-2.6
Total urinary keto acid (μM/day)	68.1	56.0	-17.8	58.2	64.2	10.3
Keto acid/g food intake	4.0	3.28	-18.8	3.97	4.1	2.8
Creatinine (O.D.* units)	35.8	32.2	-10.0	34.1	35.6	4.4
Total Bratton-Marshall amines (O.D. units)	48.7	41.2	-15.4	34.2	42.6	24.6
Diazotized sulfanilic acid positive substances (O.D. units)	76.5	64.0	-16.3	73.6	77.8	5.7
Phenolic substances/g food intake (O.D. units)	1.08	1.22	13.0	—	—	—
5-hydroxyindole acetic acid (O.D. units)	29.5	46.5	57.6	—	—	—

*Optical Density.

TABLE II

Metabolic Effects of JB 516 and Chlorpromazine
(dose 40 mg/kg)

Metabolic Entity	JB 516			Chlorpromazine		
	Control	Experimental	% Change	Control	Experimental	% Change
Food intake (g)	15.2	3.4	-77.6	13.9	1.4	-89.9
Creatinine mg/day	21.2	9.6	-54.4	21.6	7.2	-66.7
Weight of feces (g)	3.8	0.9	-76.3	3.36	0.71	-78.8
Total urinary N*	20.8	17.9	-14.1	20.4	20.0	- 2.0
Urea N (% urinary N)	64.4	60.2	- 6.5	—	—	—
Total phenolics*	8.5	9.9	16.6	7.6	8.2	7.9
Diazotized sulfanilic acid positive substances*	4.0	2.9	-27.5	4.4	2.4	-45.4
Nitrosonaphtol-. positive substances*	0.165	0.157	- 4.8	0.138	0.231	67.4
Bratton-Marshall total amines*	0.41	0.35	-14.6	0.39	0.33	-15.4
Ninhydrin-positive substances (calculated as glutamic acid*)	48.8	69.8	43.0	46.0	59.8	30.0
Urea*	30.7	23.1	-24.7	29.5	27.5	-67.7
Keto acid*	3.58	2.90	-19.0	3.09	2.27	- 26.5
Inorganic phosphate*	32.0	70.9	121.6	32.0	46.9	46.6

*Excretion of substance calculated per mg of creatinine excreted in the urine.

TABLE III

Metabolic Effects of JB 516 and Chlorpromazine
(dose 10 mg/kg)

Metabolic Entity	JB 516			Chlorpromazine		
	Control	Experi-mental	% Change	Control	Experi-mental	% Change
Food intake (g)	15.15	3.14	-79.3	15.21	13.59	-10.65
Weight of feces (g)	3.19	1.73	-45.76	3.59	3.37	- 6.12
Creatinine (mg)	21.3	14.45	-32.15	22.2	21.6	- 2.70
Urea N (mg)	319	176	-44.8	331	315	- 4.8
Urea N*	15.15	12.4	-18.1	15.2	14.8	- 2.6
Bratton-Marshall total amines	10.45	6.68	-36.1	12.21	11.0	- 9.9
Bratton-Marshall amines*	0.496	0.471	- 5.0	0.553	0.513	- 7.2
Inorganic phosphate (μM/day)	723.7	579.5	-19.2	737	831	12.7
Inorganic phosphate*	33.9	40.9	20.6	33.4	38.3	14.7
Keto acid*	4.26	3.22	-24.4	4.10	4.08	- 0.5
Ammonia*	3.59	3.24	- 9.7	3.56	3.47	- 2.5
Urinary N*	30.9	15.2	-50.8	—	—	—
Ninhydrin-positive substances*	89.0 89.0	87.6 87.6	- 1.6 - 1.6	73.7 73.7	89.0 89.0	20.8 20.8
Diazotized sulfanilic acid positive substances*	4.15	2.68	-35.4	3.76	3.19	-15.1
Nitrosonaphthol-positive substances*	0.12	0.09	-25.0	0.13	0.10	-23.1

*Excretion of substance calculated per mg of urinary creatinine.

and control animals was quite large in some of the experiments (Table II). Urine and feces were carefully collected according to a standardized procedure of rinsing the cages by the same person. The procedure employed for washing was the same from day to day with respect to the amount of water used to wash the cages and with respect to rinsing the cages and other operational details.

Urine, while being collected, was preserved from microbial decomposition by the use of 3 ml of hydrochloric acid. The urine and feces were collected for two days without administration of any drug. These specimens served as controls. After the two days, each rat received the drug each day by the intraperitoneal route. The amounts used were as follows: LSD 500 μg per animal. BOL 500 μg per animal, JB 516 40 mg/kg in one set of experiments and 10 mg/kg in another set, and chlorpromazine 40 mg/kg in one set and, 10 mg/kg in another set of experiments. After the administration of the drug, urine and feces were collected exactly as before for two more days. The collections for each day were kept and analyzed separately.

The feces were dried in a steam oven. The urines were made up to volume and analyzed for total urinary nitrogen and ammonia according to standard procedures using Kjeldahl digestion and Nessler's reagent methods. Inorganic phosphate was estimated according to Fiske and Subba Row [2] and total keto acids according to Friedman and Haugen [3]. Creatinine was estimated by reacting it with picric acid followed by an alkali [4]. Urea was estimated gravimetrically by precipitating as the xanthydrol derivative. Total amines were estimated by the Bratton-Marshall test [5]. Phenolic substances were estimated with the Folin phenol reagent after the addition of the alkaline copper solution (reagent C) of Lowry et al. [6]. The nitrosonaphthol-positive substances were estimated according to the procedure described by Udenfriend and his associates [7]. The diazotized sulfanilic acid positive substances [8] and 5-hydroxyindole acetic acid were assayed according to methods described in the literature [9]. For purposes of calculation, the individual data for each rat were first calculated and then were divided by the number of rats to compute the average.

RESULTS

The values presented in Tables I, II, and III represent the average for the animals in each group. The effects of LSD on the intact rat include piloerection, rigidity of the limbs, increased sensitivity to stimuli, a crawling-like gait, etc. However, this condition disappears in two to three hours, and the rat begins to behave normally. On the other hand, the administration of BOL does not produce any of these symptoms. Furthermore, in the two-day experiment period we did not notice any increased tolerance to LSD. This is probably owing to the short experimental period.

While LSD and BOL did not decrease the food intake of the rat drastically, chlorpromazine at a level of 40 mg/kg and JB 516 even at 10 mg/kg have done so. This effect of JB 516 is interesting in view of the enhanced activity of the animal after the administration of JB 516. This effect is probably comparable to the action of amphetamine, which is structurally related to JB 516. We have shown the similarity of action of amphetamine and JB 516 on liver alcohol dehydrogenase [10]. A striking difference between the action of LSD on the one hand and of JB 516 and chlorpromazine on the other is that the effect of LSD lasts only a few hours. So, in the 24-hour metabolic experiment the animal is under the acute influence of LSD for only a few hours, while the effects of JB 516 and of chlorpromazine are longer lasting.

The urinary creatinine level is supposed to fall in diseases affecting the muscular system. In the present experiment the decrease in the urinary creatinine after the administration of both JB 516 and chlorpromazine (Table II) is marked in spite of the fact that one drug causes sedation and the other excitation with increased movements. At the lower dose of chlorpromazine (Table III) and in the experiments with LSD and BOL (Table I) the effect of the drug on the excretion of creatinine is not marked.

In view of the extreme decrease in food intake following JB 516 and chlorpromazine, all values in Table II and some in Table III have been expressed as amounts excreted per milligram of urinary creatinine. Actually, in the experiment cited in Table II, the urinary nitrogen was higher in many cases after the administration of the drug than the nitrogen ingested in the food. This shows catabolism of the tissue nitrogen after a higher dose of JB 516 and chlorpromazine. However, the relative amounts of urea excreted are affected by LSD and by JB 516 only. We have previously discussed the effect of LSD on urea excretion [1]. In view of the inhibitory effect of JB 516 on the oxidation of ethyl alcohol and vitamin A alcohol by liver alcohol dehydrogenase [10], it is plausible to postulate altered functioning of the liver and changes in the metabolism of visual pigments subsequent to the administration of JB 516.

Another interesting metabolic aspect is the excretion of inorganic phosphate. LSD, as shown in Table I, decreases total urinary inorganic phosphate output. Chlorpromazine enhances this output (Table III). JB 516 decreases the total amount of urinary phosphate. But if expressed as micromoles per milligram creatinine, the effect of chlorpromazine at lower levels diminishes while JB 516 actually enhances the amount (Table III). Thus, there seems to be a relation between behavioral aspects as related to activity of the animal and the excretion of creatinine and phosphate.

Keto acid excretion is decreased by LSD, JB 516, and chlorpromazine, a finding suggesting that this aspect may not have a direct bearing on the action of the drug. However, as in some other estimations, in the present study determination of the total level of a group of compounds (for example, amines, keto acids, amino acids) may tell us only a part of the story. Experiments on the determination of the urinary levels of individual compounds, like noradrenalin or indole acetic acid, are in progress. An interesting result in this connection is the increased excretion of 5-hydroxyindole acetic acid after the administration of LSD to the rat (Table I). This may indicate increased metabolism of 5-hydroxytryptamine in the LSD-treated rat and corroborates our investigations on the effect of psychoactive drugs on the levels of serotonin in different parts of the brain and body (Table IV). The experimental details of the study presented in Table IV have been presented elsewhere [8]. The question whether the effect of LSD in mobilizing serotonin is specific to serotonin only or whether LSD increases the levels of other neurohormones, like noradrenalin and acetylcholine, is being further investigated.

The excretion of nitrosonaphthol-positive substances increases much more after chlorpromazine than after JB 516 (Table II). The results cited in Table III show that while chlorpromazine does not affect the excretion of Bratton-Marshall positive amines significantly, JB 516 causes an appreciable decrease. But, if expressed on the creatinine basis, this decrease diminishes to a large extent. This may suggest a positive correlation (direct proportionality) in the excretion of creatinine and these amines. On the other hand, JB 516 caused a decrease (Table III) in the urinary inorganic phosphate from 723.7 μM to 579.5 μM. When

TABLE IV

Effect of Some Psychoactive Drugs on Serotonin Levels in the Rabbit
(per cent change over control)

Organ Tissue	Effect of		
	LSD	BOL	Chlorpromazine
Liver	50.6	28.7	3.4
Lung	43.1	37.3	17.6
Kidney	71.2	100.0	5.8
Spleen	30.8	- 8.9	25.3
Heart	188.1	-28.4	-50.7
Brain			
Cerebrum	-6.25	-37.5	-54.2
Cerebellum	38.7	- 4.8	- 4.8
Stem	38.7	- 2.8	-27.4
Rest of brain	28.8	-21.2	-38.5

expressed on the basis of creatinine, these values become 33.9 and 40.9 respectively. This may denote a negative correlation between the excretion of creatinine and inorganic phosphate. Since creatine and phosphate (as phosphocreatine and adenosine triphosphate) are intimately involved in muscular activity and since animals receiving chlorpromazine and JB 516 differ greatly in their motor activity, the effect of these drugs on enzymes involved in muscular activity should be of interest.

DISCUSSION

The metabolism of phosphate seems to be related in more than one way with the effects of LSD. This may, as mentioned earlier, have a bearing on the hallucinogenic action of LSD or may simply be a reflection of the stress created in recipient animals. We have also investigated the effect of LSD, BOL, insulin, and glucagon on rabbit serum inorganic phosphate content. For this purpose, blood was drawn from a rabbit by means of a heart puncture, and the rabbit was then administered the drug by the intravenous route. After an hour, blood was drawn from the animal by the same method. This way, each experimental animal served as its own control. Details of this experiment will be published elsewhere. However, the results concerning the phosphate levels are presented in Table V.

TABLE V

Effect of Insulin, LSD and BOL on Rabbit Serum Inorganic Phosphate (values expressed as change over control)

Drug	No. Animals	% Change
Insulin	6	-24.4
LSD	6	64.3
BOL	3	3.7

TABLE VI

Blood Inorganic Phosphate Content in Schizophrenic Children (mean values)

Test	Schizophrenic			Nonschizophrenic			
	No. Cases	Average	S.D.*	No. Cases	Average	S.D.*	P†
Plasma inorganic phosphate ($\mu M/ml$)	78	0.27	0.30	29	0.16	0.15	0.01
RBC inorganic phosphate ($\mu M/g$ hemoglobin)	80	5.15	4.28	26	2.8	1.34	less than 0.01

*Standard deviation.
†Significance.

It may be seen that insulin decreased the amount of inorganic phosphate, while LSD increased it. The action of insulin may be due to increased esterification of inorganic phosphate to form glucose-6-phosphate and possibly further production of high-energy phosphate compounds. It has been reported by Abood and his co-workers [12] that LSD uncoupled oxidative phosphorylation. This action of LSD may explain the increased levels of inorganic phosphate in the serum of rabbits administered LSD. It is of interest to note that BOL did not show a similar effect (cf. Table V).

It is possible that the effect of LSD may be related to its psychotomimetic action in so far as the inorganic phosphate content of both serum and erythrocyte hemolyzates is elevated in childhood schizophrenia, as shown in Table VI. The differences between the schizophrenic population and the control hospitalized children are statistically significant. Thus, it is possible that one of the biochemical malfunctions both in psychosis and in psychotomimetic action may be related to the metabolism of phosphate and dependent exergonic processes of the organism.

REFERENCES

1. Siva Sankar, D. V., and Bender, L.: Biochemistry of lysergic acid diethylamide psychosis. in Wortis, J., Ed.: Recent Advances in Biological Psychiatry, Vol. II, Grune & Straton, Inc., New York, 1960, p. 363.

2. Fiske, C. H., and Subba Row, Y.: The colorimetric determination of phosphorus, J. Biol. Chem. 66:375, 1925.

3. Friedemann, T. E., and Haugen, G. E.: Pyruvic acid II. The determination of keto acids in blood and urine, ibid. 147:415, 1943.

4. Hawk, P. B., Oser, B. L., and Summerson, W. H.: Practical Physiological Chemistry, Blakiston Company, New York, 1954.

5. Ravel, J. M., Eakin, R. E., and Shive, W.: Glycine, a precursor of 5(4)-amino-4(5)-immidazole carboxamide, J. Biol. Chem. 172:67, 1948.

6. Lowry, O. H., Rosebrough, N. J., Farr, A. L., and Randall, R. J.: ibid. 193:265, 1951.

7. Udenfriend, S., Weissbach, H., and Clark, C. T.: The estimation of 5-hydroxytryptamine in biological tissues, ibid. 215:337, 1955.

8. Siva Sankar, D. V., Phipps, E., Gold, E., and Sankar, Barbara D.: in Some Biological Aspects of Schizophrenic Behavior, Ann. N. Y. Acad. Sci., vol. 96, 1962.

9. Udenfriend, S., Titus, E., and Weissbach, H.: The identification of 5-hydroxy-3-indole acetic acid in normal urine and a method for its assay, J. Biol. Chem. 216:499, 1955.

10. Siva Sankar, D. V., Gold, E., Sankar, Barbara D., and MacRorie, E.: Effect of psychopharmacological agents on DPN-dependent enzymes, Fed. Proc. 20:394, 1961.

11. Sankar, D. B., Siva Sankar, D. V., Gold, E., and Phipps, E.: Effect of LSD, BOL, and chlorpromazine on serotonin levels, ibid. 20:344, 1961.

12. Abood, L. G., and Romanchek, L.: Ann. N. Y. Acad. Sci. 66:812, 1957.

Interaction of Monoamine Oxidase Inhibitors with Imipramine and Similar Drugs

By WILLIAMINA A. HIMWICH, Ph.D.

Over the past two years we have been studying the effects of imipramine (Tofranil) given with tranylcypromine (Parnate) in dogs in hopes of elucidating the mechanism responsible for the toxic effects of this combination and also the basic mechanism of action of imipramine. Detailed descriptions of the behavioral reaction have been published elsewhere [1, 2]. More recently, clinical reports of disastrous results of the use of imipramine with a mono-amine oxidase inhibitor (MAOI) have appeared [3–6].

MATERIALS AND METHODS

Normal mongrel males of medium weight (10 to 15 kg) well acclimated to laboratory conditions and personnel were given one of the two following dosage schedules:

Daily for 4 days: 10 mg/kg imipramine im
5th day: 10 mg/kg imipramine im followed
                   by 2.0 mg/kg tranylcypromine iv

Daily for 4 days: 10 mg/kg chlorpromazine im
5th day: 10 mg/kg chlorpromazine im followed
                   by 2.0 mg/kg tranylcypromine iv

Thirty-five dogs out of forty tested reacted strongly in terms of behavior to the combination of imipramine and tranylcypromine. Of this group, ten were chosen for recording of cortical electro-encephalograms, blood pressure, heart rate, and rectal temperature when receiving the imipramine and tranylcypromine. These tests

We would like to thank Geigy Pharmaceuticals and Smith, Kline & French Laboratories for the generous supplies of Tofranil and Parnate and the Upjohn Co. for the heparin used.

were performed under three conditions: (1) without anesthesia,
(2) lightly anesthetized with Nembutal, and (3) curarized. At least
three weeks were allowed between each test.

The animals under curare were anesthetized with thiopental
and maintained at the surgical level long enough to permit the
necessary surgery and intubation of the trachea. They were then
placed on artificial respiration and slowly curarized as the thiopental wore off. The curare was given throughout the experiment
by slow intravenous injection from a perfusion pump. The cortical
electroencephalogram was also studied after imipramine given
alone both in multiple (chronic) and in single doses and after
tranylcypromine alone. Two dogs showing marked behavioral
effects after imipramine and the MAOI were also studied for gross
behavioral changes with 5-hydroxytryptophan (5HTP) 4 mg/kg and
tranylcypromine 2.0 mg/kg, given as described previously [7] to
distinguish the behavioral changes from those due to increased
serotonin in the brain.

Since in our experience animals given chlorpromazine (Thorazine) and tranylcypromine showed little or no behavioral effects
due to these drugs, only the cortical electroencephalogram in unanesthetized and anesthetized animals has been studied.

RESULTS

Behavioral

The essential behavioral changes have been previously described [1]. As we worked with a larger group of dogs we discovered that although rhythmical hindleg movements occurred in
all animals given imipramine and tranylcypromine as described
above, not all males disclosed sexual activation. Those animals
who failed to show this syndrome had instead generalized muscle
twitching which interfered seriously with the recording of the EEG
in the unanesthetized or lightly anesthetized animals. Even under
curare some muscle twitching persisted.

The comparison of the effects of increased brain serotonin
with those of imipramine and tranylcypromine was made in dogs
No. 5 and No. 40. The former showed sexual activation with imipramine and MAOI while the latter did not. The symptoms resulting from the two drug schedules (Table I) illustrate the differences
in the two syndromes.

Cardiovascular Changes

The intramuscular injection of the fifth dose of imipramine in
either the anesthetized or curarized animal resulted in a transient

increase in heart rate followed by a return to normal in less than 30 minutes. Tranylcypromine alone or after imipramine in the curarized animal produced an increase in heart rate and a tendency for the blood pressure to rise for about 15 minutes. In the anesthetized dog both blood pressure and heart rate were lower one hour after the injections of imipramine and tranylcypromine, although results were more consistent at this time in the anesthetized than in the curarized animals. After three to four hours, blood pressure and heart rate were still significantly below normal in the anesthetized animals while in those under curare both measurements tended to return to normal by this time.

Rectal Temperature

In the unanesthetized dog given imipramine and tranylcypromine, the rectal temperature often increased 10 to 12 F. and the animals had to be placed in a refrigerated room to save their lives. With light Nembutal anesthesia the temperature still rose but not as much, the maximum increase being 7.8 F. These animals all survived without refrigeration. When the same animals were

TABLE I
Gross Behavioral Changes in Dogs

Symptoms	Drugs Administered	
	5-HTP + MAOI	Imipramine + MAOI
Aggressiveness	+	-
Hyperactivity	+	-
Steppage gait	+	-
Extension of toes	+ +	+
Rhythmic movement of hindlegs	-	+
Sexual activity	-	+
Muscle twitch	-	+
Hyperthermia	+	+ +
Salivation	+	+

curarized, the rectal temperature tended to fall and in no instance was there a marked increase in body temperature.

Electroencephalographic Findings

A single dose of imipramine (10 mg/kg) im in a curarized animal caused the transient appearance of large amplitude slow waves for as long as ninety minutes after the injections (Fig. 1). The recordings taken on the morning of the fifth day in the animals chronically receiving imipramine, that is, twenty-four hours after the fourth dose of imipramine and before the fifth dose, were normal (Fig. 2). The injection of the fifth dose of imipramine resulted in a slower wave pattern with greater amplitude in all animals. This pattern lasted for less than two hours, and during this time the animal could not be aroused by an auditory stimulus such as a loud clap.

A single injection of tranylcypromine alone resulted in little change in the EEG in the unanesthetized dog, while in the curarized dog the recording was faster and lower in amplitude (Fig. 1). Behaviorally the unanesthetized dog appeared more restless and tense for about 30 minutes after the tranylcypromine.

The injection of the fifth dose of imipramine and tranylcypromine resulted in an EEG which after one hour had a marked increase in amplitude and a slowing of the waves (Figs. 3 and 4); such an animal failed to alert to auditory stimuli. Between two to three

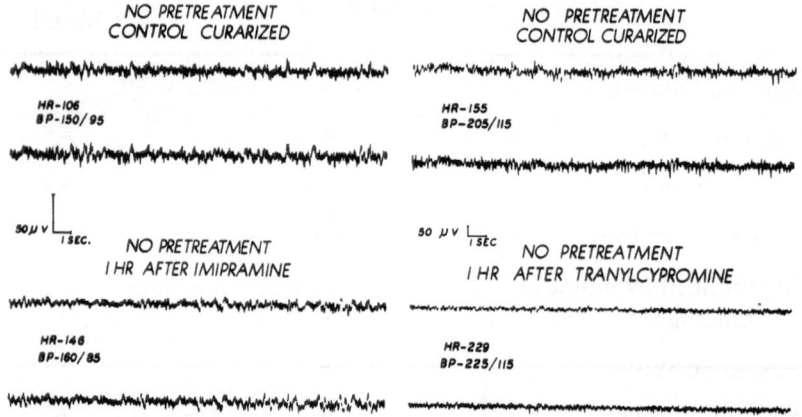

FIG. 1. Left: The effect of a single injection of imipramine, 10 mg/kg im, on cortical EEG of curarized dog with no pretreatment. Right: Cortical EEG of curarized dog with no pretreatment after a single injection of tranylcypromine, 20 mg/kg im.

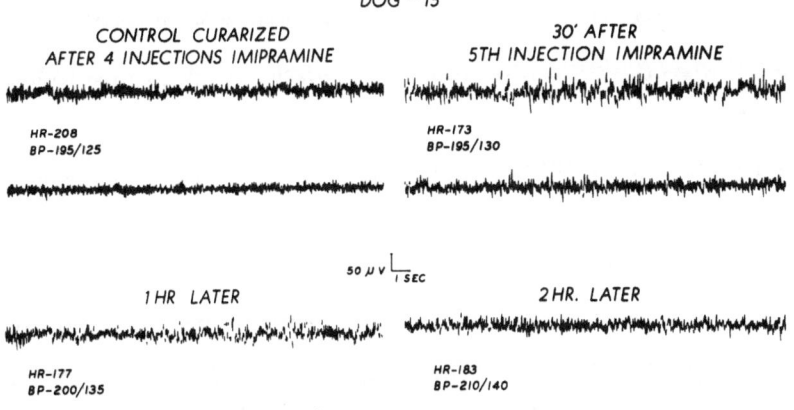

FIG. 2. Effect of fifth injection of imipramine on motor cortex of curarized dog pretreated with imipramine for four days.

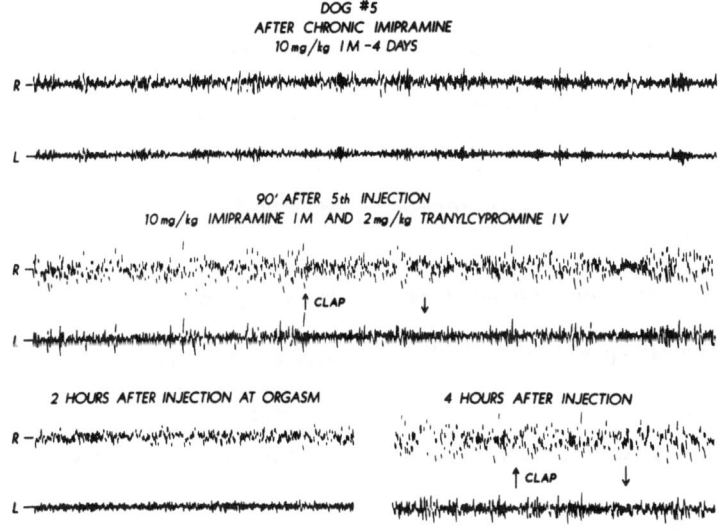

FIG. 3. Effect of imipramine and tranylcypromine on cortical EEG of unanesthetized dog who showed marked sexual behavioral response.

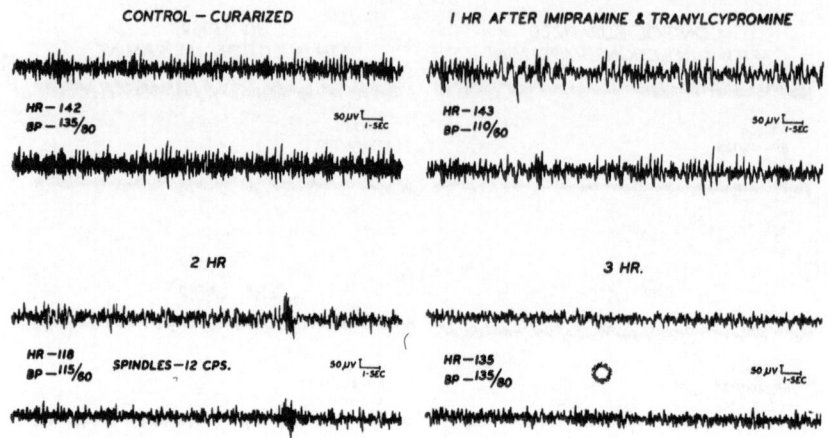

FIG. 4. Effect of imipramine followed immediately by tranylcypromine on right and left motor cortex of curarized dog. The animal was premedicated for four days with imipramine.

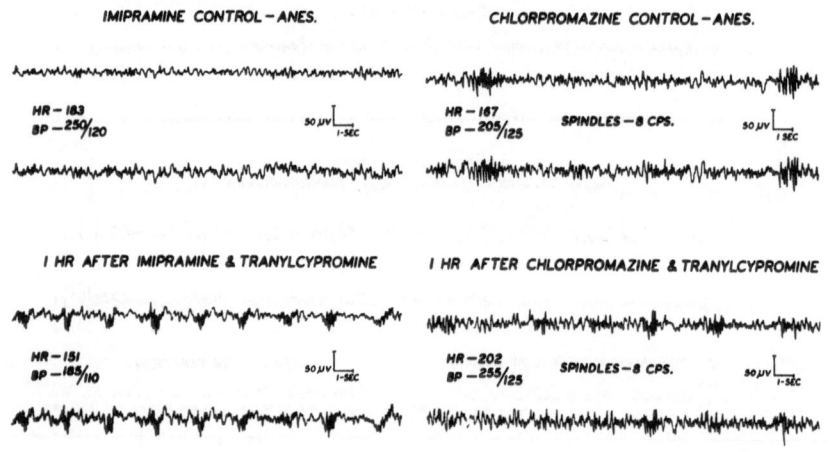

FIG. 5. Comparison of the effect of tranylcypromine on EEG of anesthetized dogs pretreated with four doses of imipramine or of chlorpromazine.

hours later, at a time when the movements of the hindlegs were most marked, some animals were having spontaneous orgasms and appeared to be oblivious to external stimuli; their EEG was markedly desynchronized. After about an hour the record again returned to the slow-wave large-amplitude pattern obtained in the early part of the experiment, and the animal again could not be alerted. Six to seven hours after the administration of the two drugs, the animals returned to normal.

Recordings such as described could be obtained only in those unanesthetized animals who did not show the muscle twitching or in the curarized animals. Animals anesthetized with Nembutal often showed enough muscle twitch to prevent the tracing of usable electroencephalograms (Fig. 5). In contrast, animals given chlorpromazine for four days showed spindling in the control record and no essential change after the fifth injection of chlorpromazine followed by tranylcypromine.

DISCUSSION

The most striking peripheral change that occurs in these animals is the rhythmic movements of the hindlegs which is accompanied either by sexual activity or by a generalized muscle twitch. In our experience only those animals in which marked muscle twitching occurred showed a large rise in rectal temperature. The possibility of a peripheral component in the hyperthermia is borne out by the failure of the temperature to rise in the curarized animal and by the comparatively moderate rise in the anesthetized animals. The peripheral component in an increase in temperature has been described [8].

The EEG after imipramine alone corresponds to that seen in rabbits treated with this drug. In this species, van Meter, Owens, and H. E. Himwich [9] have shown that the reticular formation is blocked by imipramine. However, the blocking in the dog, as suggested by the cortical record, is transient unless tranylcypromine is also given. These data indicate that tranylcypromine potentiates the imipramine effect. During the period of slow, large-amplitude activity the animal does not alert and appears to be unconscious of his surroundings. With the development of rhythmic movements of the hindlegs, the EEG becomes desynchronized although the dogs appear still to be unaware of external stimuli. It may, therefore, be argued that the alerting is due to the increased peripheral stimuli arising from the hindleg movements and the concomitant syndromes. This explanation is probably not complete, for when the movements are suppressed by curare, the EEG shows an abnormal pattern, and the animal still alerts. Stimuli arising in the periphery, however, would not be blocked by curare.

We have been interested in trying to determine the importance of the chronic treatment with imipramine in producing this syndrome. Two lines of evidence suggest that imipramine must be given for several days: one, the failure of the EEG to show a change after a single dose of imipramine intramuscularly in the curarized animal and, two, the failure of dog No. 5 to show more than fleeting behavioral symptoms if tranylcypromine was given followed alone 3 hours later, at the height of the MAOI activity, by a single dose of imipramine.

No significant data can be found for changes in either the catecholamines or serotonin [1] in these animals. Even in the rat, chronic imipramine treatment followed by tranylcypromine has little effect on the neurohormones [10]. Moreover, the behavioral effects of increased serotonin owing to 5HTP and MAOI are quite different from those caused by the combination of imipramine with MAOI. Our data lead us to believe that chronic imipramine treatment promotes the accumulation of some substance in the brain which is normally destroyed along a pathway blocked by tranylcypromine. When the metabolite can no longer be destroyed because of the action of tranylcypromine, it produces toxic effects. Such a metabolite has been proposed by Sulser et al. [11] to explain the ability of imipramine to antagonize the action of reserpine in rats. It is interesting that although we consider the period of maximum activity of tranylcypromine as far as the accumulation of serotonin is concerned in the dog brain [7] to be 4 to 6 hours after the injection, the maximum activity here occurs 2 to 4 hours after the injection. It is possible, therefore, that in this case tranylcypromine is blocking an enzyme or group of enzymes other than the amine oxidases. Clinical studies would suggest that other monoamine oxidase inhibitors also possess similar effects when combined with imipramine.

SUMMARY

The EEG changes which occur in animals receiving a single dose of tranylcypromine or of imipramine have been compared with those in animals chronically receiving imipramine followed on the fifth day by tranylcypromine. The data indicate that tranylcypromine potentiates the imipramine. Theoretically this effect could arise if a metabolite formed by imipramine accumulates in the presence of tranylcypromine.

REFERENCES

1. Himwich, Williamina A., Costa, E., and Himwich, H. E.: Brain serotonin in relation to imipramine interaction with a monoamine oxidase inhibitor. in Rothlin, E., Ed.: Neuropsychopharmacology, Vol. II, Van Nostrand, New York, 1960.

2. Himwich, Williamina A., and Petersen, J. C.: Effect of the combined administration of imipramine and a monoamine oxidase inhibitor, Am. J. Psychiat. 117:928, 1961.

3. Singh, H.: Atropine-like poisoning due to tranquilizing agents, Am. J. Psychiat. 117:360, 1960.

4. Davies, G.: Side-effects of phenelzine, Brit. M. J. 2:1019, 1960.

5. Luby, E. D. and Domino, E. F.: Increased drug.toxicity resulting from large doses of imipramine (Tofranil) and an MAO inhibitor in a patient with suicidal intent, in press.

6. Ayd, F. J., Jr.: Toxic somatic and psychopathologic reactions to antidepressant drugs, in press.

7. Himwich, Williamina A., and Costa, E.: Behavioral changes associated with changes in concentrations of brain serotonin, Fed. Proc. 19:838, 1960.

8. Benedict, F. G., and Cathcart, E. P.: Muscular work. A metabolic study, with special reference to the efficiency of the human body as a machine, Carnegie Inst. of Washington, No. 187, 1913.

9. Meter, W. G. van, Owens, H. F., and Himwich, H. E.: Effects of Tofranil, an antidepressant drug, on electrical potentials of rabbit brain, Canadian Psychiat. Assoc. J. 4:S113, 1959.

10. Morpurgo, C.: Personal communication.

11. Sulser, F., Watts, J. F., and Brodie, B. B.: Blocking of reserpine action by imipramine, a drug devoid of stimulatory effects in normal animals, Fed. Proc. 20:321, 1961.

CHAPTER 25

Correlation of the Cerebral Biochemical and Functional Effects of Monoamine Oxidase Inhibitor Antidepressants

By AMEDEO S. MARRAZZI, M.D., E. ROSS HART, PH.D.,
JOSE M. RODRIGUEZ, M.D., MELVYN I. GLUCKMAN, PH.D.,
AND ZOLA P. HOROVITZ, PH.D.

One group of so-called antidepressants belongs to the monoamine oxidase (MAO) inhibitors. It therefore seemed instructive to examine the correlation between the chemical and functional changes induced in the brain by monoamine oxidase inhibitors and to ask how these are related to an antidepressant action.

On the basis of the cerebral synaptic inhibitory action of minute doses of serotonin, we proposed it in 1955 as a cerebral inhibitory neurohumor [1]. We supported this in 1957 by demonstrating the similar action of an intracarotidly injected MAO inhibitor, which caused a fall in the titer of the cerebral MAO in the ipsilateral (or "injected") hemisphere and a presumed accumulation of serotonin corresponding to the cerebral synaptic inhibition in the ipsilateral cortex [2]. Thus an antidepressant that is a MAO inhibitor might induce profound enough changes in the cerebral synaptic neurohumoral mechanism to significantly modify the distorted synaptic neurohumoral equilibrium which we have postulated as a potential mechanism in some forms of mental disturbance [3, 4]. If such an influence can be verified, it becomes important to understand what role it plays in the reported clinical antidepressant effect.

MATERIALS AND METHODS

To insure cerebral actions only minimally complicated by other effects, the MAO inhibitors iproniazid* and phenylisopropyl hydrazine (JB 516)† were introduced by close arterial (intracarotid)

---

*Kindly supplied by Dr. G. Zbinden of Hoffman-LaRoche, Inc.
†Kindly supplied by Dr. J. H. Biel of Lakeside Laboratories.

injection in the cat lightly anesthetized with sodium pentobarbital.
Because intracarotid injections expose the carotid sinus and
carotid body to comparatively high concentrations of the substances being studied, it became necessary to determine the
influence, if any, of local intracarotid effects upon the transcallosally evoked cortical potentials that were used as the index of
synaptic transmission. This was accomplished by: (1) denervating
the carotid sinus and (2) bypassing the region. The lack of effect
of denervation is illustrated in Fig. 1, which shows that the cerebral
synaptic inhibitory action of serotonin, as evidenced by the reduction of the transcallosally evoked cortical potential, is not changed
by carotid sinus denervation either unilaterally or bilaterally. The
blood pressure tracing in the upper left hand corner of this figure
illustrates the reactivity of the innervated sinus on occlusion of
the common carotid arteries below the sinuses.

It is possible to bypass the baro- and chemo-receptor areas in
the common carotid artery by injecting above the region, i.e.,
above the level of the lingual artery, as illustrated in Fig. 2. By
occluding the common artery above the sinus region, i.e., above
the lingual artery, which is left open, it is possible to perfuse the
carotid sinus and carotid body region without allowing access to
the brain. Figure 3 shows the utilization of these devices to
demonstrate that the effect of intracarotidly injected serotonin

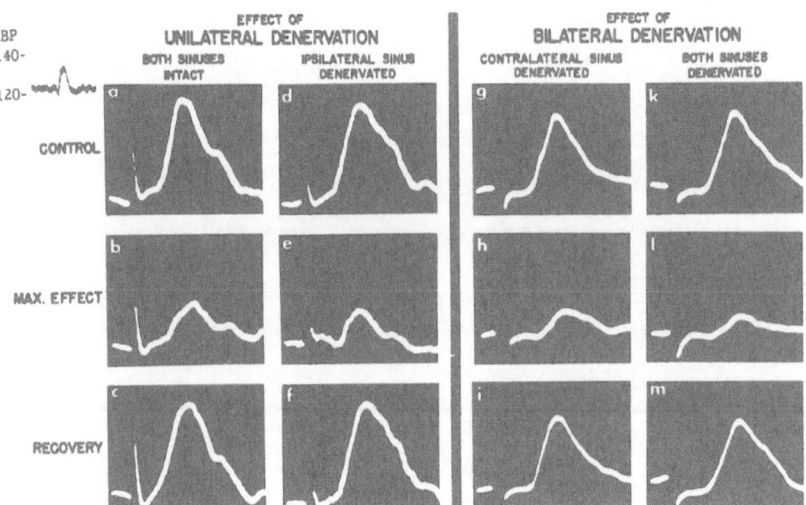

FIG. 1. Serotonin inhibition of transcallosally evoked cortical potentials with carotid sinus
intact and denervated. Injections in left common carotid-pentobarbitalized cats.

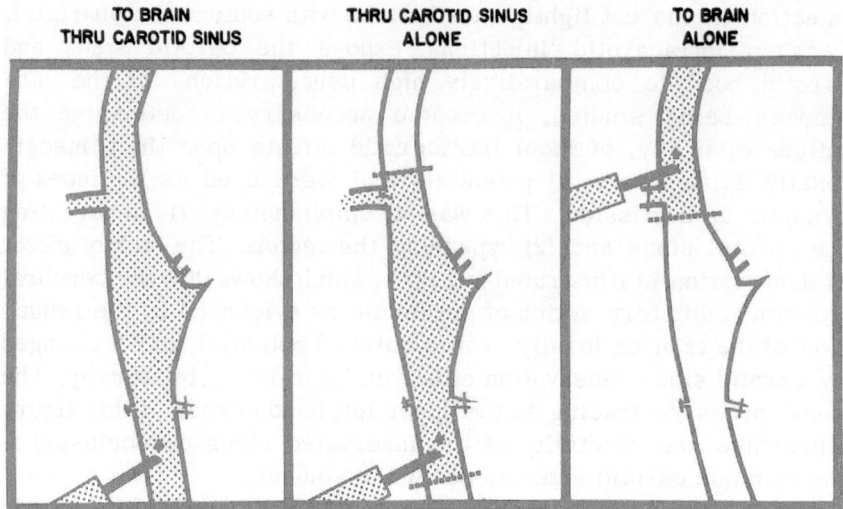

FIG. 2.   Selective access to brain, carotid sinus, or both.

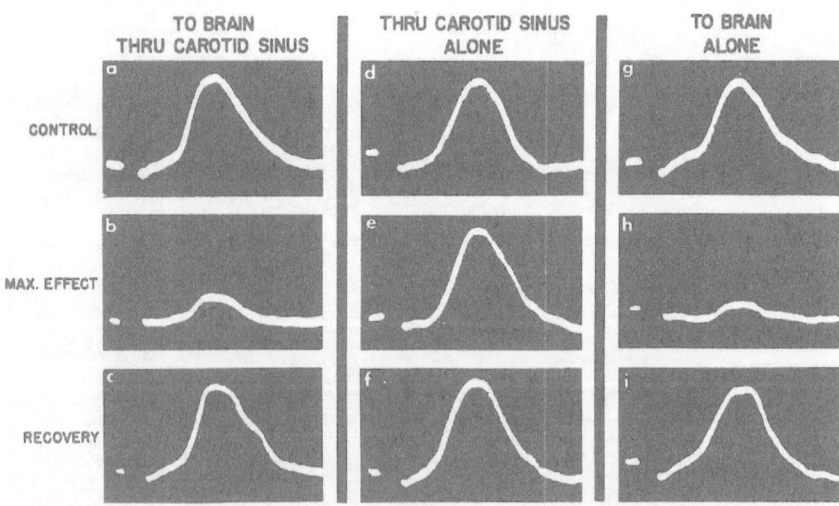

FIG. 3.   Nonparticipation of carotid sinus in serotonin inhibition of transcallosally evoked cortical potentials. Serotonin 10 μg/kg in pentobarbitalized cats.

does not differ when it is delivered to the brain alone or to the brain through the carotid sinus and, further, that perfusing the carotid sinus and carotid body region alone with serotonin produces no effect on the transcallosally evoked cortical potentials. It is therefore clear that in these experiments the carotid sinus and carotid body do not contribute to the action of the intracarotidly injected substances on the evoked cortical responses.

Before going any further, it seems wise to bring out that the cerebral synaptic inhibitory action of the compounds, whose relation to MAO inhibition we propose to examine in detail, is not manifested by a close chemical analogue, isoniazid, which is, however, almost devoid of monoamine oxidase inhibition. The chemical formulas pictured in Fig. 4 show the structural closeness of isoniazid and iproniazid. However, isoniazid, in keeping with its low MAO inhibitory potency, does not produce any effect on cerebral synaptic transmission in doses comparable to that of effective amounts of iproniazid.

To obtain a more detailed correlation between the presence of MAO inhibitors in the brain and the biochemical and functional effects, it was necessary to determine in the ipsilateral hemisphere the cerebral concentration of the MAO inhibitors, the inhibition of MAO, the concentration of serotonin, and the ability of cerebral synapses to transmit test impulses. Simultaneous curves of these data would allow point-to-point comparison to establish a degree of correlation. The MAO inhibitors used are hydrazine derivatives, and a method was developed in these laboratories [5] for measuring them by adapting to a colorimetric assay a spot test described by Feigl [6] using a phosphomolybdic acid reaction with hydrazine. MAO activity was measured by the ammonia microdiffusion method of Cotzias and Dole [7]. Serotonin was extracted by the butanol method of Bogdanski, Pletscher, Brodie, and

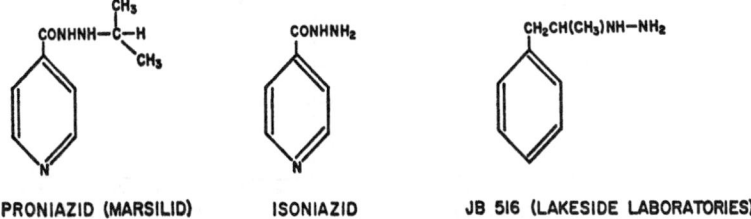

IPRONIAZID (MARSILID)   ISONIAZID   JB 516 (LAKESIDE LABORATORIES)

FIG. 4.   Formulas for iproniazid, isoniazid, and JB 516.

Udenfriend [8], separated by acidification, and read in the Aminco-Bowman spectrophotofluorometer at a fluorescence wave length of 540 mμ and an activation wave length of 295 mμ. Cerebral synaptic transmission was measured by evoking transcallosally, with constant submaximal stimuli, potentials recorded from the surface of the suprasylvian or lateral gyri in the manner customary in these laboratories [9].

These determinations were carried out in two series of cats in which the ipsilateral hemisphere was removed (and frozen immediately with liquid nitrogen) at various times after the intracarotid injection of iproniazid in one series and phenylisopropyl hydrazine (JB 516) in the other series.

RESULTS AND CONCLUSION

The simultaneous curves of the four values determined in each series are displayed in Fig. 5. The curves exhibit a convincing

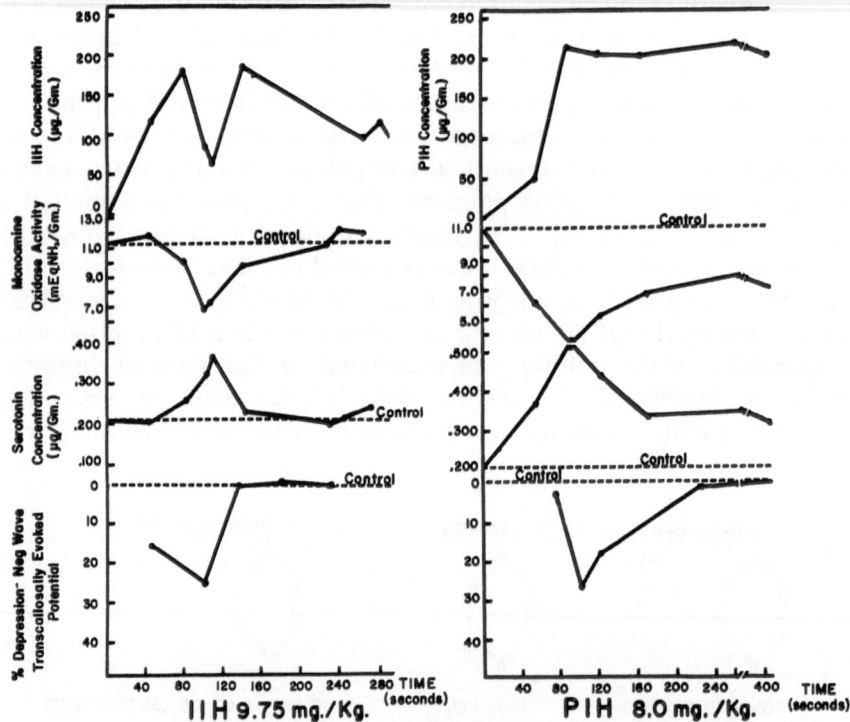

FIG. 5. Correlation of biochemical and functional data at cerebral synapses. MAO inhibitors by intracarotid injection in cat. Chemistry and evoked potentials from ipsilateral hemisphere.

correlation between a rise in cerebral concentration of MAO inhibitor and a fall in cerebral MAO titer, i.e., inhibition of MAO, a resulting rise in cerebral serotonin concentration, and a consequent reduction in cerebral synaptic transmission, as indicated by the reduction of the height of the transcallosally evoked cortical potentials. All four curves exhibit sufficiently close correlation in onset, rise to peak, fall and termination of effects to warrant the conclusion that the synaptic functional change observed was, in fact, due to *in situ* serotonin liberated by presynaptic (transcallosal) stimulation and preserved by the action of MAO inhibitors.

The data clearly demonstrate that serotonin accumulated *in situ* exercises the synaptic inhibition that was predicted on the basis of the cerebral neurohumoral inhibitory role we had previously ascribed to it [1, 2]. All but one of the criteria established for qualifying as a cerebral neurohumor are now satisfied for serotonin. It has been demonstrated that: (1) it exists in the cerebral cortex, (2) it exhibits a high potency in producing cerebral synaptic inhibition, and (3) this effect can be produced by natural serotonin when accumulated *in situ*. The last remaining criterion is the difficult one of creating the severe artifact of accumulating enough serotonin *in situ*, by excessive stimulation and by interference with its destruction, so that it can be collected in the effluent from the site. The localized perfusion required for this procedure is difficult to achieve in the brain. Nevertheless, the data presented are considered very strong evidence that serotonin is, indeed, a cerebral synaptic inhibitory neurohumor along with adrenalin, noradrenalin, and perhaps others.

DISCUSSION

The two MAO inhibitors with the powerful effects on cerebral synaptic transmission described are currently popular antidepressants. It is, therefore, highly pertinent to consider the role of such modification of cerebral synaptic transmission and of the synaptic neurohumoral equilibrium in the mechanism of the antidepressant effect.

To do so, it is necessary to understand the kind of effects that can be brought about by the synaptic action, in this case the synaptic inhibitory action of serotonin accumulated by the restraint of its destruction through the inhibition of MAO. The situation becomes clear when it is realized that the only modification in function that cells are capable of is an increase (excitation) or a decrease (inhibition) of those functions with which they are endowed and which, in the last analysis, follow from the properties of protoplasm. As diagrammed in Fig. 6, each of the primary actions, i.e., excitation and inhibition, can, when operating in a suitable network, produce secondary effects—through action on depressor rather than on activator cells—which are the opposite of the primary ones. In the case of inhibition this means that inhibition of suppressor neurons, or disinhibition, releases the final neuron to exhibit a secondary excitation.

We will recall now that we have demonstrated [, 10–12] that exogenous psychotogens like lysergic acid diethylamide (LSD-25), mescaline, bufotenin, harmaline [13], etc. produce a distortion of the cerebral synaptic equilibrium in the direction of excessive inhibition through the addition of the inhibitory action of the exogenous psychotogens to that of the normally operating neurohumoral inhibitors; and we have postulated that endogenous psychotogens may act in a similar manner. Assuming that the latter is the case in some forms of mental disturbance, it becomes evident that the preservation of serotonin through the inhibition of monoamine oxidase would aggravate the distortion of cerebral synaptic neurohumoral equilibrium that already exists in the direction of excessive inhibition. How does this fit the reported clinical findings? When iproniazid and JB 516 and the potent MAO inhibitors in general are successful, the amelioration they induce is most evident in chronic catatonic patients, who become more communicative

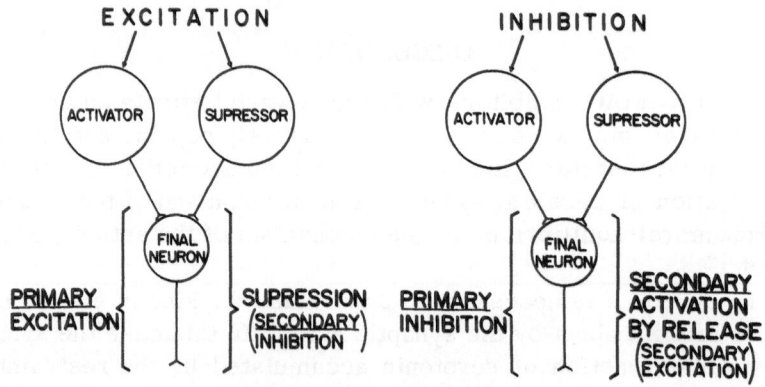

FIG. 6.   Kinds of effects due to synaptic actions.

and thereby more accessible to other therapies, particularly those dependent upon the success of interviews. Regarding catatonia as a form of inhibition, the effect would then be consistent with the inhibition of inhibition or a release or secondary activating effect of locally accumulated serotonin, as diagrammed in Fig. 6. It would thus seem that, in this instance, the illness is merely being moved from one phase of inhibition to another, which, since it happens to improve communication, makes the patient seem better and may make him, in fact, more amenable to other therapy. That such aggravation of the underlying process, interpreted here as excessive cerebral synaptic inhibition, can indeed occur is illustrated by the fact that the symptomatology in acute schizophrenia is uniformly reported as being enhanced or worsened by this type of antidepressant [14, 15].

We need to emphasize that a distortion of cerebral synaptic neurohumoral equilibrium could equally well result from an excess of excitation. This could be actual, or it could be a relative excess due to a deficiency of a neurohumoral inhibitor like serotonin. In either case the increase at the synapse of a neurohumoral inhibitor would tend to correct this condition and restore neurohumoral equilibrium. This, then, would be another possible way in which an antidepressant could act to more directly relieve the situation in that segment of the mentally disturbed population where the underlying cause is a disturbance of neurohumoral equilibrium owing to an excess of excitatory neurohumor.

Finally, because certain reportedly effective antidepressants have no significant MAO inhibitory action, the possibility needs to be entertained that the antidepressant effects of even those antidepressants that are powerful MAO inhibitors might be unrelated to the MAO inhibitory action.

SUMMARY AND CONCLUSIONS

1. The possible mode of action of antidepressants with powerful monoamine oxidase inhibitory effects has been considered in view of the possible relation between the demonstrated increase in cerebral serotonin due to such antidepressants and the disturbed cerebral synaptic neurohumoral equilibrium postulated as the underlying mechanism in some forms of mental disturbance.

2. The close correlation between the chemical changes induced, especially the increase of *in situ* serotonin, and function at cerebral

synapses has confirmed and strengthened the cerebral synaptic neurohumoral role attributed to serotonin.

3. These data make possible three alternative explanations for the mechanism of action of antidepressants which are potent monoamine oxidase inhibitors. These are:

(a) Augmentation of the existing distortion of synaptic equilibrium in the direction of inhibition by extending inhibition to sites that result in release phenomena or secondary activation.

(b) Counteraction of excessive excitation due to existing distorted cerebral synaptic neurohumoral equilibrium by the inhibitory action of the locally accumulated serotonin.

(c) An action unrelated to the monoamine oxidase inhibitory effects of these antidepressants.

These three alternatives are not necessarily contradictory, since they may apply to three different forms of mental disturbance whose underlying mechanism is characterized in one case by excessive synaptic inhibition, in another by excessive synaptic excitation, and in a third by some other as yet not clearly visualized mechanism.

REFERENCES

1. Marrazzi, A. S., and Hart, E. R.: The relationship of hallucinogens to adrenergic cerebral neurohumors, Science 121:365, 1955.

2. Gluckman, M. I., Hart, E. R., and Marrazzi, A. S.: Cerebral synaptic inhibition by serotonin and iproniazid, ibid. 126:448, 1957.

3. Marrazzi, A. S.: Psychosis as a function of disturbed chemical regulation of cerebral synaptic transmission. Rinkel, M. P., and Denber, H. C. B., Eds.: in Chemical Concepts of Psychosis, Proc. Symp. Second Internat. Congr. Psychiat. McDowell-Obolensky, New York, 1958, p. 305

4. Marrazzi, A. S.: A theory of hallucination on a neuropharmacologic basis. in Wortis, J., Ed.: Recent Advances in Biological Psychiatry, Vol. II, Grune & Stratton, New York, 1960, p. 333.

5. Horovitz, Z. P.: A Biochemical and Pharmacological Correlation of the Effects of Certain Monoamine Oxidase Inhibitors, Thesis, Univ. of Pittsburgh, 1960.

6. Feigl, F.: Spot Tests in Organic Analysis, Elsevier Publishing Co., Amsterdam, 1956, p. 469

7. Cotzias, G. C., and Dole, V. P.: Microdetermination of monoamine oxidase in tissues, J. Biol. Chem. 190:665, 1951.

8. Bogdanskı, D. F., Pletscher, A., Brodie, B. B. and Udenfriend, S.: Identification and assay of serotonin in the brain, J. Pharmacol. Exp. Therap. 117:82, 1956.

9. Marrazzi, A. S.: Methodological problems in neuropharmacological research, in Wortis, J., Ed.: Recent Advances in Biological Psychiatry, Vol. II, Grune & Stratton, New York, 1960. p. 379.

10. Marrazzi, A. S.: The effects of certain drugs on cerebral synapses. in The

Pharmacology of Psychotomimetic and Psychotherapeutic Drugs, Ann. N.Y. Acad. Sci. 66:496, 1957.

11. Marrazzi, A. S.: Synaptic and behavioral correlates of psychotherapeutic and related drug actions. in Some Biological Aspects of Schizophrenic Behavior, ibid., 96: 211, 1962.

12. Marrazzi, A. S.: Inhibition as a determinant of synaptic and behavioral patterns. in Pavlovian Conference on Higher Nervous System Activity, ibid., 92: 990, 1961.

13. Unpublished data from these laboratories.

14. Bailey, S. d'A., Bucci, L., Gosline, E., Kline, N. S., Park, I. H., Rochlin, D., Saunders, J. C., and Vaisberg, M.: Comparison of iproniazid with other amine oxidase inhibitors. in Amine Oxidase Inhibitors, ibid. 80: 643, 1959.

15. Goldman, D.: Clinical experience with newer antidepressant drugs and some related electroencephalographic observations, ibid. 80: 687, 1959.

Discussion of Chapters 14, 23, 24, and 25
by Harold E. Himwich, M.D.

I have been assigned the pleasant duty of opening the discussion on these four important papers but in the short time allotted I am forced to limit my remarks. In regard to the paper of Dr. Siva Sankar and associates, it is interesting that the metabolic changes induced by LSD were not duplicated by BOL, the brom derivative of LSD. Although both LSD and BOL are equally able to block the peripheral effects of serotonin, BOL is much inferior to LSD as a psychotomimetic drug. Even comparatively large amounts of BOL evoke less behavioral disturbance than much smaller doses of LSD. In this regard the parallelism between the slight behavioral and minimal metabolic changes with BOL is suggestive.

It is comforting to an investigator to know that his findings have been confirmed and amplified by other workers using entirely different techniques. Dr. Siva Sankar and his group noted increased urinary excretion of 5-hydroxyindole acetic acid after the administration of LSD. Freedman and Giarman [A] have found that LSD increases the serotonin content of the brain and presumably elsewhere in the body, and these experiments present one cause for the increased urinary output of the serotonin product observed in the present paper.

In reviewing the biochemical effects of such agents as mescaline and LSD, it is apparent that these drugs are not only psychotomimetic behaviorally but also mimic the metabolic disturbances observed in psychotic patients. For example, normal human subjects given LSD sufficient to produce psychotic symptoms showed a reduction in the excretion of inorganic urinary phosphate as compared with control values found in the same subjects. During the period of action of LSD, ACTH also markedly enhanced the excretion of inorganic phosphates. These effects of LSD and ACTH are evident not only in nonpsychotic human subjects but also in animals. Urinary phosphate excretion in normal guinea pigs [B] was markedly decreased by the administration of 50 mg of LSD, and these results are confirmed in the present paper for another species, namely, rats. Moreover, when ACTH and LSD were given simultaneously, the action of the latter was blocked.

Most interesting are the results that show that the levels of plasma and erythrocyte inorganic phosphate are higher in schizophrenic children. In the first place, Hoagland and co-workers [C] reported a decreased excretion of phosphates in adult schizophrenic patients as compared with normal controls in the resting state, but a greater than normal output in the patient group after the administration of ACTH. That effect of ACTH of course suggests that there is a greater retention of phosphate in the adult, a retention which results in a greater output after ACTH. In view of the difficulty in making the diagnosis of childhood schizophrenia, these correlations between adult and child metabolic alterations are especially significant. I would appreciate greatly hearing Dr. Sankar's views on this question.

The important findings reported by Dr. Williamina Himwich possess an interesting history. She had been observing the untoward effects of this combination of two different types of antidepressant drugs for over a year before the first clinical reports appeared. We all feel that it is not safe to extrapolate from one species to another and least of all to man because of his highly developed central nervous system. But in this case the exception proves the rule. We now have several clinical reports with the bad results coming from the use of imipramine (Tofranil) with monoamine oxidase inhibiting drugs. The patients exhibit profuse sweating, extreme restlessness and hyperexcitability, generalized convulsions, and hyperpyrexia, and one of these patients had a lethal exitus with a temperature of 109 F. It seems that any monoamine oxidase inhibitor yields the same results: phenelzine (Nardil), nialamide (Niamid), tranylcypromine (Parnate), iproniazid (Marsilid), isocarboxazid (Marplan), and a mixture of trifluperazine 1 mg and tranylcypromine 10 mg (Parstelin). All these monoamine oxidase inhibitors produced untoward effects when given with imipramine.

As Dr. Williamina Himwich has indicated, the mechanism involved is obscure but the message is clear. It is unwise to try to accelerate recovery from depression by using a mixture of these two different types of antidepressant drugs. I would like to ask Dr. Himwich, from the viewpoint of her observations, what special advice she can give to the clinician who has used this unfortunate combination of drugs.

The papers of Dr. Aprison and Dr. Marrazzi and co-workers were concerned with the interactions between serotonin and acetylcholine. In general, there are two fundamental processes in the passage of the nerve impulse, conduction along a nerve and transmission at a break of continuity such as synapse. This break involves the function of a chemical neurotransmitter and acetylcholine has been demonstrated to be liberated at the terminations of parasympathetic nerves, by the motor nerve in the neuromuscular junction and in synapses of the spinal cord. Similarly, noradrenalin is liberated at the terminations of sympathetic nerves. Suggestions have come that acetylcholine and noradrenalin may serve as neurotransmitters in the brain. B. B. Brodie has made the hypothesis that serotonin may be the neurotransmitter in place of acetylcholine in the brain and especially in the hypothalamus, where he also suggests that noradrenalin is active as a neurotransmitter.

There are many similarities between serotonin and acetylcholine. For example, just as there is an acetylcholine esterase to inactivate acetylcholine, so there is a monoamine oxidase to inactivate serotonin; and just as there is an anticholinesterase to cause a pile-up of acetylcholine in the brain, so there are monoamine oxidase inhibitors to cause a pile-up of serotonin. This similarity however is only superficial and does not hold on deeper analysis. Acetylcholine is found in the cell membrane and is released at specific synaptic sites. Serotonin, in contrast, is held bound in intracellular granules. Acetylcholine can exert an action on the postsynaptic membrane while serotonin is released within the cell. Acetylcholine esterase occurs in the cell membrane where acetylcholine is inactivated. Monoamine oxidase, however, occurs with mitochondria intracellularly. Thus, acetylcholine, which occurs in the periphery of the cell, is liberated there and is inactivated in the same site.

Serotonin is found within the cell, and is inactivated intracellularly. It would be difficult indeed to imagine that serotonin could mediate transmission, for it would first have to travel to the surface of the cell to effect transmission and then return within the cell for inactivation. Finally, it should be said that a monoamine oxidase inhibitor does not necessarily duplicate the same changes as those induced by an excess of serotonin. This has been shown again by the paper of Dr. Himwich.

Gertner [D] has shown that serotonin affects the function of acetylcholine in the process of transmission of the nervous impulse. Dr. Aprison offers the theory that serotonin acts as an anticholinesterase, thus preventing the destruction of acetylcholine and therefore increasing its concentration. In general, he presents two different kinds of data, *in vitro* and *in vivo*. He shows that *in vitro* serotonin can act as an anticholinesterase and offers in support a beautiful analysis of the kinetics involved in this action. It is true that Dr. Aprison offers some *in vivo* evidence as he finds that the death rate from acetylcholine poisoning is increased with the administration of serotonin. But it will still be necessary for him to show that serotonin acts as an anticholinesterase *in vivo* causing a reduction in acetyl-choline esterase activity and increasing the concentration of acetylcholine in the brain.

Dr. Marrazzi has attacked the same problem of the interaction of serotonin and acetylcholine in a different way. Many years ago Dr. Marrazzi showed that adrenalin peripherally blocks the transmission effected by acetylcholine. We have already mentioned experiments of Gertner in which he disclosed that a monoamine oxidase inhibitor blocks transmission through the superior cervical ganglion, a ganglion which releases serotonin on perfusion. Thus, the best work shows definitely that neurotransmission effected by acetylcholine can be blocked by adrenalin and by serotonin in the peripheral portions of the nervous system. Dr. Marrazzi, however, took a big step forward when he assumed the peripheral effect as a model for the central effect. He has shown us a beautiful slide where he correlates the degree of cerebral oxidase inhibition with the titer of monoamine oxidase activity, the serotonin content and intensity of cerebral synaptic transmission initiated by a constant test signal in the transcallosal system. But we have already said that a monoamine oxidase inhibitor may not only block many biogenic amines but may also exert other actions. Dr. Marrazzi must rule out other changes wrought by monoamine oxidase inhibitor drugs before he can pin this blocking at the trans-callosal synapse entirely on serotonin.

REFERENCES

A. Freedman, D. X. and Giarman, N. J.: Fed. Proc. 19:266, 1960.

B. Bergen, J. R. and Beisaw, N. E.: Fed. Proc. 15:15, 1956.

C. Hoagland, H., Rinkel, M., and Hyde, R. W.: A.M.A. Arch. Neurol. Psychiat. 73:100, 1955.

D. Gertner, S. B.: Nature 183:750, 1959.

CHAPTER 26

Studies on Mescaline XII: Effects of Prior Administration of Various Psychotropic Drugs

By PAUL RAJOTTE, M.D., HERMAN C. B. DENBER, M.D., AND DOROTHY KAUFFMAN, R.N.

In comparing the blocking action of different psychotropic drugs on the mescaline-induced state, chlorpromazine and triflupromazine were found to be the most active, prochlorperazine and thiopropazate moderately so, while diethazine accentuated the mescaline response. Promazine and promethazine were ineffective, a finding concurring with that in clinical practice. The intramuscular injection of these drugs after mescaline did not influence the continuous fall of amino acids and eosinophils [1].

The halogen on the phenothiazine nucleus was felt to be related to the antipsychotic effect, since chlorpromazine was far superior to promazine. There was no apparent explanation, however, for the marked blocking activity of the nonpiperazine phenothiazines against mescaline as opposed to those with a piperazine side chain. This seemed to contradict the results in daily clinical practice, for halogenated piperazine derivatives have a more rapid action on hallucinatory syndromes than chlorpromazine; the latter is particularly effective in anxiety states.

Why do barbiturates block the mescaline-induced state completely yet have no direct or immediate action in the psychoses? Does mescaline simply produce a biochemical anxiety stress[2] which can be neutralized by any sedative agent? Could the prior administration of some psychotropic drugs inhibit the mescaline-induced state in a fashion analogous to their clinical activity? If so, this might serve as a simple screening device for new drugs [3].

THE SETTING

The patients chosen for this study were treated in the research division ward of Manhattan State Hospital, a 3000–bed institution of the New York State Department of Mental Hygiene. The ward has 55 acute and chronic female patients, most of them schizophrenic, and is run along the principles of a therapeutic community [4, 5]; all patients are fully aware of its particular nature. The staff carries on various research activities and, in addition, performs the hospital service functions.

MATERIALS AND METHODS

There were 39 trials in 38 patients (Table I) receiving a drug or saline followed by mescaline or saline. They had not been taking any medication for at least ninety-six hours before and were fasting on the morning of the test. The following compounds administered intramuscularly were unknown to the observer: 50 mg of chlorpromazine (five patients), 200 mg of diethazine (seven patients), 250 mg of Sodium Amytal (six patients), 20 mg of amphetamine* (eight patients), 5 mg of haloperidol (five patients), 3 mg of thioperazine (five patients), and 5 cc of physiological saline solution (three patients). One-half hour afterwards 500 mg of mescaline sulfate dissolved in 20 cc of physiological saline was injected intravenously. Saline (20 cc) was substituted for mescaline in the controls.

Before a patient received mescaline, she was told: "You will have a test once or, perhaps, more than once, depending on the

*d,l-amphetamine sulfate.

TABLE I

Clinical Diagnoses

Diagnosis	No. Cases
Schizophrenia	
Paranoid	15
Catatonic	6
Mixed	6
Simple	2
Hebephrenic	1
Psychoneurotic	6
Manic-Depressive	2
Total	38

results. Tomorrow I will give you an injection and you will simply
tell me how it makes you feel. We will also take blood a few times.
I will stay with you all the time. If you have any questions, you can
ask me now or talk with the other patients who have already had
the test. But whatever you hear, remember that nobody reacts
exactly the same way."

The immediate effects of the drugs (or saline) were considered
as either (1) producing drowsiness or (2) being ineffective. The
clinical reactions to mescaline were observed during four hours
and tabulated under four headings: (1) verbal, (2) motor, (3) neurovegetative, and (4) perceptual. The reactions in each group were
graded as either marked, moderate, or mild. They were termed
marked (3+) when the mescaline effects were present at least two-
thirds of the observation period, moderate (2+) when the symptoms
lasted more than one-third and less than two-thirds of the four-hour
observation time, minimal (1+) when the symptoms occurred over
a duration of time totaling less than 75 minutes. Appraisal of the
total response was made by the sum of the separate reactions. In
this way, unequal reactions in any one or all of the above categories
were taken into account. Where the additive scores of all four groups
totalled 4+ or less, the grading was one of a total mild response.
A total moderate response was 5+ to 8+, and more than 8+ constituted a total marked response.

All patients were interviewed the next day to obtain additional
information or to clarify the meaning of some ambiguous findings.

RESULTS

The immediate effect of a single dose of chlorpromazine produced drowsiness in four of five patients. Diethazine gave the same
effect in four of seven patients, and Sodium Amytal in two of six.
Amphetamine increased the verbal productivity in seven of eight
patients. The other drugs were without effect.

Chlorpromazine proved to be the most effective inhibiting agent
of the mescaline-induced state (Table II). There were four marked
responses in the diethazine group. These patients had a very severe
reaction to mescaline in the verbal, motor, and perceptual spheres.

There were one marked, five moderate, and two mild responses
in the amphetamine group. Sodium Amytal had little effect upon the
sequence of events in five of six patients. The saline sample (three
patients) was too small to allow any conclusions.

TABLE II

Response to Mescaline According to the Preinjected Blocking Agents
(39 trials in 38 patients)

Blocking Agent	Intensity of Response			Total No. Cases
	Mild	Moderate	Marked	
Chlorpromazine	4	1	0	5
Thioperazine	0	4	1	5
Haloperidol	1	4	0	5
Diethazine	2	1	4	7
Saline	1	1	1	3
Amytal	1	2	3	6
Amphetamine	2	5	1	8

The neurovegetative reactions were minimal with chlorpromazine, haloperidol, and in four of five patients receiving thioperazine
but were moderate or marked with amphetamine, diethazine, Sodium
Amytal and saline. Perceptual changes were absent in all cases
pretreated with chlorpromazine and thioperazine but were present
to varying degrees in the others. The changes were not always
verbalized but could be inferred from the patient's behavior. When
a mute subject lengthily examined her hand, turning it around with
a bewildered look, it was interpreted as a perceptual change. The
following day's interview always confirmed the clinical observations.

It made little difference for the end result with chronic schizophrenic patients if a neuroleptic or other drug was given (Table III).
The schizophrenic patients in remission showed one marked and
five moderate responses with a neuroleptic, while there were six
marked and five moderate responses with nonneuroleptics.

The blocking effect produced by the injection of a drug before
mescaline was much less pronounced than when given afterwards.
A complete block was never obtained, and even with a minimal
response some mild autonomic changes were noted during the first
half-hour. The duration and intensity of the mescaline-induced

TABLE III

Response to Mescaline According to Diagnostic Groups and Comparing the Action of Preinjected Neuroleptic and Nonneuroleptic Substances

Diagnostic Groups	Mild		Moderate		Marked	
	Neuroleptic	Nonneur.	Neuroleptic	Nonneur.	Neuroleptic	Nonneur.
Acute schizophrenia	0	1	1	2	0	0
Remitted schizophrenia	1	1	5	5	1	6
Chronic schizophrenia	3	3	0	1	0	1
Psychoneurosis	1	1	3	0	0	1
Manic-depressive psychosis	0	0	0	1	0	1
Total (38 patients)	5	6	9	8	1	9

state were decreased in general, and after an hour or so the response was already waning. There was one marked response with a neuroleptic blocking agent* in 15 cases, whereas nine such responses occurred among 23 patients given other drugs. This was in distinct contrast to the observations made when mescaline was given alone; the one-hour postmescaline period corresponded with the appearance of varied and intense signs and symptoms [3].

With the prior administration of a neuroleptic, instead of the sharp verbal and motor expressions of anxiety and discomfort one frequently heard complaints such as, "This whole thing is boring... it is too long...I wish I could be back on the ward." It was necessary to terminate the mescaline-induced state with the aid of chlorpromazine only once because of uncontrollable symptoms, when a neuroleptic was used for initial blocking action. On the other hand, this was done four times with diethazine, twice each with saline and amphetamine, and once with Amytal.

*Chlorpromazine, thioperazine, and haloperidol.

DISCUSSION

While we were unable to assert definitely that diethazine aggravated the response to mescaline (since the summed action of both drugs was being observed), the evidence is very suggestive, inasmuch as four of the ten marked responses occurred in this group.

Amphetamine did not enhance the mescaline-induced state, with two mild, five moderate, and one marked response. When four of these patients received saline-mescaline in a third series of trials, three had identical reactions (moderate), while the fourth had a severe response.*

It has been indicated elsewhere that the clinical state induced by mescaline is neither an intoxication, a neurosis, nor a psychosis but a state of being in which the clinical spectrum runs from sleep to murderous rage and from normality to thoroughly disorganized states [6]. Schizophrenic subjects react to mescaline in a manner about inversely proportional to the length of their illness [7]. It is difficult to attribute the results in an acutely ill psychotic subject to either the drug or the illness. When the drug is given in a phase of remission, the psychosis is reactivated for the test period; administered to a chronic schizophrenic subject, it hardly produces any reaction. Eight patients had chronic schizophrenia (average duration of present hospitalization 47.1 months), and six of these had a mild response. Twenty-two belonged to the schizophrenic group in remission (average duration of present hospitalization 4 months), and of these two had a mild reaction as opposed to seventeen with a moderate or marked response (Table III).

There were five moderate responses with neuroleptic and nonneuroleptic drugs in the remitted schizophrenic group. Since the nonneuroleptic compounds should not have had an inhibitory effect upon the mescaline-induced state, the material was analyzed further. Three of the group having had a moderate reaction received amphetamine before mescaline. Biochemical studies have shown that intravenous mescaline caused an immediate fall in the level of ninhydrin-positive substances, and significance was achieved by one-half hour [2]. The fall of ninhydrin-positive substances and the intensity of the clinical reactions were correlated; the levels of the former fell as the mescaline-induced reaction became more intense. Immediately following amphetamine there was a rise in these levels,

*This was not the same patient who had a marked response in the original trials.

while the fall after mescaline was delayed, not attaining significance until two hours afterwards [3]. In view of these findings and as suggested by the clinical results, it can be inferred that there is some biochemical antagonism between amphetamine and mescaline.

The neurovegetative signs and clinical reactions with amphetamine were dissociated, with the former moderate to marked and the latter mild to moderate. This suggests that the autonomic reactions function independently of the cortical responses in this case.

What could be the nature of the mescaline stress? In schizophrenia, mescaline generates anxiety as the foremost symptom and other emotions are noticeably absent. The anxiety could result from the patient's changed apperception of the world and his body. The schizophrenic subject may view this as a destructive event with loss of and/or transformation of the body or its parts. Because he does not know how far these changes will proceed, terror becomes more and more marked. The intense anxiety leads one to wonder if the patient is not equating them to changes in the world and self. Theoretically, if this goes far enough, it could lead to symbolic death, explaining to some degree the severe psychological and motor reactions with mescaline. The neurotic patients, on the other hand, recognize the boundaries of the mescaline-induced state, and their anxiety does not have the devastating effects seen with schizophrenic patients. The former ofttimes tend to describe their reaction as "thrilling."

Perceptual changes were found only once with chlorpromazine and thioperazine. The presence of perceptual distortions is indicative of a disorganization of those central functions subserving man's relation in time and space. Mescaline seems to remove the normal protective filter mechanisms that prevent the organism from being overwhelmed by a flood of sensory stimuli. When these restrictions no longer exist, there is a state of confusion with perceptual discrimination no longer possible. Thus, like the patients of Davie and Freeman [8], they confused various peripheral stimuli. ("There is my father in the doorway. He'll kill me.") The patient responds with the autonomic nervous system to the drugs since this is probably a more primitive response, but when protected (chlorpromazine and thioperazine) the reaction is stopped. Where the contrary is true (diethazine, Amytal, and saline), the autonomic reaction is followed by the symptoms due to mescaline. Chlorpromazine and thioperazine, which protect against the perceptual changes due to mescaline, do the same in clinical practice.

Our data yield no reason for the greater clinical effectiveness of piperazine phenothiazines as opposed to their decreased ability to block mescaline. The measurement of the ninhydrin-positive substances during the mescaline-induced state seems to offer a more reliable index of the drug's clinical activity than the clinical responses. As our studies continue with increased numbers in each group, some of these questions will probably be answered.

The mescaline stress has some specificity with regard to those compounds that will block the different symptoms. Sodium Amytal, with its sedative properties, was ineffective, yet chlorpromazine, also sedative but antipsychotic, was very effective. It is difficult to say why intravenous barbiturates administered after mescaline will block its effects [9] while prior intramuscular injection does not. The route of administration may be a factor, and further studies will test this.

In view of the relationship between the blocking effects of different drugs on the induction of the mescaline-induced state and their correlation with results in clinical psychiatric practice, we are led to believe that the drug-induced condition can be considered as an analogy of the endogenous psychosis without at the same time suggesting any specificity. Only continued investigation will either demonstrate the validity of such a hypothesis or show it to be a fallacy [10].

SUMMARY AND CONCLUSIONS

1. Chlorpromazine, thioperazine, haloperidol, Sodium Amytal, d,l-amphetamine sulfate, diethazine, and saline were administered in 39 trials to 38 patients before mescaline. Chlorpromazine was most potent, followed by thioperazine and haloperidol, in blocking the induction of the mescaline-induced state.

2. There was little differentiation in the end result with a chronic schizophrenic subject if a neuroleptic or other drug was given. On the other hand, for the schizophrenic patients in remission, the neuroleptics were able to block most of the symptoms, while the other drugs could not.

3. There is a certain antagonism between amphetamine and mescaline, which is supported by the biochemical and clinical data.

4. Some theoretical considerations have been made about the nature of the mescaline stress.

REFERENCES

1. Denber, H. C. B., and Merlis, S.: Studies on mescaline VI: Therapeutic aspects of the mescaline-chlorpromazine combination, J. Nerv. Ment. Dis. 122:463, 1955.

2. Denber, H. C. B.: Studies on mescaline XI: Biochemical findings during the mescaline-induced state with observations on the blocking action of different psychotropic drugs, Psychiat. Quart. 35:18, 1961.

3. Denber, H. C. B., Teller, D. N., Rajotte, P., and Kauffman, D.: Studies on mescaline XIII: The effect of prior administration of various psychotropic drugs on different biochemical parameters: a preliminary report. Ann. N.Y. Acad. Sci. 96:14, 1962.

4. Denber, H. C. B.: A therapeutic community: analysis of its operation after two years. in Denber, H. C. B., Ed.: Research Conference on Therapeutic Community, Springfield, Charles C. Thomas, 1960.

5. Denber, H. C. B.: A study of the therapeutic community. in Masserman, J., and Moreno, J. R., Eds.: Progress in Psychotherapy, New York, Grune & Stratton, Inc., 1960.

6. Denber, H. C. B.: Clinical considerations of the mescaline-induced state. in Rinkel, M., and Denber, H. C. B., Eds.: Chemical Concepts of Psychosis, New York, McDowell Oblensky, Inc., 1958.

7. Merlis, S.: The effects of mescaline sulfate in chronic schizophrenia, J. Nerv. Ment. Dis. 125:432, 1957.

8. Davie, J., and Freeman, T.: Disturbances of perception and consciousness in schizophrenic states, Brit. J. M. Psychol. 34:33, 1961.

9. Hoch, P. H.: Psychosis producing and psychosis relieving drugs. in The Brain and Human Behavior, ARND, Baltimore, Vol. 36, The Williams & Wilkens Company, 1958.

10. Hollister, L.: Drug-induced psychoses and schizophrenic reactions: a critical comparison, Ann. N. Y. Acad. Sci. 96:80, 1962.

Discussion by Sidney Merlis, M.D., F.A.C.P.

The data presented by Drs. Rajotte and Denber and Miss Kauffman are at once provocative and novel. To my knowledge, it is one of the first attempts using a well-defined consistent research design to establish an answer to a question which has been in the minds of all of us whose interest and work have had to do with the psychotomimetic drugs. Much has been written about mescaline and LSD-25 and related compounds. Reports have ranged from basic well-prepared physiological reports to fanciful clinical reports suggesting promising clinical and therapeutic activity which for the most part has been disappointing.

It is only in very recent times that these drug effects have been removed from the category of being considered as producing a schizophrenic-like condition and are now more accurately described as a toxic state. The early hopes and expectations that researchers felt with the introduction of these compounds have to a very large extent not materialized. The compounds have not been unequivocally accepted as therapeutic agents. They have not fulfilled the promise of giving us major insight into the dynamics and physiology of schizophrenia. Dr. Denber and his associates are among the few investigators who have continued their clinical research activities with mescaline and over the past few years have significantly contributed to our understanding of the physiological and psychodynamic correlations relative to this drug-induced state.

The work involves a rather interesting concept, namely, the attempt to correlate clinical effectiveness of various psychotropic agents to alterations of the mescaline response. It is an effort to present information which is so necessary to bridge the gap that exists between the use of psychotomimetic drugs as experimental agents and the psychotic disturbances that we see clinically in our patients.

There are several points in this report which require some comment. In essence, the data represent an effort to study the psychotropic drug effect by means of a human bioassay method utilizing mescaline as the standard. Pharmacologists are ordinarily reluctant to use bioassay methods unless no other means are available. To this extent the procedure is justified in the paper just read. The criteria, however, for reliability of any bioassay method, because of its inherent variability, can only be discounted by adequate experimental trials and the use of suitable statistical methods. This the authors have indicated will eventually be done. The final evaluation of the suitability of this procedure must await additional trials.

The obstacles of natural patient variability and diverse clinical responses to so complex a drug as mescaline is not so easily discounted. Subjects who receive mescaline show a great variety of reactions to the drug. What is even more significant and to a large extent not too often described is that individual subjects show different responses to mescaline on different days. To further complicate the picture, it is known that various psychotomimetic drug antagonists when used alone can also show highly individualized and equally diverse reactions.

Further considerations require a more specific clarification of the distinction between a true pharmacological antagonism (blocking) and actual suppression. We must differentiate more precisely between evidence of specific blocking with rather modest doses of a compound and a masking or suppression secondarily related to impaired awareness in heavily premedicated individuals. It would appear, for example, that the barbiturates act by such a suppressive action.

While the psychological changes in the mescaline state are less easily predictable and thus more subject to errors in individual evaluations, the physiological reactions are somewhat more characteristic and thus may be used to some degree as a parameter of drug effect. One must always remember that the physiological responses are compatible with a general bodily response to external stress and are not specific for mescaline alone.

Lastly, I would like to point out that the thesis presented by the authors is an analogical argument. Namely, the program of research here described is inferring a further degree of resemblance from an already observed degree. The doctrine of signatures formerly so prevalent in therapeutic medicine is being implied with the psychotomimetic drugs. In the past, walnuts were prescribed for brain diseases because they physically so resembled a brain and bear grease was used for baldness because bears are so hairy. Mescaline has been used in the same manner because of the seeming resemblance of its effect to schizophrenia. Dr. Denber and his associates are acutely aware of the problems relative to this type of research. He uses good judgement and considerable restraint in presenting his data. He is particularly aware of the limitations imposed, and because of this awareness the data presented must be considered as most meaningful. I, for one, shall look for additional reports in this most interesting series of studies.

CHAPTER 27

Effects and Interactions of Imipramine, Chlorpromazine, Reserpine and Amphetamine on Self-Stimulation: Possible Neurophysiological Basis of Depression

By LARRY STEIN, Ph.D.

Neural theorizing about the affective disorders has been given substance by recent discoveries of brain systems for positive and negative reinforcement. Brain loci for negative motivation were demonstrated by Delgado, Roberts, and Miller [1] in experiments that followed up the early work of Hess [2]. These investigators showed that electrical stimulation of certain thalamic and hippo-campal sites in the cat could be substituted for painful stimulation for the motivation of several forms of learning, including the conditioning of anxiety. Shortly thereafter, Olds and Milner [3] reported that electrical stimulation of the septal region and parts of the hypothalamus had the effect of a powerful reward. This was ingeniously demonstrated by a "self-stimulation" experiment in which rats with permanent electrodes were trained to stimulate their own brains thousands of times per hour by pressing a lever. These findings have been generalized to a number of species and have been extended even to man. In the human studies, subjective reports of pleasure and pain have been obtained after electrical stimulation of specific subcortical regions [4].

From this work it is not unreasonable to infer the presence of centers for reward and aversion whose function is to provide feedback to motor programming circuits based on the consequences of on-going behavior. The feedback is positive in the case of reward or negative in the case of punishment—go or stop. Presumably these

Recipient of the A. E. Bennett Award for research in biological psychiatry.

motivational centers are in delicate balance and reciprocally inhibit each other.

As a first guess, we have tentatively taken the view that agitations and depressions result from disturbances in the balance between the motivational centers. Put simply, agitations result from pathological overactivity of reward function (too much go), and depression from underactivity (too little go). Olds [5, 6] originated the hypothesis with respect to the agitations and documented it with pharmacological findings. Chlorpromazine, which successfully controls psychotic agitation, inhibited self-stimulation of reward structures at low doses, while other central depressants, like meprobamate and pentobarbital, which are not specific for the control of agitation failed to inhibit self-stimulation at comparable doses.

This paper is concerned with the explication and experimental test of the part of the hypothesis that deals with depression. Briefly, it is suggested that the depressed patient suffers from insufficient positive reinforcement. Even normal people, of course, become depressed during periods of low "pay-off." The depressive, however, despairs even when the environment supplies a normal amount of reinforcement. In neural terms we assume the reward system of the depressive is pathologically hypoactive despite a normal input. We propose further that this hypoactivity may be due either to some defect within the reward system, or may result from the inhibition of this system by the excessive activity of the antagonistic anxiety-aversion system. We are tempted in the former case to speak of withdrawn or passive depression and in the latter case of agitated depression.*

Like Olds [5, 6], we will attempt to document our speculations with pharmacological evidence obtained from self-stimulation tests, using drugs that have known clinical actions. In this presentation, we report the effects, and particularly the interactions, of two

---

*Experimental models of the two conditions are suggested by well-established findings in experimental psychology. Withdrawn or passive depression, the case where reward function is intrinsically weak, may be viewed as analogous to experimental extinction. In experimental extinction, the reinforcement for a previously rewarded response is withheld. After a number of nonrewarded responses are emitted, the trained behavior gradually drops out. Agitated depression, the case where essentially normal reward centers are suppressed by the excessive activity of aversion centers, may have a model in the conditioned suppression situation of Estes and Skinner [7], and Hunt and Brady [8]. In these experiments, ongoing, positively reinforced, operant (lever-pressing) behavior is suppressed in the presence of a stimulus that, through previous conditioning, evokes an anxiety or conditioned fear reaction. Thus the same result, depression of positively reinforced behavior, may be achieved by quite different means and also may be accompanied by different "secondary" or associated reactions.

antidepressant drugs, imipramine and amphetamine, and two tranquilizing or depressant drugs, chlorpromazine and reserpine.* Particular attention has been paid to the comparison of imipramine and chlorpromazine. These chemically similar compounds appear to differ qualitatively in their clinical actions, but published experimental data have provided little basis as yet for this qualitative difference [9]. We will present evidence indicating opposite psychopharmacological actions for these drugs.

MATERIALS AND METHODS

Adult male rats were implanted stereotaxically with permanent bipolar platinum electrodes in the hypothalamus or midbrain tegmentum. Some typical positively reinforcing locations and their stereotaxic coordinates are indicated in Fig. 1. The platinum wires were 0.01 in. in diameter, twisted together and insulated except at the tips. In early studies the stimulus was a paired-pulse waveform described by Lilly et al. [10]. The intensity of the Lilly waveform was varied between 5 to 10 ma. For most of the work reported here the stimulating waveform was a square pulse of 0.2-msec duration presented at 100 pulses/sec through a cathode follower output stage and an isolation transformer to the electrodes [11]. The intensities

*The term "antidepressant" is used here loosely to designate compounds having either antidepressive or euphorigenic activities. Stricter usage would reserve this term for the present for imipramine, its derivatives, and monoamine oxidase inhibitors. Amphetamine (and related phenethylamine derivatives) is more properly classified with cocaine and caffeine as a psychostimulant. See Stein [19] for further discussion of these classifications.

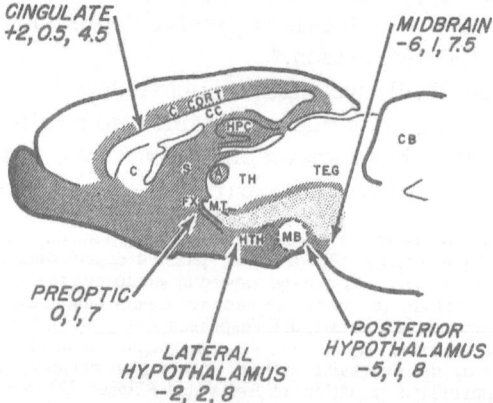

FIG. 1. Map of reward areas (shaded) and punishment areas (stippled). The stereotaxic coordinates are given in millimeters in the following order: antero-posterior from bregma, lateral from midline, depth from surface of brain (after Olds [5]).

of this waveform ranged from 0.25 to 0.5 ma. Both stimulating conditions were relatively noninjurious and thus allowed the self-stimulation base lines to be stable for many months.

In the present experiments a modified version of the self-stimulation technique was used, which we have described in detail elsewhere [12]. This technique has the animal automatically trace its threshold for the rewarding stimulation continuously for periods of 6 hours or more. In preliminary training the animals learn to obtain brief (0.15 second) trains of current of fixed intensity by operating a lever. After the rates of self-stimulation have stabilized, the automatic threshold schedule training is begun. The procedure is illustrated in Fig. 2. The animal works in a two-lever chamber, as shown to the right. To obtain the rewarding electrical stimulation, the animal must operate the lever marked "stim." Each successive brain shock, however, is reduced in intensity by a small step. Our best results have been obtained when 15 to 20 equal current steps are available between a moderately rewarding top value and zero. The second lever can be operated at any time to reset the current to the top step. The reset lever never gives brain shocks. In this procedure, then, the animal operates the stimulation lever until the current is driven down to a nonrewarding or unsatisfactory level, and then tells the experimenter what this level is by operating the reset lever.

The projected detail shows how this set of events is recorded. The short horizontal bars on the ordinate indicate the 18 current steps that are available. The recording pen, following the decreasing brain shocks, starts at the top and moves downwards one step with

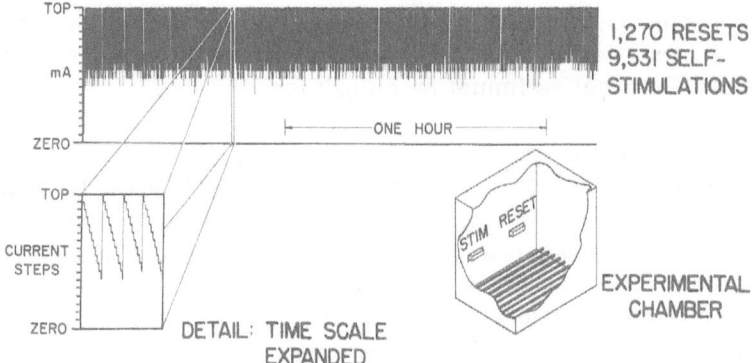

FIG. 2. Method of recording the performance in the automatic threshold procedure and diagram of the two-lever chamber.

each response at the stimulation lever. When the current is driven below the reward threshold, the reset lever is activated, causing the stimulator and the recording pen to reset to the top. The animal then starts the next stimulation series. The jagged edge of the curve at the bottom gives, in sequence, the current intensities at which resets occurred and thus traces the reward threshold.

An actual record of performance for a highly trained animal appears in the upper section of the slide. The stability of the performance is evident. With a week's rest between sessions, records like this one can be obtained for many months. These chronic preparations have the great advantage of permitting the comparison of many different drugs within the same animal.

Pharmacological tests were not begun until the individual self-stimulation performances had clearly stabilized. Also, on each test day we would allow sufficient time for the base line to stabilize before making the injection. As a rule, we would attempt to follow the entire action through to recovery whenever possible. Frequently, however, the recoveries only were partial.

At least a week was allowed between dosings of the drugs to permit the effects to wear off. All doses are expressed in terms of the total salt except for reserpine. For this drug the doses are given in terms of the base. All injections were intraperitoneal.

RESULTS

Drug-induced changes in the excitability of the stimulated structures may be discerned by a glance at the records. Sensitizing drugs lower the threshold and cause resetting to occur at lower current steps. Conversely, inhibiting drugs elevate the threshold and cause resetting to occur at higher current steps; in large doses, they may inhibit self-stimulation altogether.

Direct Effects of the Drugs

In the discussion above we assumed, with Olds, that the tranquilizing drugs, chlorpromazine and reserpine, act by inhibiting the brain structures mediating reward effects. In our test these drugs were expected to elevate the reward threshold and cause resetting to occur at higher current steps. Figure 3 shows this to be the case for a representative animal with an electrode in a reward area of the midbrain tegmentum. A control injection of saline produced no important effect. Shortly thereafter, a 2-mg/kg dose of chlorpromazine caused resetting to occur at higher current steps, starting

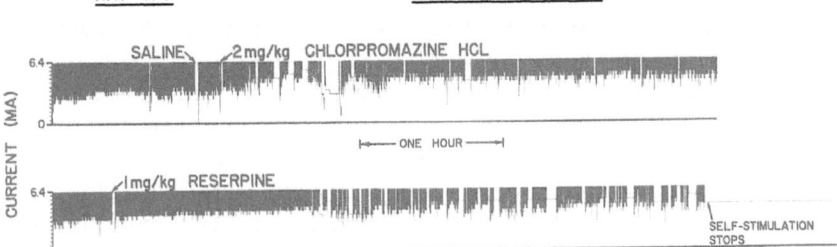

FIG. 3.   Effects of chlorpromazine and reserpine on self-stimulation threshold performance.

about 10 minutes after the injection. At the peak of the effect self-stimulation was inhibited completely for brief periods, indicated by the white spaces. Reserpine at 1 mg/kg elevated the threshold slightly after about 45 minutes; then it produced pausing for approximately 2 hours; and finally it inhibited self-stimulation altogether for the rest of the day. When this animal was tested again three days later the base line was abnormally high. Recovery to the prereserpine level required twelve days.

A similar effect and a similar pattern of recovery from a single dose of reserpine (0.6 mg/kg) may be seen in Fig. 4 in another

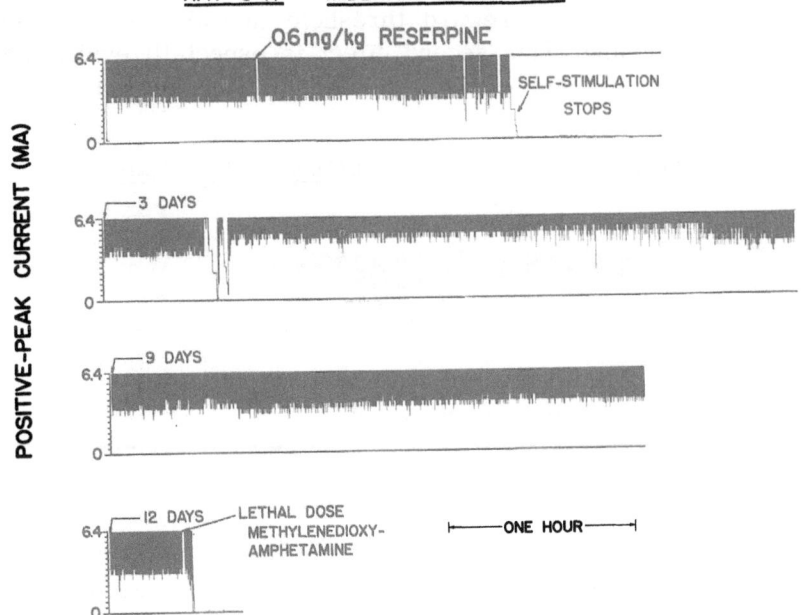

FIG. 4   Effects of a single dose of reserpine traced for twelve days.

rat with a midbrain electrode. This animal, the most stable per-
former we ever had, was killed by an unfortunate overdosing of
methylenedioxyamphetamine twelve days after the reserpine injection. Close inspection of the predrug base line in the top and
bottom records suggests, however, that recovery from the effects
of the reserpine dosing was complete after twelve days.

One important aspect of the inhibitory effects of both chlorpromazine and reserpine should be made clear. The animals were
carefully observed at the height of the drug effects, during the
time that self-stimulation was inhibited altogether. No obvious
impairment of motor functions could be seen. It just seemed that
the animals were no longer interested in brain stimulation.

Opposite effects on reward thresholds were predicted for the
antidepressant drugs, amphetamine (or methamphetamine) and
imipramine. These drugs were expected to facilitate the activity
of the reward structures and thereby cause resetting to occur at
lower current steps. Figure 5 shows this to be true in the case of
methamphetamine but not of imipramine. This animal, implanted in
the lateral hypothalamus had a characteristically "spotty" base line
performance due to frequent pausing between bursts of self-stimulation. After a brief period of warm-up, however, the base line level
of resetting may be seen to be stable. D-methamphetamine at
2 mg/kg lowered the reward threshold and also decreased the
amount of pausing. This second effect is especially evident after
the threshold-lowering effect had worn off. The session was ter-

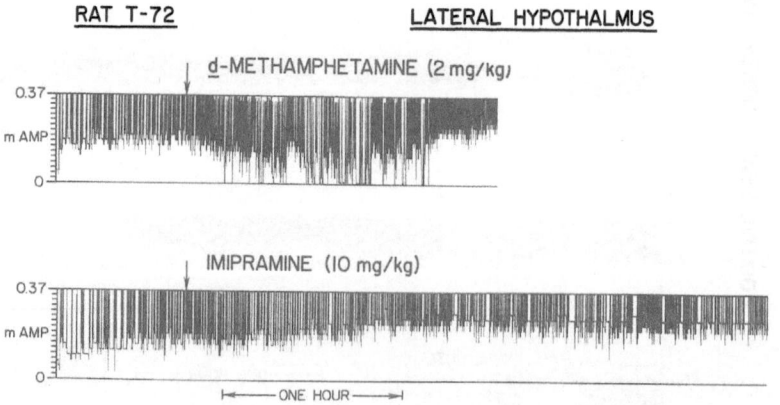

FIG. 5. Effects of d-methamphetamine and imipramine on self-stimulation threshold performance.

minated before this unexpected action of methamphetamine had dissipated. (A better demonstration of this effect may be seen in Fig. 6.)

Contrary to prediction, imipramine (10 mg/kg) raised the threshold for reward (Fig. 5). Lower doses of this drug had no effect, and larger doses produced greater inhibition; these tests indicate that imipramine, given by itself, has the same qualitative action as chlorpromazine on self-stimulation. Chlorpromazine was found to be about ten times more potent as an inhibitor. These results coincide with published pharmacological findings [13].

The effect of d-amphetamine on pausing is demonstrated for an animal with a midbrain electrode in Fig. 6. After the drug wears off, the pausing returns. The 0.5-mg/kg dose of d-amphetamine was too small to produce lowering of the threshold in this animal. It appears that amphetamine can make a spotty animal dependable, while chlorpromazine or reserpine can make a dependable animal spotty.

Interaction of the Drugs

If the two classes of drugs act in opposite ways on the same brain system, as assumed in the discussion above, it should be possible to demonstrate antagonisms and reversals between their effects. Furthermore, members of the same class might be expected to augment each other's actions.

Figure 7 shows that the inhibiting effect of chlorpromazine (1 mg/kg) can be reversed by d-amphetamine (0.75 mg/kg). This animal, like others with posterior hypothalamic electrodes, was especially sensitive to both drugs. The sensitivity is evidenced by

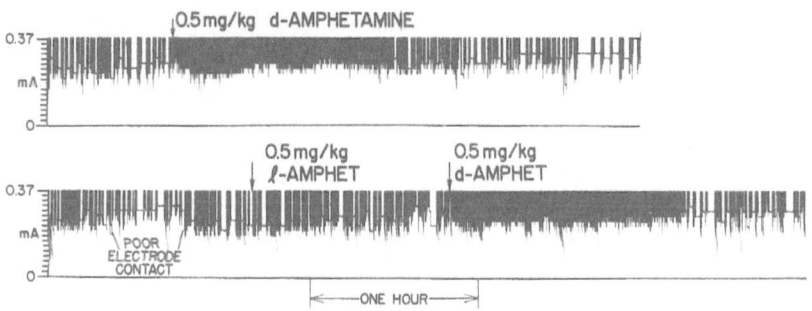

FIG. 6. Elimination of pausing (white spaces) by d-amphetamine. Note the slight effect of l-amphetamine and the reproducibility of the d-amphetamine effect.

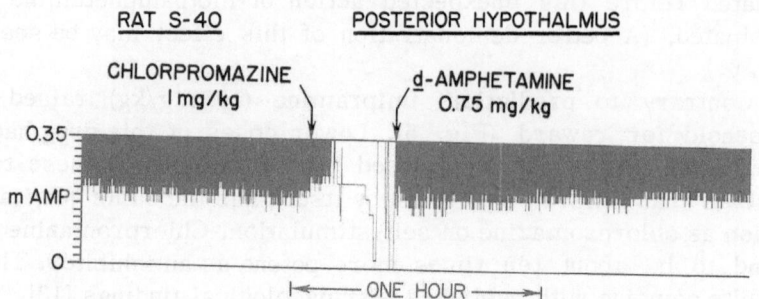

FIG. 7. Reversal of chlorpromazine-induced inhibition of self-stimulation by d-amphetamine.

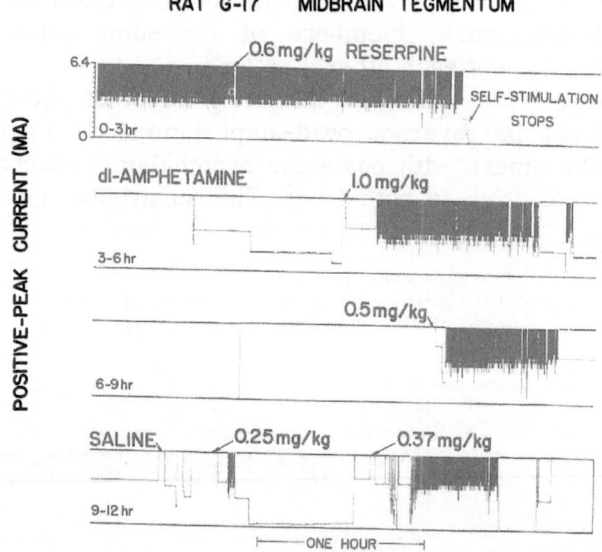

FIG. 8. Graded durations of reversal of reserpine inhibition of self-stimulation by various doses of dl-amphetamine.

the low doses of the drugs required for the effects and the rapid onsets of their actions.

The reversal of reserpine-induced inhibition of self-stimulation by various doses of dl-amphetamine is depicted in Fig. 8. A single, continuous, 12-hour record of performance is shown, broken into four equal sections for ease of presentation. After a control hour of the recording of responses to establish the base line, a single dose (0.6 mg/kg) of reserpine was injected (top section). The drug took effect after approximately one hour and would have eliminated the self-stimulation behavior for the rest of the day if amphetamine were not given. Four injections of dl-amphetamine, ranging from 0.25 to 1.0 mg/kg, were administered at intervals during the day. Self-stimulation was restored after each amphetamine injection and the duration of the recovery was related to the amount injected. A test injection of saline failed to restore self-stimulation. (The small amount of apparent activity after saline represents several "free" stimulations given by the experimenter.)

Even more interesting were the interactions between the anti-depressant drugs, imipramine and methamphetamine. The effects of pretreating with either imipramine or chlorpromazine on the response to methamphetamine are compared in Fig. 9. The upper curve shows the effect of 1-mg/kg dose of d-methamphetamine. A moderate lowering of the threshold lasting for about an hour may be noted. The dose was chosen deliberately to produce a small but reliable effect. The middle curve shows the effect of pretreating with chlorpromazine 20 minutes before the methamphetamine

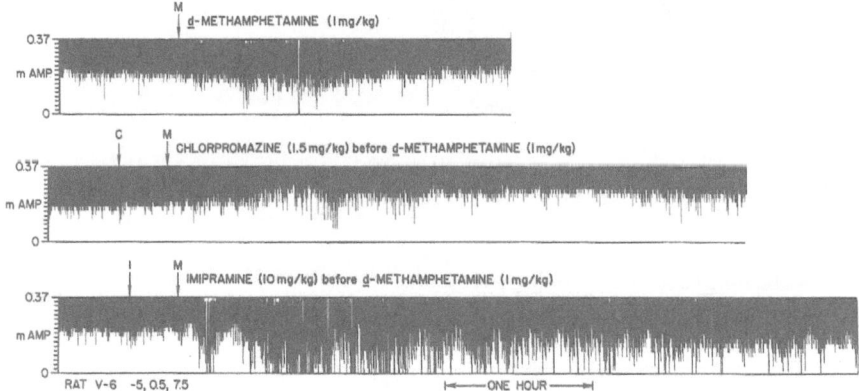

FIG. 9. Opposite effects of chlorpromazine and imipramine on the threshold-lowering effect of d-methamphetamine.

injection. The inhibitory effect of this dose of chlorpromazine evidently was somewhat stronger than the facilitating effect of the methamphetamine so that the net effect produced was an elevation of the threshold that lasted for more than three hours. The bottom curve shows the profound augmentation of the methamphetamine response that is produced by pretreatment with imipramine. Both the magnitude and the duration of the methamphetamine effect are clearly enhanced. This demonstration of opposite pyschopharmacological effects of imipramine and chlorpromazine is consistent with their different clinical actions.*

Figure 10 compares the strength of the imipramine augmentation with the effect of doubling the amphetamine dose. This experiment was performed on a rat with an electrode in the midbrain tegmentum. Comparing the middle record and the bottom one, it is clear that the degree of augmentation induced by 10 mg/kg of imipramine far exceeds the increase produced by doubling the amphetamine dose.

Next, we explored further the interrelations of imipramine, amphetamine, and chlorpromazine. Figure 11 furnishes evidence that chlorpromazine can diminish, or block altogether, the augmenting effect of imipramine on amphetamine. Three experiments are depicted here for a midbrain animal. In the experiment shown at the top, chlorpromazine was given first, then imipramine, and finally

*The facilitating effects of amphetamine on conditioned avoidance behavior also are potentiated by imipramine [14].

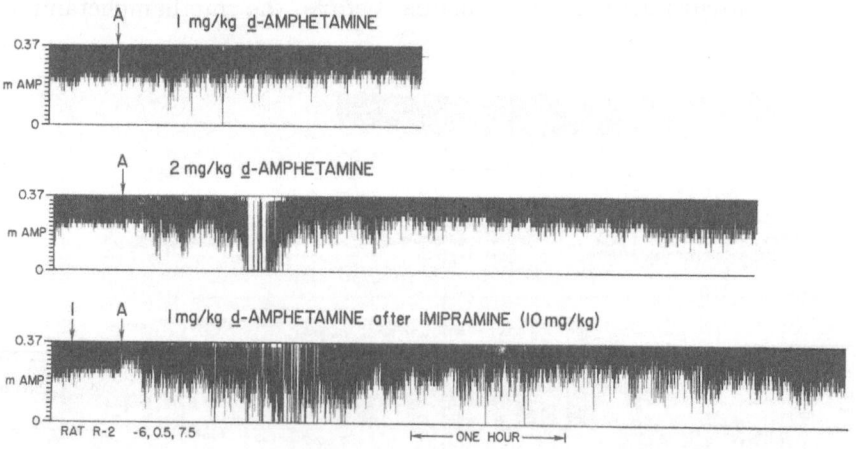

FIG. 10. Comparison of imipramine potentiation of amphetamine with the effect of doubling the amphetamine dose.

amphetamine. The second record shows a similar experiment with the order of the chlorpromazine and imipramine injections reversed. Comparing these records with the record at the bottom, we see that chlorpromazine may be given either shortly before or shortly after imipramine to block its augmenting effect on amphetamine.

These effects also may be demonstrated with the regular self-stimulation procedure. It will be recalled that under this procedure the animal operates a single lever to obtain fixed-intensity brain shocks. The method is made more sensitive by making available only a minimal current level, usually in the vicinity of the threshold for self-stimulation.

Figure 12 presents cumulative records of self-stimulation of a rat with a midbrain electrode in six weekly experimental sessions under various drug conditions. The slope of the curves gives the rate of self-stimulation; flat sections of the curve indicate periods of no response. The depressed base line rate of self-stimulation generated by the threshold current intensity is seen in Fig. 12a. A small dose of d-methamphetamine (0.25 mg/kg) produced a clear increase in rate beginning about 15 minutes after the injection (Fig. 12b). Pretreatment with 3 mg/kg of chlorpromazine antagonized the facilitative effect of the methamphetamine on self-stimulation (Fig. 12c). In contrast, pretreatment with 5 mg/kg of imipramine hydrochloride greatly augmented the increase in the self-stimulation rate induced by methamphetamine (Fig. 12d). This dose of imipra-

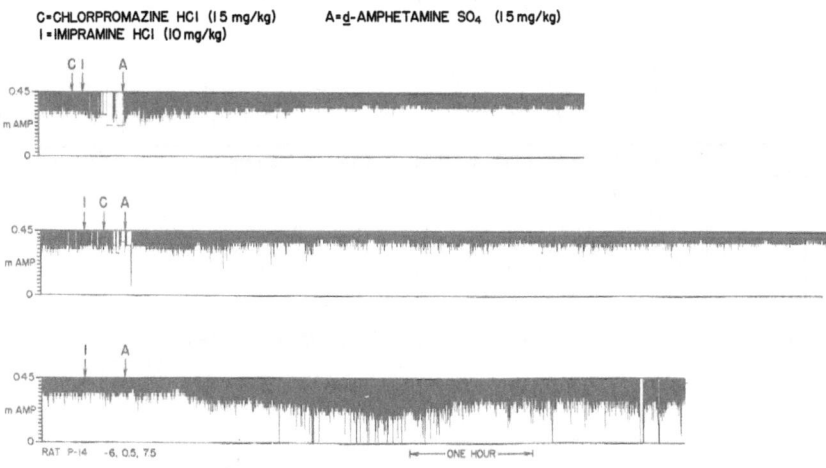

FIG. 11. Blocking of imipramine potentiation of amphetamine by chlorpromazine (given either before or after imipramine).

mine has no apparent effect of its own on self-stimulation. Greater augmentation is seen to result from a 15-mg/kg dose than from a 5-mg/kg dose (compare Figs. 12d and 12e). The latency of the methamphetamine response also was decreased by imipramine pretreatment; the effect on latency appeared to be dependent on the dose of imipramine. Finally, it may be seen that chlorpromazine antagonized the augmenting effect of imipramine on methamphetamine (compare Figs. 12e and 12f). These results are entirely consistent with the threshold findings.

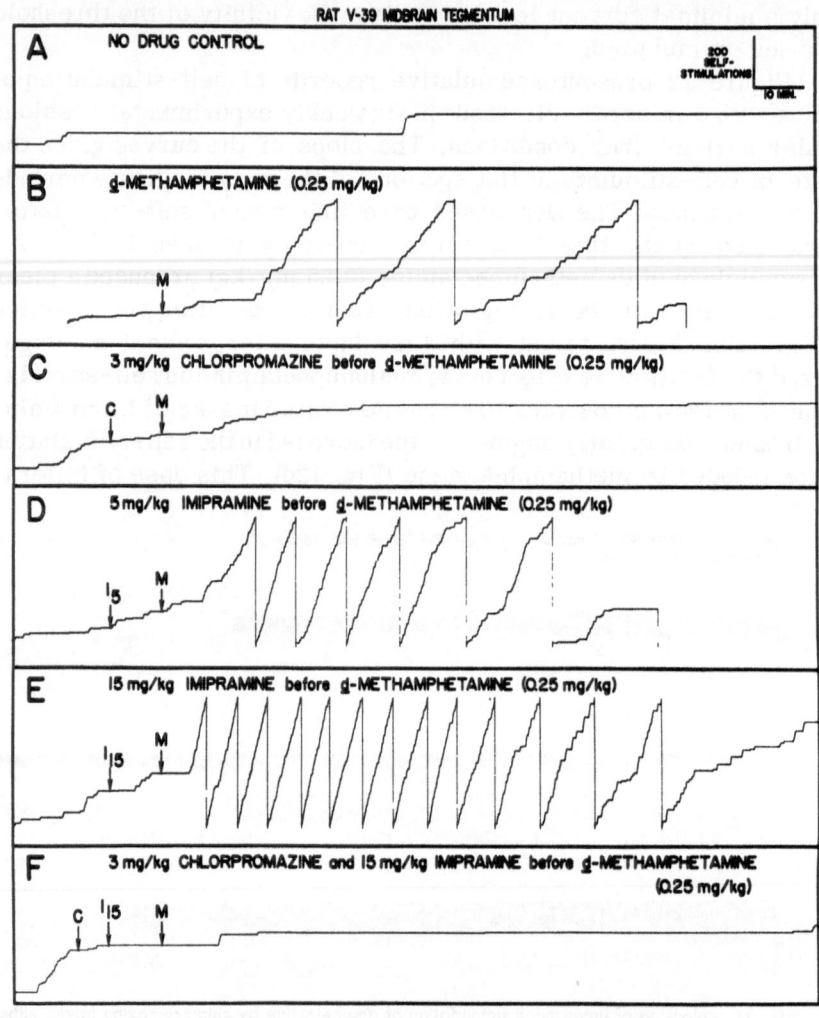

FIG. 12. Effects and interactions of drugs on the rate of self-stimulation.

We are attempting to characterize the nature of the ampheta-mine-augmenting property of imipramine. This work is only be-ginning. As a start we have compared the effects of imipramine and atropine, as imipramine is known to have a distinct anticholi-nergic property. Figure 13 portrays this comparison for a rat implanted in the posterior hypothalamus. The middle curve shows that atropine pretreatment produced a noticeable augmentation of the amphetamine effect. However, the atropine augmentation appears only modest in comparison to that produced by imipramine. At the peak of the effect produced by imipramine and methamphetamine the animal was so stimulated that it continued to operate the stimu-lation lever for zero current.* In view of the difference between imipramine and atropine in activity, and since the dose of atropine is estimated to be at least 20 times as potent *in vitro* in anticholi-nergic action than the imipramine dose, we conclude that the anti-cholerinergic property is not crucial.

In order to validate the amphetamine potentiation test as a device for measuring antidepressive activity, it should be shown

*This effect can be understood by assuming that stimuli (visual, propioceptive, etc.) generated by the lever-pressing behavior have acquired a conditioned reward value by previous association with the positively reinforcing brain stimulation. At the height of the drug effect, this conditioned reinforcement is sufficient to maintain lever pressing even after the current has been driven down to zero. The author has demonstrated that reward value may be established in originally neutral stimuli by paired presentations with re-warding brain stimulation [15].

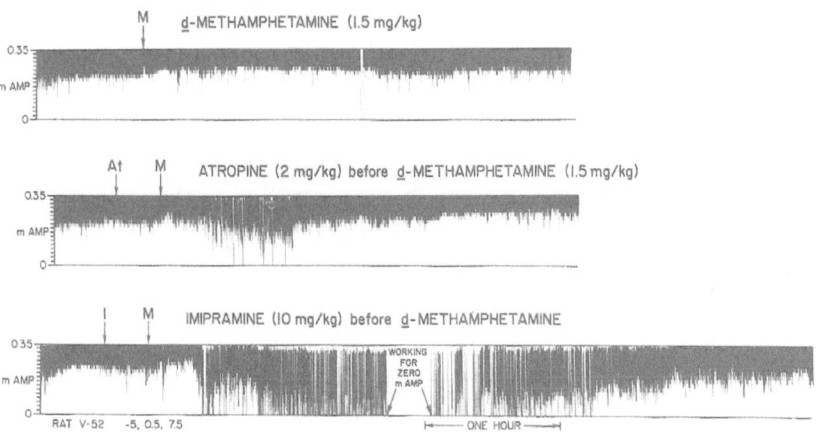

FIG. 13. Comparison of effects of imipramine and atropine on the response to d-metham-phetamine. The white spaces at the top of the imipramine — methamphetramine record are merely recording artifacts and result when a new sequence of self-stimulation is started before the pen fully resets.

that other antidepressant agents also have this activity. To our knowledge, the only other compound that has been determined clinically to have an imipramine-like, antidepressive activity is amitriptyline (Elavil). Figure 14 shows the results of a comparison between amitriptyline and imipramine for their ability to augment the response to amphetamine. Amitriptyline does in fact have activity in our test, readily seen by comparing the top and bottom records. This increases our confidence in the test. Amitriptyline appeared to be less potent than imipramine. Although twice the dose was used, 20 mg/kg of amitryptyline vs. 10 mg/kg of imipramine, a smaller and shorter-lived effect was obtained.

The next data to be presented suggest that the interactions between chlorpromazine and amphetamine are more complex than we have indicated so far. In addition to its action of diminishing the magnitude of the response to amphetamine, chlorpromazine sometimes will prolong the duration of the amphetamine effect. Figure 15 presents one such observation. The effect of d-methamphetamine against the pausing of a "spotty" midbrain animal is shown in the top record. The white spaces, indicating pauses, were eliminated for about an hour by the 0.5-mg/kg dose and returned when the drug wore off. The two lower records show that pretreatment with

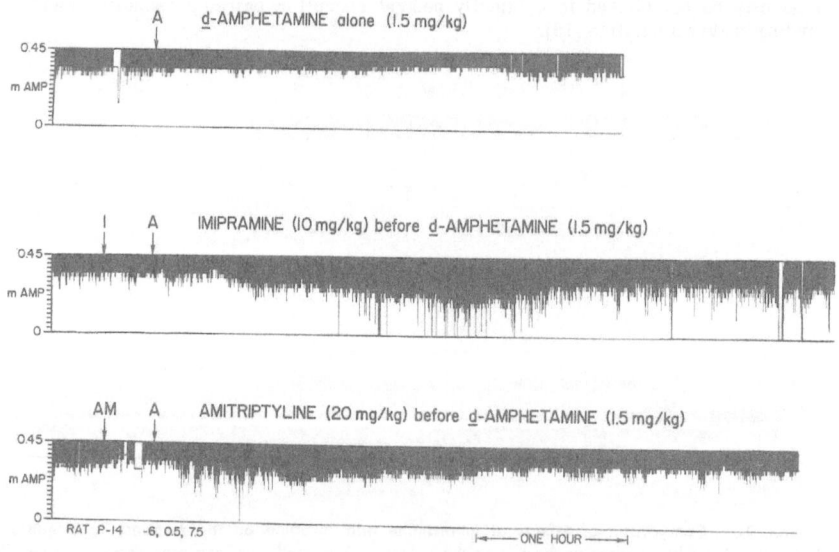

FIG. 14. Comparison of the effects of imipramine and amitriptyline on the response to d-amphetamine.

chlorpromazine can double the duration of the methamphetamine effect against pausing. It is possible that this apparently paradoxical finding is related to the work of Martin, Riehl, and Unna [16], who reported that chlorpromazine prolonged the pressor response to norepinephrine. This finding tempts one to view chlorpromazine and imipramine as belonging to the same psychopharmacological family. Both have an antidepressive action (seen as amphetamine potentiation or prolongation) at lower doses and an ataractic component (seen as inhibition of self-stimulation) at higher doses. In imipramine, the antidepressive component is pronounced and well separated in dose from the ataractic component; in chlorpromazine, the ataractic component is strong and poorly separated, if at all, from the antidepressive component.

Preliminary Data with Electroconvulsive Shock

It is well established clinically that electroshock is an effective treatment in depression. In some cases, it is the only effective treatment. From our hypothesis relating depression to reward activity, we suppose that electroshock exerts some kind of beneficial effect on the brain reward centers. By facilitating the activity of these brain centers, the depression is alleviated.

This notion is easily tested by means of the regular self-stimulation experiment. Establish a low base line rate of self-stimulation by a proper selection of the stimulating current and then administer

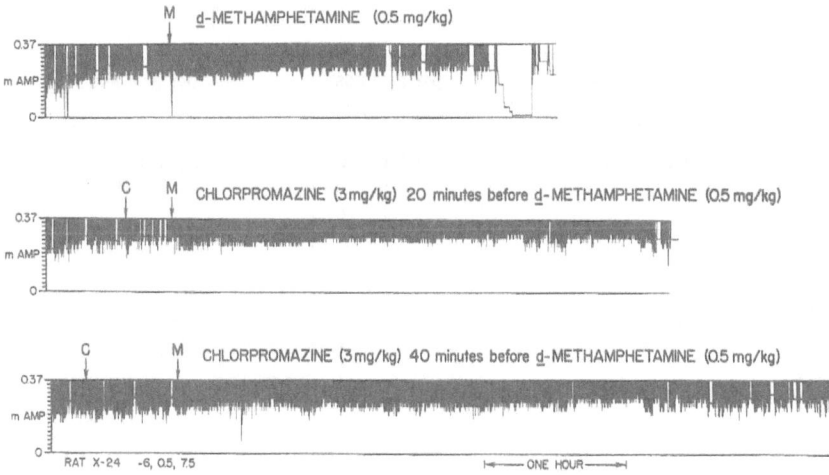

FIG. 15. Paradoxical prolongation of amphetamine effect against pausing by chlorpromazine.

a series of electroshock treatments. If the activity of rewarding brain sites is enhanced by convulsive therapy, the rate of self-stimulation will increase.

Figure 16 shows a positive result for one animal of four tried so far on a preliminary basis. Each cumulative record segment shows the self-stimulation output for a 40-minute experimental session. In the top row are three pre-electroshock records. The first two show the low-rate base line typical of this animal. The third shows that this animal was very responsive to methamphetamine; a 0.5-mg/kg dose was administered 10 minutes before the start of the session.

The middle two rows of records give the performance during the electroshock series. Two convulsions were elicited each day, one in the morning shortly after the self-stimulation test and the second late in the afternoon. This schedule permitted a 16-hour recovery period between any self-stimulation test and the last previous convulsion. No effect is seen during the first three days. On the fourth day, after six treatments, a moderate increase in the

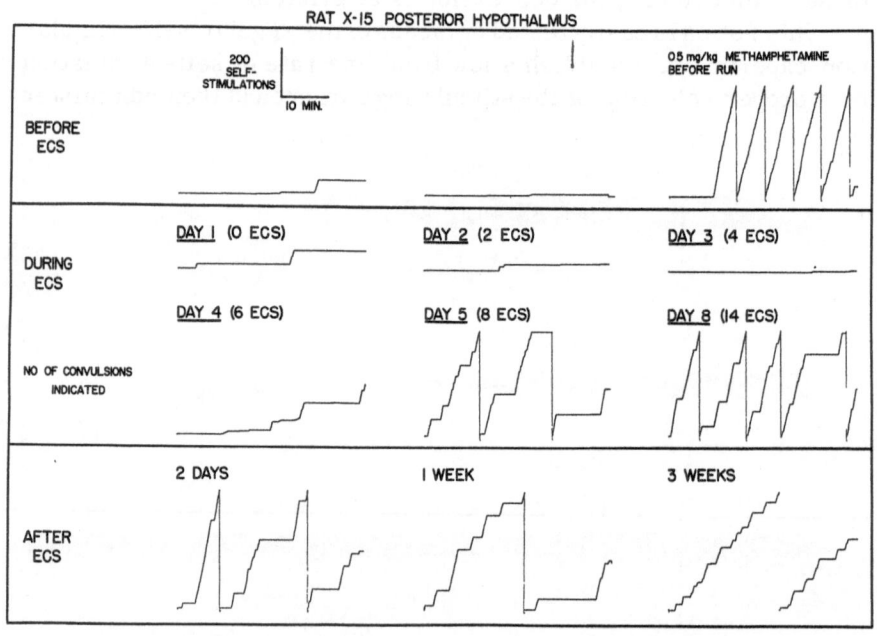

FIG. 16. Beneficial effect of electroconvulsive shock (ECS) on the rate of self-stimulation.

self-stimulation rate was obtained. Two more treatments produced a substantial rate increase on the fifth day. The peak increase in rate was obtained on the eighth day after 14 treatments. On the next day a somewhat lower rate was obtained. For this reason we stopped the treatment series after giving one more on that day, making a total of 17 electroshocks.

The bottom row shows the posttreatment records—two days, one week, and three weeks—after the last electroshock. Obviously the effects of the treatment persist. [Note added in proof: In further testing, electroconvulsive shock did not improve the self-stimulation performance of six additional rats.]

DISCUSSION AND CONCLUSIONS

Our results, to a surprising extent, may be taken to support the hypothesis that depression results from a hypoactivity of reward processes in the brain. Chlorpromazine and reserpine, which sometimes produce depression in the clinic, were found to inhibit reward structures. On the other hand, amphetamine, which sometimes produces euphoria in patients, was observed to facilitate the activity of reward structures. Also in line with prediction was the observation that amphetamine can counteract the depressing effects of chlorpromazine and reserpine.

The findings with imipramine are more difficult to interpret. When administered alone, this drug had a weak inhibiting action, contrary to the effect predicted for an antidepressant. Unlike chlorpromazine, however, imipramine did not antagonize the facilitating effects of amphetamine on self-stimulation. Indeed, it strongly potentiated them. Such a potentiation suggests that imipramine may act in some indirect augmenting capacity rather than through direct stimulation of reward structures. This seems to accord with the suggestion of Sigg [3] that imipramine acts by exerting a "sensitizing" effect on adrenergic synapses (in a manner similar to that proposed for cocaine). An alternative theory would state that imipramine blocks the compensating mechanisms that are activated when reward structures are (over)stimulated.

Sigg also proposed that a common denominator for antidepressant activity consists of an activation of central adrenergic synapses. We find this suggestion compatible with our findings in

the light of two considerations: (1) the work of Vogt [17] showing
that structures of the reward system have an unusually rich distribution of norepinephrine and (2) the suggestions of Brodie and Shore
[18] that amphetamine acts centrally by mimicking norepinephrine
and that chlorpromazine acts centrally by blocking norepinephrine.

After assuming, in addition, that self-stimulation is facilitated
by the enhancement of adrenergic activity in the reward system, we
offer the following as best guesses to account for our results:

1. Chlorpromazine (and reserpine) inhibit self-stimulation by
   blocking (or depleting) endogenous catechol amine.
2. Amphetamine facilitates self-stimulation by mimicking or
   releasing endogenous catechol amine.*
3. Amphetamine counteracts chlorpromazine-induced inhibition
   of self-stimulation by mimicking or releasing catechol amine,
   thereby shifting the chlorpromazine-catechol amine "equilibrium" in favor of catechol amine; amphetamine counteracts reserpine-induced inhibition by substituting for the depleted catechol amine or releasing it from partially depleted
   stores.
4. Imipramine in high doses weakly inhibits self-stimulation by
   a mild chlorpromazine-like blocking of catechol amine.
5. Imipramine in moderate doses potentiates and prolongs the
   effects of amphetamine by some as yet unspecified biochemical mechanism. A promising lead, however, is perhaps provided by *in vitro* studies of Goldstein and Contrera [20] which
   demonstrate that imipramine inhibits the hydroxylating enzyme, dopamine β-oxidase, responsible for the conversion
   of dopamine to norepinephrine. Thus, imipramine could
   enhance the central effects of amphetamine by preserving
   dopamine (on the assumption that amphetamine acts by mimicking or releasing dopamine). Or amphetamine itself may
   be preserved by imipramine, as its metabolism seems to
   involve hydroxylation of the ring or sidechain [20, 21].
6. Electroconvulsive shock therapy is beneficial in depression
   by facilitating, in some way, the activity of neural reward
   centers. While our data are only fragmentary, our hunch is
   that electroshock selectively suppresses the activity of
   punishment centers and thereby frees previously inhibited

---

*The general term "catechol amine" is used to avoid a specification of a particular
catechol amine. However, dopamine seems more likely to be involved in these effects
than either norepinephrine or epinephrine.

reward centers. The findings of Hunt and Brady [8] support this notion.

SUMMARY

1. Two tranquilizers, chlorpromazine and reserpine, and two antidepressants, amphetamine and imipramine, were studied for their actions and interactions on the sensitivity of "rewarding" hypothalamic and midbrain tegmentum brain sites. A modified self-stimulation technique permitted a continuous tracing of reward thresholds.
2. Chlorpromazine and reserpine raised thresholds for electrical reinforcement and, in large doses, inhibited self-stimulation altogether. Amphetamine lowered thresholds for reinforcement and also increased the rate of self-stimulation. Imipramine had weak inhibitory effects on self-stimulation.
3. The inhibitory effects of chlorpromazine and reserpine were reversed by amphetamine. The facilitating effects of amphetamine were antagonized by chlorpromazine.
4. Imipramine had a profound potentiating effect on the response to amphetamine in doses which had no apparent effects of their own. A clear differentiation was thus provided between imipramine and chlorpromazine.
5. These results were interpreted as evidence in support of a neurophysiological theory of depression. The theory assumes that depression results from pathological hypoactivity of reward activity of the brain. The results also were discussed from a chemical viewpoint that related the actions of the drugs to influences on endogenous catechol amine in the reward system.

REFERENCES

1. Delgado, J. M. R., Roberts, W. W., and Miller, N. E.: Learning motivated by electrical stimulation of the brain, Am. J. Physiol. 179:587, 1954.

2. Hess, W. R.: The Functional Organization of the Diencephalon, Grune & Stratton, Inc., New York, 1957.

3. Olds, J., and Milner, P.: Positive reinforcement produced by electrical stimulation of septal area and other regions of rat brain, J. Comp Physiol. Psychol. 47:419, 1954.

4. Heath, R. G., and Mickle, W. A.; Sem-Jacobsen, C. W., and Torkildsen, A.: in Ramey, E. R., and O'Doherty, D. S., Ed.: Electrical Studies on the Unanesthetized Brain, Paul B. Hoeber, Inc., New York, 1960, chs.

5. Olds, J.: Studies of neuropharmacologicals by electrical and chemical manipulation of the brain on animals with chronically implanted electrodes, in Bradley, B. P. et al., Eds.: Neuro-Psychopharmacology, Elsevier Publ. Co., Amsterdam, 1959.

6. Olds, J., and Travis, R. P.: Effects of chlorpromazine, meprobamate, pentobarbital, and morphine on self-stimulation, J. Pharmacol. Exp. Therap. 128:397, 1960.

7. Estes, W. K., and Skinner, B. F.: Some quantitative properties of anxiety, J. Exp. Psychol. 29:390, 1941.

8. Hunt, H. F., and Brady, J. V.: Some effects of electro-convulsive shock on a conditioned emotional response ("anxiety"), J. Comp. Physiol. Psychol. 44: 88, 1951.

9. Costa, E., Garattini, S., and Valzelli, L.: Interactions between reserpine, chlorpromazine, and imipramine, Experientia 16:461, 1960.

10. Lilly, J. C., Hughes, J. R., Alvord, E. C., Jr., and Galken, T. W.: Brief noninjurious electrical waveform for stimulation of the brain, Science 121:468, 1955.

11. Brodie, D. A., Moreno, D. M., Malis, J. L., and Boren, J. J.: Rewarding properties of intercranial stimulation, ibid. 131:929, 1960.

12. Stein, L., and Ray, O. S.: Brain stimulation reward "thresholds" self-determined in rat, Psychopharmacologia 1:251, 1960.

13. Sigg, E. B.: Pharmacological studies with Tofranil, Canadian Psychiat. Assoc. J. 4:575, 1959.

14. Carlton, P. L.: Augmentation of the behavioral effects of amphetamine by atropine, Pharmacologist 2:70, 1960.

15. Stein, L.: Secondary reinforcement established with subcortical stimulation, Science 127:466, 1958.

16. Martin, W. R., Riehl, J. L., and Unna, K. R.: Chlorpromazine III. The effects of chlorpromazine and chlorpromazine sulfoxide on vascular responses to l-epinephrine and levarterenol, J. Pharmacol. Exp. Therap. 130:37, 1960.

17. Vogt, M.: The concentration of sympathin in different parts of the central nervous system under normal conditions and after the administration of drugs, J. Physiol. 123:451, 1954.

18. Brodie, B. B., and Shore, P. A.: A concept for a role of serotonin and norepinephrine as chemical mediators in the brain, Ann. N. Y. Acad. Sci. 66:631, 1957.

19. Stein, L.: New methods for evaluating stimulants and antidepressants, in Nodine, J. H., Ed.: Sixth Hahnemann Symposium: Psychosomatic Medicine, Lea & Febiger, 1962.

20. Goldstein, M. and Contrera, J. F.: Inhibition of dopamine β-oxidase by imipramine, Biochem. Pharmacol. 7: 278, 1961.

21. Axelrod, J.: Metabolism of epinephrine and other sympathomimetic amines, Physiol. Rev. 39: 751, 1959.

Discussion by Harold E. Himwich, M.D.

The fame of the A. E. Bennett Award has grown with the years, as indicated by the quality of the papers received by the committee and the submission of one paper each from England and Austria. The opinions of the four members of the committee—Dr. Seymour S. Kety, Dr. Warren S. McCulloch, and Dr. George N. Thompson—were divided and each member chose a different paper for first place. Only one paper maintained high ratings with all four members, and this one was that of Dr. Larry Stein.

The results presented by Dr. Stein show that imipramine has special characteristics different from those of its chemical cousin, chlorpromazine, and illustrate the chief advantage contributed by the use of the new psychoactive drugs, namely, their specificity of action. The sedatives used before the tranquilizers did not exhibit specificity in regard to psychotic symptoms and could not relieve schizophrenic hyperactivity and calm the patients or reduce the intensity of hallucinations and delusions without inducing sleep. Similarly, imipramine seems to be specific for the endogenous depressions. Depressed patients become more active after the administration of amphetamine, but they are also worse off, for they reveal agitation. The nonspecific action of imipramine (Tofranil) and amitriptyline (Elavil) is sedative both in animals and in nondepressed human subjects. In fact, in our studies imipramine produced a desirable sedation in some schizophrenic patients. Yet, remarkable to say, only in depressed patients does it exert its specific antidepressant action. Dr. Stein's paper presents an analysis which affords a basis for the specificity of the chemical action of imipramine.

VI MISCELLANEOUS STUDIES

CHAPTER 28

Neural Correlates of Psychophysiological Developments in the Young Organism

By ARNOLD B. SCHEIBEL, M.D.

The present data represent one phase of a long-term investigation of the brain stem reticular core and its relation to certain ego functions in which the investigator and his wife have been involved for some years [1–5]. The immediate goal of this study has been an examination of those structural-functional substrates which might underlie psychophysiological development in the newborn. More specifically, and of greater pertinence to the neuropsychiatrist, we have sought developmental clues to mechanisms subserving awareness and the selection of certain sensory data from much more extensive presentations. Although answers to the second problem are not yet obvious, it appears that the form and degree of maturity of the brain significantly determine its ability to respond to, or ignore, certain modes of stimuli. Additionally, with maturation may come loss of ability to react to certain types of stimuli, a suggestion which has been advanced in a different context and on purely clinical grounds by some psychoanalysts [6].

Since this study was initiated, in the spring of 1958, several reports of somewhat similar nature have appeared [7–10]. Differences in selection of data and in conclusions drawn from such studies reflect variation in choice of techniques, in animal species used, and in orientation of the observers. Because of limitations of space, only a few significant aspects of our study will be presented, with fuller reports to appear in the future.

Supported in part by grants from the National Institute of Neurological Diseases and Blindness, U. S. Public Health Service.

TECHNIQUE

Fifty neonatal kittens were operated within 3 to 12 hours of delivery. Minute amounts of intraperitoneal Nembutal (30 mg/kg) were used as basal anaesthesia supplemented by ether with the animal held steady in a specially constructed head-holder. On the basis of previously prepared control measurements, fine tripolar depth electrodes were introduced through burr holes and fixed in position with quick-drying dental cement. The diameter of the sharpened electrode tips averaged 80 to 100 μ and projected 5 to 8 mm beyond the thin central supporting staff to produce minimal damage at the recording-stimulating sites, which included mesencephalic reticular formation, nonspecific (reticular) thalamic nuclei, specific thalamic relay centers, hippocampus, entorhinal cortex, and caudate nucleus. Cortical surface sites were recorded through stainless steel watchmaker screws, and all lead-off wires were soldered to microminiature Winchester 7 and 14 pin "female" plugs, also fixed to the skull with dental cement. The kittens were returned to their litters after all ether was blown off, and in most cases the mother continued to care for them. Otherwise, they were kept in warm boxes and fed by means of doll baby bottles.

Histological data were obtained from litter mates sacrificed at intervals and the specimens stained by modified rapid Golgi methods and controlled by the usual Nissl or Klüver material.

DISCUSSION OF RESULTS

The development of electrocortical rhythms has been discussed by a number of investigators and will be described only briefly. Maturation of the electrocerebellogram and electroreticulogram will be discussed elsewhere. At birth and for the first day or two thereafter, irregular 4- to 6-per-second rhythms alternated with slower patterns, presumably as the level of consciousness varied. Potential amplitudes seldom exceeded 50 μv. Faster rhythms approaching alpha frequencies gradually developed over the first ten days to two weeks, commensurate with the degree of maturity of the animal, and adult rhythms were achieved between the third and fifth weeks of life. One of the first signs of maturation was the appearance of isolated spindle bursts between fifth and seventh days, interpreted as early physiological evidence of developing synaptic relations between nonspecific corticipetal fibers and still immature apical dendrites (Fig. 1).

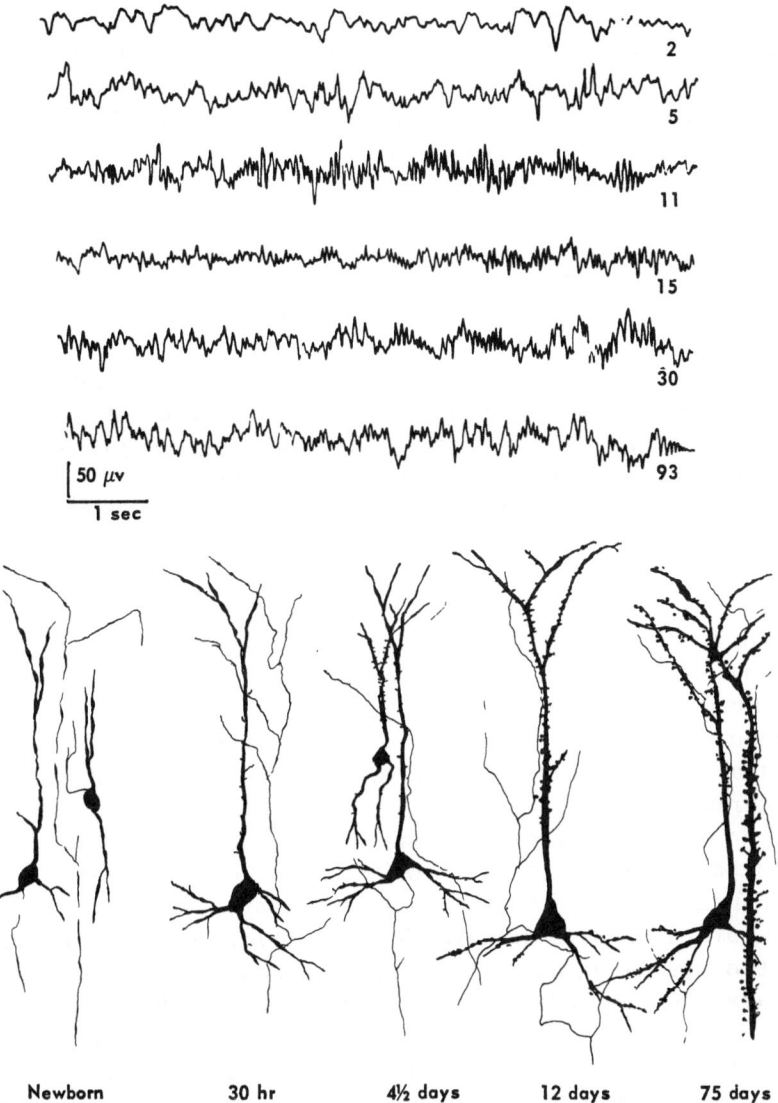

FIG. 1. Correlated structurofunctional maturation of the neocortical EEG. Upper: Progressive development of the electrocorticogram from irregular 3- to 6-per-second perinatal activity to essential maturity by the end of the first month. Spindle bursts are very obvious by the middle of the second week, as is the beginning of alpha activity. Further development includes restriction of spindling and increase in regularity of alpha patterns with better differentiation between periods of sleep and wakefulness. Lower: Structural changes in pyramidal cells include, besides the obvious maturation of apical dendrites and growth of basilar dendrite system, the development of dendrite spines and the establishment of synaptic contact between these elements and corticipetal nonspecific (thalamic reticular) fibers.

Several investigators have attempted to relate functional developments to specific structural changes [5, 7, 8]. The methods of visualization will of course determine the nature of the observations. Thus, utilization of aniline stains and/or reduced silver will emphasize soma size and arrangement and the proximal portions of dendrites. The Golgi-Cox method will reveal dendrite masses, dendrite membrane detail (within certain limits), and some geographical features. However, as has previously been pointed out, neural elements such as somata and dendrites do not exist *in vacuo* but in the most intimate relations with neuroglia, terminal axons, other dendrites, etc. [10]. For these reasons, a more comprehensive technique such as the rapid Golgi method (or the electron microscope at a different order of magnitude) is indicated for more complete evaluations of the structural changes in progress.

Using the rapid Golgi method, it has been possible to watch changes of apparent significance occurring simultaneously in the apical dendrites of pyramids, in the terminal fibers developing synaptic relations along their surface, in the basal dendrites of these cells, in the horizontal cell-fiber plexus of the first and sixth layers, and in the short-axoned cells of the second and fourth layers. It seems unlikely that we are wise enough to spot any one of these changes as specifically causal to a specific functional element. However, it seems likely that in the interplay of their mutual developmental patterns may lie the substrate of functional maturation.

Rapid repetitive stimulation of the reticular tegmentum at frequencies of 300 per second has been shown optimally effective for producing cortical activation in the adult animal [11]. Slow frequencies are ineffective. However in the newborn kitten and for a week or two after birth, fast frequencies are usually without effect on the cortex while slow frequencies of the order of 10 per second are likely to produce short runs of cortical low-voltage fast activity. Correlative to this observation is our inability to produce more than one or two sequences of activation at any one time without doubling or tripling the stimulating voltage. Some hours of "recovery" are necessary between attempts at cortical activation (Figs. 2 and 3).

It may be premature to attribute these peculiarities of cortical response to specific factors. Structural analyses reveal that nonspecific corticipetal fibers have already reached most layers of the neocortex although their ultimate structural forms and relations

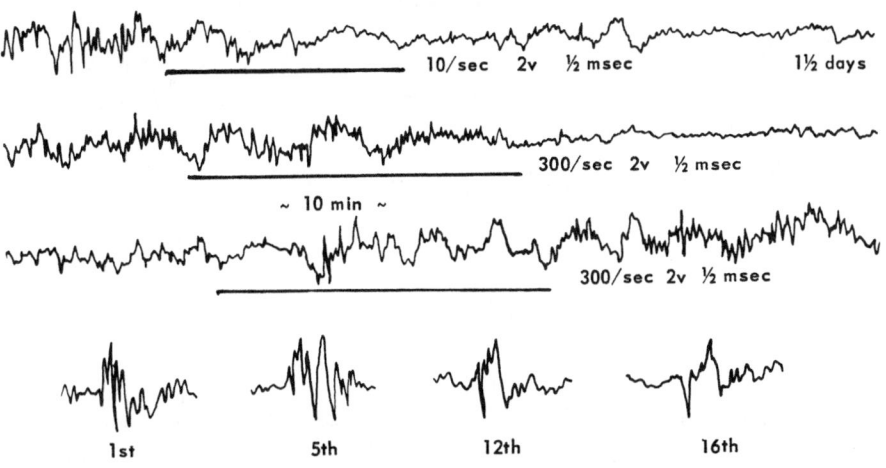

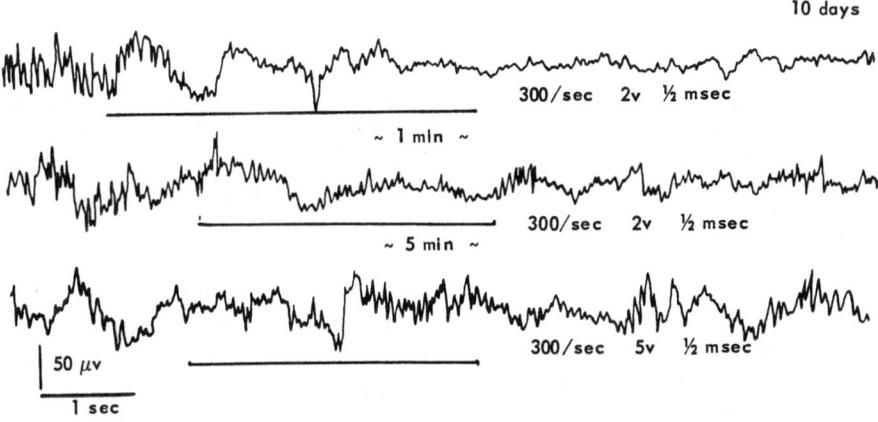

FIG. 2. Upper and lower series of three traces. Upper: Fatigue or adaptation effects caused by mesencephalic reticular activation of cortex. The first trace shows that at one and a half days of age, 10-per-second stimulation is maximally effective as an activating frequency if attempted once. A subsequent stimulation at 300 per second is also moderately effective once (though this frequency is often completely ineffective at this age). Ten minutes later, another attempt at 300-per-second activation fails. Lower: At the age of ten days this kind of fatigue phenomenon still obtains, with 300-per-second stimulation of mesencephalic reticular formation proving effective once but not a second time (one minute later) or a third time (five minutes later). The central group of individual records indicates that evoked cortical responses to specific sensory stimuli (light flashes) may be repeated a number of times. At this age (one and a half days) responses are surface negative, though with developing fatigue initial positivity of unknown significance develops.

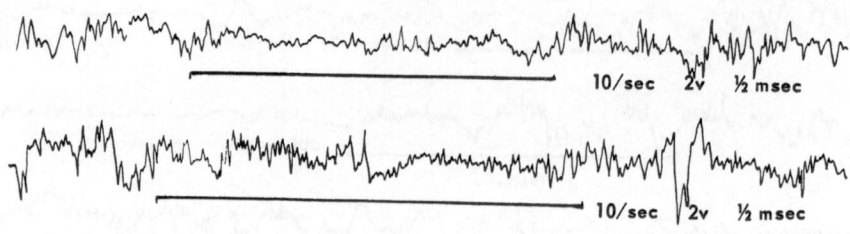

16 days

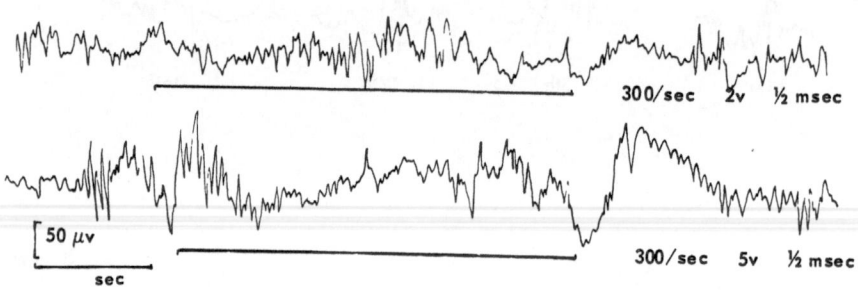

FIG. 3. Normal activation patterns have still not appeared by the sixteenth day of postnatal life. Upper: 10-per-second activation of mesencephalic reticular formation produces transient activation of cortex during period of stimulation but is ineffective when attempted a moment later. Lower: in this animal (No. 31) 300-per-second activation is still virtually completely ineffective at 2- and 5-v stimulation. (One week later this frequency had become moderately effective while 10-per-second frequencies had become ineffective.)

are far from realized. It is very difficult to demonstrate contacts between these axons and the apical dendrites of third and fifth layer pyramids, nor have the characteristic short-axon collaterals yet appeared. The postsynaptic apical dendrites are also immature, showing either the diffuse "hairlines" of primitive neurons or the relatively smooth and knobless surface characteristic of the early postnatal period. Coincident with the appearance of appreciable numbers of dendrite spines toward the end of the first postnatal week or early in the second, axodendrite contacts begin to be noticeable along with an increase in complexity of the presynaptic axons, giving an appearance of winding or climbing along the dendrites. The first appearance of these features appears to be correlated with the beginning of spindling patterns in the cortex and the first signs of alpha activity. Increasing maturation of this synaptic system in the late second and third weeks coincides in time with (1) increasing effectiveness of fast reticular frequencies in producing cortical activation, (2) decreasing effectiveness of slow frequencies in producing this effect, and (3) rapid waning of the "habituation" or "fatigue" effect following one or two reticular stimulations.*

Histological maturation of the axodendrite apparatus might seem to offer one obvious basis for these changes. However, it is not easy to explain why any activation effects are then possible before these structural changes are obvious. In the relatively small number of kittens successfully implanted within one to three hours of birth, we have noticed marked variation even within these limits, and gross and microscopic observation have similarly revealed wide variation in cortical maturation at birth. Such changes have also been noted by Ellingson [15] and others.

Some neonates showed small, virtually lissencephalic hemispheres while others showed almost adult gyral patterns and greater brain size. Microscopic analysis of Golgi impregnations also showed wide variations from poorly differentiated neurons, looking more like late neuroblasts than cortical pyramids, to rather well-developed elements with advanced apical and basal dendrites and the early appearance of spines. We must infer that early activation effects even at 10-per-second frequencies represent early axodendrite interaction where some functional articulation already exists. Greater efficacy of slow over rapid frequencies in the early days of development might then reflect physiological peculiarities of the immature nonspecific corticipetal axon, still of relatively small diameter and poorly myelinated relative to its adult state. Whatever the reasons for this change of sensitivity to reticular-stimulation frequency, and they may be multiple, the phenomenon

---

*Until recently, the role of dendrite spines or gemmules has been an anomalous one in the neurological literature. First described by Ramon y Cajal [12], who believed that they were part of the synaptic mechanism of dendrites, the most common argument of their detractors has been that they represent silver or methylene blue artifacts owing to deposition of stain in extracellular spaces along dendrites or else are caused by fixation shrinkage of the tissue. Protagonists of these structures felt that, even if artifacts, they probably represent the remains of some type of specialized structure along the dendrites, while the more daring suggested that their presence in vivo served to increase the available postsynaptic surface area. Recent investigations by Gray [13] with the electron microscope have clearly delineated the dendrite spine on cortical shafts and a specialized structure within characterized by sacs and dense bands. Analogous structures have more recently been demonstrated by Fox [14] on the tertiary branchlets of Purkinje cells in the cerebellum, deeply indenting the adjacent parallel fibers. Such findings would seem to indicate that the spine system is a specific synaptic mechanism whose progressive maturation in the early stages of postnatal development bears an important relationship to functional development.

offers an interesting example of a loss of sensitivity in cortical response to one type of input as maturation proceeds. Some analysts have suggested that the infant is selectively sensitive to the immediate surrounding emotional climate and may respond to affective attitudes of which the parents themselves are unaware [6]. Receptive abilities of this type might represent at a much higher level of psychological organization another example of a receptive parameter lost with maturation.

The development of refractoriness in cortical activation responses following only one or two episodes of reticular stimulation may be related to immaturity in synaptic mediator systems. The investigations of Desmedt and La Grutta [16] have implicated nonspecific cholinesterases as one group of substances possibly involved in cortical activation phenomena, and it is possible that delayed resynthesis of such transmitter substances by immature enzyme systems may be involved in the long refractory periods here described. A similar explanation is proposed by Purpura et al. [8] for prolonged absolute refractory periods in the activity cycles of superficial cortical responses in the perinatal cortex.

In contrast to nonspecific systems projecting upon the cortex, specific sensory relay systems appear capable of producing relatively larger numbers of consecutive cortical-evoked responses before showing obvious signs of fatigue. A gradual loss of the evoked response does occur with repetition, bearing a rough relationship to the frequency with which the cortical responses are evoked. In the immediate postnatal period cortical responses to flashes of light are highly variable in pattern but usually marked by a surface negative component (Fig. 2) followed by smaller positive and negative components, occasionally forming trains of diminishing amplitude. Usually by the middle of the second week a small surface positive component appears, preceding the negative wave, and with maturation grows in size to occupy an increasingly significant proportion of the evoked response. Similar progressions are reported by Marty et al. [17] and by Ellingson [15] although auditory responses are reported as always showing initial positive responses by Grossman [18] and by Rose et al. [19].

Structural correlates of this progression of functional patterns are still under study. Purpura et al. [8] attribute initial surface negativity in the perinatal organism to activity predominating in the apical dendrite system. "A reasonable interpretation is that the synaptic activity generated in the cortical depths at this stage is relatively weak and likely to be swamped by summated axodendritic PSP's developing in superficial cortical regions." They suggest that an extension of the basilar dendrite system of pyramids during the second postnatal week and afterwards accounts for the increasing depth activity and consequent change in evoked patterns.

There is no question that basal dendrite systems are progressively elaborated during the second and third weeks following birth, thereby appreciably increasing the available synaptic receptor area for these neurons. However, and in contradistinction to less revealing histological methods, the rapid Golgi technique shows that simultaneous changes are occurring in two other closely adjacent elements which must be considered of equal or greater importance. One is the elaboration of the terminating presynaptic bushy arbor of the specific thalamocortical relay; the other is the elaboration and maturation of the short-axoned components (Golgi type II cells) of the second and fourth layers. At birth, termination of the specific thalamocortical relay fibers is usually quite simple, characterized by a restricted number of bifurcations in the fourth and fifth layers. Most of these terminal collaterals appear to bear blunt enlargements or "growth cones" and by the end of the first week have produced sufficient terminal reduplications to form a fairly heavy plexus engulfing the granules of the fourth layer and the initial portions of the apical dendrites of the fifth layer pyramids. Simultaneously, though at a somewhat slower rate, the Golgi type II cells show developmental change, progressing from simple bipolar patterns at birth to widely branching dendrite systems and from insignificant axon filaments to dense networks filling the somal surroundings (Fig. 4). Temporal patterns here are less obvious because of problems with differential impregnation, but we have the distinct impression that short-axon elaboration may continue in the cat during the first six to eight weeks of life.

On the basis of these developments, we suggest that initial surface negative responses are indeed due to superficial dendrite activity responding to the relatively unimpeded advance of the activity front ascending from still simple terminal mechanisms in the fourth and fifth layers. The developing complexity of the terminal arbors and then of the local granule cell axon plexus produces neuropil fields of growing complexity whose activity is increasingly manifest by initial surface positivity. This probably represents not only a masking of the previously seen initial negativity but an actual displacement of it caused by the interposi-

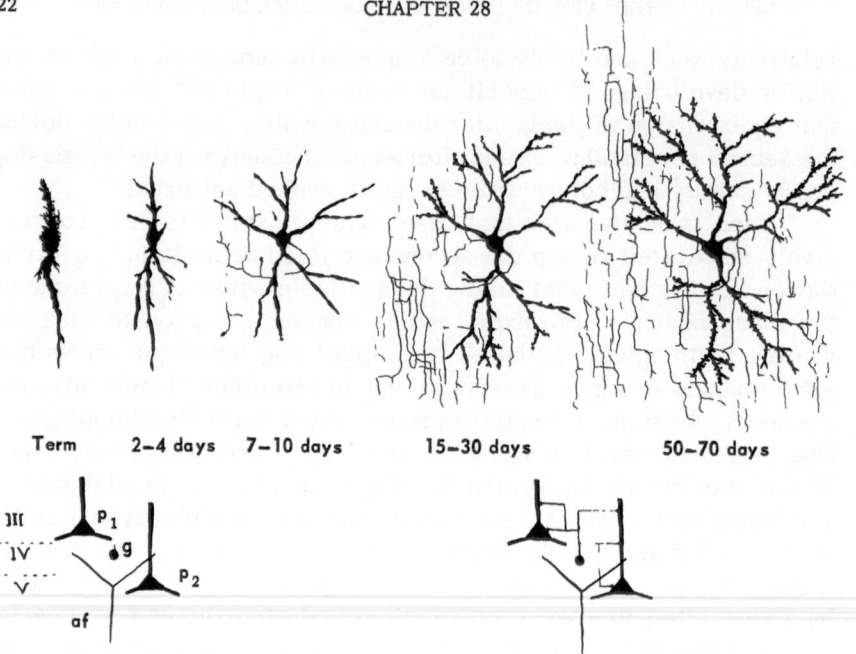

Term   2–4 days   7–10 days   15–30 days   50–70 days

FIG. 4. The development of the short-axoned Golgi type II (granule) cell of the second and fourth layers in cortex reconstructed from many Golgi impregnations. As the short-axon plexus matures during the late first and second months, it is suggested that this effectively serves to interpose a new circuit element into cortical loops between the corticipetal specific afferent, af, and the pyramids of layers III, p₁ and V, p₂.

tion of a short-axoned neuropil buffer between the specific afferent system and the pyramidal components of the cortex.

It may not be overstating the case to suggest that an entirely new neuropil field is interposed between corticipetal radiations and the cortical pyramid system between the fourth and sixth week of life by the maturation of the Golgi type II axon system. The appearance of such a field must greatly enrich and complicate cortical circuitry and enhance the range of possible response patterns of postsynaptic components as well as increasing, by one synapse at the very least, the specific sensory pathways through the cortex. It seems not unlikely that widespread depolarization phenomena, already described as characteristic of neural activity transmitted into richly arborized terminating presynaptic systems [20], develop in the axonal neuropil formed by specific cortical afferents and especially by the enmeshed short-axoned cells of the fourth layer. This activity probably reflects in the initial surface positivity of the maturing or adult cortex, a phenomenon followed by developing negativity as the active process is transferred to and decrementally ascends apical dendrites.

Despite much conjecture, the functional significance of short-axon cells is still only inferred. Contemporary thinking largely reflects Ramon y Cajal's suggestion that an increase in numbers of these cells as the phylogenetic scale is ascended is related to the increasing complexity of psychoneural function, the possible physiological bases of these effects being sketched by Eccles [21] and his co-workers. Possible clinical validation of these ideas may be found in the repeated demonstration of the Vogts [22] that the thickness of the short-axoned second and fourth cell layers in the cortices of individuals with unusual sensory "gifts" were appreciably greater than that of those in ungifted control subjects. Thus, an individual who maintained the ability of intense eidetic recall during life showed unusual thickness of these layers in visual cortices, while a musician known for the excellence of his "perfect pitch" showed similar changes in auditory receptive areas [22]. In each case the difference appeared to lie in a much greater number of these cells, as seen in thionine sections, and a presumably more extensive neuropil field.

Space limits the description of conditioning procedures attempted in newborn and young animals. Figure 5 summarizes one type of procedure attempted in a number of the kittens. Starting at the beginning of the tenth week of life, kitten No. 13 was called by her name, Po-po-jo, and each call was followed by about one minute of feeding from a doll bottle. Only three to six presentations were attempted each day during a single 30-minute recording period. The first pair of traces in Fig. 5 show that at the sixty-eighth day of life (three days after the beginning of the conditioning procedure) no electroencephalographic responses were noted in neocortical (occipital to frontal) or entorhinal stations nor was there any behavioral response. By the one hundred seventeenth day of life, well-developed responses were seen in both leads.

The second pair of tracings shows a differential response to the examiner's voice, which first used a nonfamiliar word ("Goldilocks") not previously associated with the conditioning procedure followed in the third pair of leads by the use of the conditioned stimulus name, Po-po-jo, and each call was followed by about one minute of in either tracing while the reinforced word produces immediate changes in both and a behavioral effect (climbing up on the side of

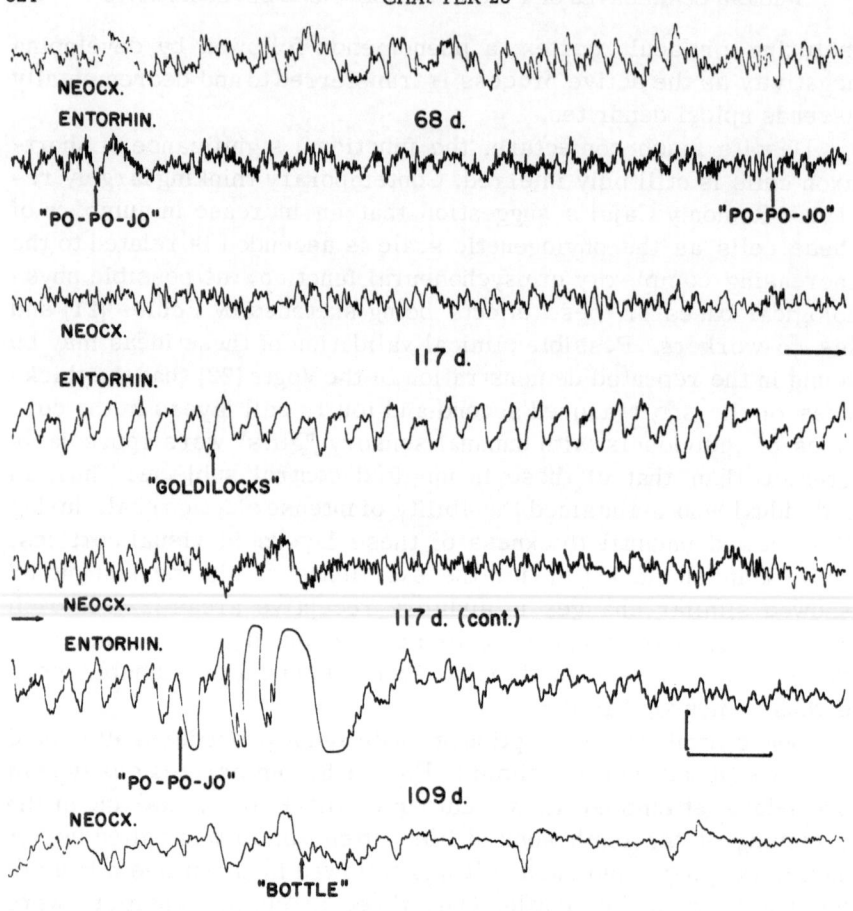

FIG. 5.   Precis of one type of conditioning procedure attempted in young kittens.

the testing box), as indicated by the movement artifact in the entorhinal lead. The occipitofrontal tracing shows an increase in frequency and decrease in amplitude over the previously awake but
resting base line, while the high-amplitude (75 to 100 μv) three per
second waves of entorhinal cortex are desynchronized. The last
tracing in Fig. 5 shows a similar experiment carried out with
another kitten (No. 18) conditioned to the word "bottle." Upon presentation of the word following a conditioning period of about one
month, the kitten immediately awakened and sought the reward.
Rapid changes from sleeping to wakeful states were consistently
noted upon presentation of the reward conditioned verbal stimulus
even though nonconditioned auditory stimuli (bells, buzzers, clicks,

etc.) produced no behavioral response and little or no EEG change in the sleeping record.

Data to be reported and documented elsewhere show that adequate differentiations can be made by the third month of life between the conditioned word spoken by the usual investigator and by a stranger. In the latter case one or two trials seem all that is necessary for the young organism to make the differentiation, thereafter disregarding the conditioned word delivered by a stranger while responding to the familiar voice of the investigator. We are trying to determine the earliest point where such discriminations can be made. Thus far we have not succeeded at establishing a point earlier than the seventh to tenth weeks of life. Most of the definitive structural changes have been effected well before this, while, as previously indicated, full maturation of the short-axon cell plexus is achieved only at this time. We therefore suggest, from the structurofunctional point of view, a possible relationship between the development of certain types of perceptive differentiating (discriminating) capabilities and the full development of the neuropil fields generated by these enigmatic neural components.

SUMMARY

1. Attempts are made to relate the maturation of the electro-corticogram in newborn and postnatal animals to maturation of the axon-dendrite complex formed by cortical projections of thalamic nonspecific (reticular) systems and the apical dendrite shafts of cortical pyramids.

2. Classical activation techniques upon the neocortex by reticular stimulation are relatively unsuccessful until the third or fourth week of life. Slow frequency stimulation is initially more effective owing probably to structurofunctional characteristics of the immature tissue.

3. Reticular activation of the cortex shows rapid "fatigue" or "accommodation" with long (10- to 12-hour) rest periods necessary between trials.

4. Evoked potentials produced by specific sensory stimulation show relatively greater resistance to "fatigue," and a progression from surface negativity to surface positivity over the first few weeks of life. Attempts are made to relate these changes to structural changes in the neuropil field, especially in the fourth layer.

5. Certain conditioning procedures are described in which kittens show the ability to discriminate between highly specific sensory

cues. Preliminary evidence suggests that certain aspects of these discriminations may be related to maturation of short-axon cell neuropil fields.

REFERENCES

1. Scheibel, A. B.: On detailed connections of the medullary and pontine reticular formation, Anat. Rec. 109:85, 1951.

2. Scheibel, M. E.: Axonal efferent patterns in the bulbar reticular formation, ibid. 121:362, 1955.

3. Scheibel, M. E., Scheibel, A. B., Mollica, H., and Moruzzi, G.: Convergence and interaction of afferent impulses on single units of reticular formation, J. Neurophysiol. 18:309, 1955.

4. Scheibel, M. E., and Scheibel, A. B.: Hallucinations and the brain stem reticular core. in West, L. J., ed.: Symposium on Hallucinations, Grune & Stratton, Inc., New York, 1961.

5. Scheibel, M. E., and Scheibel, A. B.: Development of reticulo-cortical control in the newborn, Am. Acad. Neurol. 29, 1959 (oral report).

6. Sullivan, H. S.: Conceptions of modern psychiatry, The William Alanson White Psychiatric Foundation, Washington, D. C. 1947.

7. Schade, J. P.: Origin of the spontaneous electrical activity of the cerebral cortex. in Wortis, J., Ed.: Recent Advances in Biological Psychiatry, Vol. II, Grune & Stratton, Inc., New York, 1960.

8. Purpura, D., Carmichael, M. W., and Housepian, E. M.: Physiological and anatomical studies of development of superficial axodendritic synaptic pathways in neocortex, Exp. Neurol. 2:324, 1960.

9. Schade, J., and Baxter, C.: Changes during growth in the volume and surface area of cortical neurons in the rabbit, ibid. 2:158, 1960.

10. Scheibel, M. E., and Scheibel, A. B.: Discussion in Symposium on Dendrites, EEG Clin. Neurophys., Suppl. No. 10, 1958.

11. Moruzzi, G., and Magoun, H. W.: Brain stem reticular formation and activation of the EEG, ibid. 5:1, 1949.

12. Ramon y Cajal, S.: Histologie du systeme nerveux de l'homme et des vertebres, Consejo Superior de Investigaciones Cientificas (reprinted), Madrid, 1952.

13. Gray, E. G.: Axo-somatic and axo-dendritic synapses of the cerebral cortex: an electron microscope study, J. Anat. 93:420, 1959.

14. Fox, C.: Personal communication.

15. Ellingson, R. J.: Cortical electrical responses to visual stimulation in the human infant, EEG Clin. Neurophys. 12:663, 1960.

16. Desmedt, J. E., and LaGrutta, G.: Control of brain potentials by pseudo-cholinesterase, J. Physiol. (London) 129:46, 1955.

17. Marty, R., Contamin, F., and Scherrer, J.: Cortical response to photic stimulation in a newborn cat, ibid. 10:761, 1958.

18. Grossman, C.: Electro-ontogenesis of cerebral activity. Forms of neonatal responses and their recurrence in epileptic discharges, A.M.A. Arch. Neurol. Psychiat. 74:186, 1955.

19. Rose, J. E., Adrian, H., and Santibanez, G.: Electrical signs of maturation in the auditory system of the kitten, Acta Neurol. Latinoamer. 3:133, 1957.

20. McCulloch, W. S., Lettvin, J. Y., Pitts, W. H., and Dell, P. C.: An electrical

hypothesis of central inhibition and facilitation, Res. Publ. Ass. Nerv. Ment. Dis. 30:87, 1950.

21. Eccles, J. C.: The Neurophysiological Basis of Mind, Clarendon Press, Oxford. 1953.

22. Vogt, C., and Vogt, O.: Personal communication.

Discussion by R. J. Ellingson, Ph.D.

This sort of correlative anatomical, physiological, and behavioral developmental study has long been needed, and I am glad that it has been undertaken by workers as well qualified to do so as the Scheibels. The ultimate significance of this work for the behavioral sciences is, I think, obvious.

I would like to make three points (inferences from limited electrophysiological developmental data), which are, I am sure, already known to the Scheibels.

1. Individual differences among very young animals of the same chronological age are often greater than those among adults. For example, the standard deviations of visual and auditory cortical evoked response latencies are considerably greater for young than for adult animals in several species studied.

2. The rate of development of various "systems" within one nervous system may differ considerably. For example, in the young kitten the visual system is by several criteria less well developed than the auditory, and reaches maturity at a later date. It would be of interest to know the degree to which anatomical indicators of maturity of the respective structures parallel the electrical findings.

3. Species differences in rate and order of development of the various parts of the nervous system may differ considerably. For example, it is not possible in kittens to record visual cortical evoked potentials until after birth, and in many until seven to ten days after birth. In humans we have recorded them (from the scalp) in premature infants as early as twenty-six weeks after conception.

This valuable work by the Scheibels opens up more research possibilities than can be handled by one group of workers. It is to be hoped that others will follow their lead.

Discussion by Williamina A. Himwich, Ph.D.

The study of the developing brain is my first love in the field of research. I am delighted to welcome to this field a worker with the wide range of talents displayed by Dr. Scheibel in his paper. Studies of this sort are necessary before we can understand the maturation of the neurophysiological responses of the brain.

We have not worked with kittens but have used one-day-old puppies. In these animals under curare and artificial respiration we find spindles, which apparently are sleep spindles separated by irregular low-wave activity. I would like to ask Dr. Scheibel if he has tried this type of preparation in his study of the kitten.

Dr. Scheibel's paper illustrates the development of the anatomical structure necessary for the production of the typical adult pattern of the EEG. This undoubtedly is also accompanied by the accumulation of the necessary biochemical substrates to support the electrical activity. Unfortunately, little has been done on this subject in the kitten. We have done some studies which suggest that in the cat as in the dog the glutamic acid level at birth and within the next few days is approximately two-thirds of the adult value. Other studies in the rat and the guinea pig would suggest that at the point where the adult-type EEG appears the protein is also about two-thirds of the adult level. Enzymatic activity is increasing rapidly, and sodium and potassium concentrations are approaching the adult level at this time. All of these events, both anatomical and biochemical, appear to be necessary for the production of electrical activity.

Dr. Scheibel did not attempt to condition the kittens to auditory stimuli before their tenth week of life. I would have expected that such conditioning could have been accomplished earlier on the basis of observations of the behavior of young kittens. Also since auditory evoked potentials mature by five to ten days of age, as shown by Ellingson, auditory conditioning might be possible as soon as the muscles are sufficiently developed. I wonder if Dr. Scheibel would care to comment on this point.

I would like to compliment Dr. Scheibel on this very elegant study of the development of the dendrites and the EEG in the kitten. I hope he will continue in this field and give us many more such valuable papers.

Answer by Dr. Scheibel

The comments of Drs. Himwich and Ellingson are very much appreciated. We have not yet determined the earliest postnatal age at which conditioning and extinction phenomena can be demonstrated. We have no reason to doubt that younger animals can show such responses. Correlation of structurofunctional studies with biochemical data should remain the goal of projects of this sort. Time did not allow presentation of some chromatographic data obtained along with the histological and physiological material. We hope to report this later.

Anatomical and physiological variation from kitten to kitten is indeed striking, as is the range of primitive response patterns, even in kittens of the same litter. This variation may be so great as to necessitate extreme conservatism in relating psychophysiological behavior of one litter mate at one developmental epoch to the Golgi picture, as revealed by a litter mate sacrificed at that same time.

Studies of Plasma Protein Factors That May Be Involved in Psychoses

By HUDSON HOAGLAND, Ph.D., ROBERT B. PENNELL, Ph.D., JOHN R. BERGEN, Ph.D., CALVIN A. SARAVIS, Ph.D., HARRY FREEMAN, M.D., AND WERNER KOELLA, M.D.

During the last five years work has been reported from four independent groups indicating the existence of a protein factor in human plasma that may be involved in psychotic behavior. In contrast to many investigations, these studies refreshingly tend to confirm each other.

REVIEW OF STUDIES: THREE GROUPS

In 1957 Heath et al.[1,2] at Tulane University reported the extraction of a protein fraction from the plasma of schizophrenic patients that, when injected into nonpsychotic volunteers, produced transient psychotic episodes. They called this substance "taraxein" and in double blind studies reported that similar fractions from nonpsychotic subjects had no effects on injection. They used an animal bioassay to test their taraxein fractions prior to tests on man, a test which consisted of observing the effects of its injection into monkeys. Active fractions were reported to produce catatonic-like states in the monkeys and also the occurrence of spiking from septal regions of the brain, as recorded from implanted electrodes in chronic preparations. The initial procedure used by the Tulane workers for the isolation of taraxein proved to be difficult to reproduce. The procedure indicated, however, the precipitability of the postulated protein by ammonium sulfate at concentrations long known to precipitate the less soluble globulins from plasma. It also showed taraxein to belong to that group of globulins which are insoluble in the absence of electrolyte, the euglobulins. The initial steps of the Tulane procedure were virtually identical with those used for many years in the preparation of gamma globulins.

Early attempts to confirm the effects of taraxein by other workers were unsuccessful. Extraction procedures similar to those used at Tulane according to Robins [3] and Siegel et al. [4], who report negative findings from several other laboratories, yielded inactive fractions; and various criticisms of the Tulane procedures and techniques have been discussed [2]. Melander and Martens [5], however, have reported that taraxein potentiates the action of some psychoactive drugs.

Taraxein is unstable. Fractions reported active at Tulane when shipped to other laboratories for testing in monkeys were found to be inactive [2].* Some taraxein fractions from schizophrenic patients were found inactive by the Tulane group. The lability of taraxein and the uncertain reliability of its extraction procedures are factors that may well account for the difficulty in obtaining confirmatory results.

During 1956 and 1957, Winter and Flataker [6] at the laboratories of Merck Sharp & Dohme studied the effects of injecting plasma samples from hospitalized psychotic patients, physically ill non-psychotic hospitalized patients, and normal control subjects into young rats of the Holtzman strain and observed the effects on their behavior. They used for a bioassay a measure of the ability of the rats to climb a 5-ft rope from the floor to a platform containing food pellets. The rats were fasted twenty-four hours before testing and were allowed to eat only briefly on the food platform before being returned to their cages. After a period of training, the rats ran up the rope in 2 to 3 seconds with great regularity and without any indication of decrement in performance throughout the course of a day, as measured by the climb time. Drugs such as lysergic acid diethylamide (LSD) and mescaline, which in man produce psychotic episodes, increase the climbing time when injected into trained rats. Usually the increases in climbing time occur within minutes after the intraperitoneal injection of an active substance, reach a maximum within half an hour, and diminish to preinjection levels by the end of an hour. Following the injection of a drug like LSD, the rats were tested at 5, 10, 20, 30, 45, and 60 minutes post-injection or until the climb time reached its preinjection values. The climbing time in seconds was plotted against the time after

*Also, personal communication.

injection in minutes and the area under the skewed bell-shaped curve, minus that under the base line, was called the climb time delay (CTD), and reported in minute-seconds. For each determination of CTD, a group of animals, usually five, was used and the value reported as mean CTD. The area under the curve has been shown to have a linear relationship to the logarithm of the drug dosage. The injection of saline has no effect on the CTD. The validity and significance of the data were established by analysis of variance.

Winter and Flataker found that the intraperitoneal injection of 1 ml of blood plasma or serum from normal and psychotic subjects increased the CTD after the manner of LSD except that the time course for serum or plasma was longer. The injection of plasma or of serum from the majority of schizophrenic patients and other psychotic patients produced a response which averaged two to three times greater than that of plasma from normal control subjects. Comparisons of the effects of plasma from 80 psychotic patients with that of 82 nonpsychotic subjects, including both general hospital patients and normal well subjects showed a marked and highly significant difference between the two groups. The CTD for the 80 psychotic patients averaged over 400 minute-seconds, while that from both 47 normal volunteers and 35 physically ill hospitalized patients averaged about 150 minute-seconds. The difference between the psychotic subjects and the other two groups was significant with a P value of less than 0.001. The plasma samples from the psychotic subjects were obtained from chronic patients of three psychiatric hospitals and included a variety of diagnoses. There appeared to be no systematic difference in the CTD values for the various categories of psychoses among the 80 patients.

Attempts to confirm these findings have been both successful and unsuccessful. Ghent and Freedman [7] were unable to find differences when they injected serum from schizophrenic and normal control subjects into rats in a CTD study. This study involved relatively few patients and controls compared to that of Winter and Flataker. Our own study [8], however, using plasma but not serum and using the same procedure as that of Winter and Flataker, has confirmed this work.

The work of the Merck Sharp & Dohme group and our studies thus indicated the desirability of fractionation procedures to obtain more information about the possible nature of the active substance involved. Accordingly, Sanders et al. [9] fractionated human serum. Their method differed somewhat from that of the Tulane group. For the preparation of globulins known to have solubilities similar to those described for taraxein, they chose the cold ethanol method of Cohn[10] with Lever's modification[11] for their separations and developed a further purification which gave them a fraction (Cohn Fraction III) similar in constituents to the taraxein-containing fraction of Heath. They found that this fraction produced some behavior changes in monkeys as well as marked CTD changes in rats. However, purification and concentration of this fraction yielded highly active fractions of plasma both from normal and psychotic donors. The greater the purity the greater the activity but the less the differentiation (with purification) between normal and patient plasma samples. Tests at various states of purification revealed that the activity of the fraction from normal plasma increased during the purification procedures, whereas activity of the fractions from psychotic plasma was apparent from the start. This led these workers to postulate that the active fractions occur normally in close association with an "inhibitor" which was presumably removed during the purification procedures. This postulate suggests that the inhibitor of the active substance affecting the rats is present in adequate amounts in normal individuals but in inadequate amounts in psychotic patients. We shall presently describe further tests made by the Merck Sharp & Dohme group and by our own group in an attempt to demonstrate the properties of this inhibitor, which appears to be removed in a discarded supernatant fraction during the course of extraction of the active fraction.

EXPERIENCES OF ONE GROUP OF WORKERS

We would like now to describe our own attempts to isolate and identify an active factor in human plasma. We found in our early studies of the effects of plasma on the rat CTD that the activity of the samples was lost quite rapidly on their standing and disappeared on their freezing. Pennell accordingly decided upon a more rapid and gentle method of fractionation, the zinc method 12 of Surgenor et al. [12], involving the precipitation of certain plasma protein constituents by zinc. This procedure divides the plasma into two fractions, one called the stable plasma protein solution (SPPS) containing primarily albumins and a number of other soluble protein constituents; and a second fraction precipitated by zinc and then redissolved that is called the plasma globulin precipitate (or PGP fraction). This consists primarily of beta, gamma, and some alpha globulins and includes the fraction in which taraxein was reported by the Tulane group.

A special value of the zinc method is that fractionating requires a shorter time to perform, three days in contrast to six days necessary for the procedures of the Tulane and Merck Sharp & Dohme groups. It is important that fractionation be prompt and as short as possible to prevent loss of activity. The zinc method also involves less drastic exposures to temperature differences and effects of solvents than do other procedures. Our method permits the detection of loss of activity, as compared to the original plasma, during the preparation of the fractions, and has brought sharply into focus the great lability of the active fractions. We have, however, also used the procedures of both the Merck Sharp & Dohme and Tulane groups to compare with our results. We have been able to confirm the effects on our rats using taraxein obtained by the Tulane technique as well as fractions obtained by the Merck Sharp & Dohme method. Our PGP fraction gives CTD effects on the rats similar to those obtained with taraxein. We have found the zinc method more reliable, in that in our hands our proportion of active fractions using this method is higher as might be expected from the nature of the procedure.

There are, however, differences to be noted in comparing our tests with those of the Tulane group. Our PGP samples are active in the rats when obtained both from normal plasma and from that of the psychotics. There is about twice the average activity, however, in the samples from the psychotic patients as in those from normal control subjects, and this difference is maintained with purification and concentration. The Tulane group reports that they do not encounter any taraxein-like action from normal plasma. We also obtain, as does the Merck Sharp & Dohme group, fractions from psychoses other than schizophrenia (involutional psychoses and manic depression) with an average high activity higher than that of control samples but below that of the schizophrenic populations. While the activity of fractions from our nonschizophrenic psychotic subjects averages higher than that from plasma of nonpsychotic subjects, the differences are not statistically significant [13], as they are when we compare samples from schizophrenic subjects with those of our nonpsychotic population. According to Heath et al. [1], their taraxein is only obtained from schizophrenic and not from other psychotic patients and never from normal persons. It should be borne in mind, however, that we are using

very different bioassay methods. Heath has used monkeys and human
subjects and we have used the rat CTD test for a bioassay.

In our CTD studies we have compared pooled plasma samples
from two psychotic patients with a sample from one normal control
subject. These samples were processed at the same time at the
Protein Foundation. This matching of patient and control for each
experiment is important because inevitably there are variations in
batches of rats from time to time and in aspects of the extraction
procedures. Blood samples of 125 ml are drawn for processing. In
one study[8] we tested only patients newly admitted to the hospital
and before diagnosis. Blood samples were drawn from these acute
cases within a few days after admission, thus obviating effects of
chronic hospitalization *per se*. Patients on ataraxic drugs were
excluded. This study consists of 36 psychotic patients, 30 of whom
later turned out to be schizophrenic subjects matched against 19
normal control subjects. Figure 1 shows the data of this experiment, indicating that the psychotics' samples averaged about twice
the amount of substance as measured by the rat CTD as did the

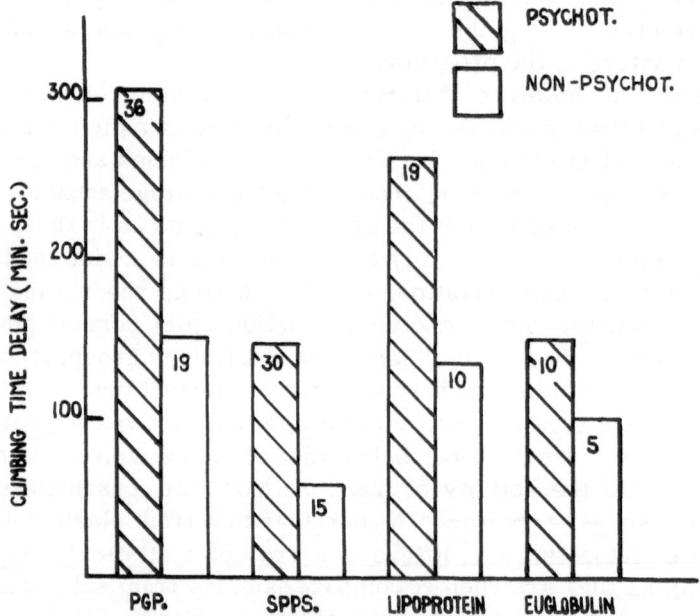

FIG. 1. Mean climbing time delay produced in trained rats by intraperitoneal injections of
plasma protein solutions from psychotic and nonpsychotic persons. Thirty of the psychotic subjects
were diagnosed as schizophrenic. Number of subjects tested shown by number in bar. (From A.M.A.
Arch. Neurol. [8])

control samples. Maximum activity was found in the PGP fractions, but significant activity was also found in the SPPS fractions. Subsequent improvement in methods of separation, however, have shown the activity to occur, to a significant degree, only in the PGP fraction and not in the SPPS fraction. In other studies we have found no average differences in the activities of plasma PGP fractions in our rat tests between these acute cases and chronic schizophrenic patients, nor have we found significant sex differences. We have tested samples from approximately 200 psychotic patients and 100 normal control subjects. We have not as yet studied a population of psychoneurotic patients.

While not shown in the subsequent tables, an analysis of variance procedures has been applied to our data [8]. The differences between patient and control groups to be described in this paper are significant for the most part at better than the 1% level of confidence. The statistics will be published elsewhere.

As mentioned, our early studies showed that all human plasma produced a significant CTD when injected intraperitoneally into trained rats. Examination of plasma fractions prepared by standard fractionating techniques soon indicated that this activity resided in globulins easily precipitated by ammonium sulfate, cold ethanol, or zinc cations. The albumins and the less readily precipitated globulins, though comprising the bulk of the total plasma protein, were esentially devoid of the ability to delay the climbing time of the trained rats.

The fraction of plasma responsible for the delay in climbing time was extremely labile. Storage of plasma and protracted fractioning techniques resulted either in complete loss of activity or in erratic, poorly reproducible results. Prompt separation of plasma from the cellular elements of blood and prompt fractionation by the simplest fractionating techniques were therefore adopted. Even so, it was impossible to retain the activity of the plasma fractions upon storage for more than a day or two. Our investigation revealed that the activity of the fractions could be retained for weeks when they were stored under hydrogen [14]. This was not true for storage under nitrogen, oxygen, or air. Although the true meaning of this observation is not evident, it led to an investigation of the importance in maintenance of increased levels of reducing agents during the fractionation procedure. Ascorbic acid, a natural constituent of plasma, was chosen. Table I illustrates the heightened activity of the zinc-precipitated globulins (PGP) prepared in the presence of

TABLE I

Activities (Disturbance of Climbing Time) of Globulins Prepared
in Presence of Varying Amounts of Ascorbic Acid

Ascorbic Acid Concentration (mM)	CTD (min-sec) Produced by Plasma Globulin Precipitate	
	Nonpsychotic	Psychotic
0.5	46	117
1.0	155	266
2.0	179	275
4.0	239	675

TABLE II

Comparison of Effect on Climbing Time of Trained Rats
of PGP and SPPS Prepared from Normal Human Plasma
in the Absence and Presence of Added Ascorbic Acid

Sample	No. Donors	No. Rats Injected	Mean CTD (min-sec)
		No added ascorbic acid	
PGP*	29	117	181
SPPS†	17	130	52
		Added ascorbic acid	
PGP†‡	32	115	549
SPPS†‡	9	20	45

*Each injection equivalent to amount of fraction in 1 to 2 ml plasma per 100 g rat body weight.
†Each injection equivalent to amount of fraction in 1 to 5 ml plasma per 100 g rat body weight.
‡Ascorbic acid concentration during isolation: 1 to 4 mM.

increasing concentrations of ascorbic acid. The activity of all the samples increases with increasing concentrations of ascorbic acid, and the ratio of the differences between patient and control samples is maintained.

In all subsequent fractionations a concentration of 4 mM ascorbic acid has been used throughout the procedure. Table II permits more extensive comparison of the CTD produced by PGP prepared with no added ascorbic acid with that prepared in the presence of an added reducing agent. It will be noted that the ascorbic acid has no effect on the CTD produced by SPPS. Storage under hydrogen likewise has no effect on the activity of SPPS.

Further purification of the active factor could be obtained by precipitation of the redissolved PGP at pH 5.8 followed by diethyl-aminoethyl cellulose (DEAE) chromatography of the resulting precipitate. The procedure in brief by which the active globulin may be prepared is as follows:

Plasma is separated promptly from the cells of whole blood by centrifugation. The plasma is diluted with an equal volume of cold (2 to 4 C) 0.15 M sodium chloride solution containing 8 mM ascorbic acid adjusted to pH 6.4. To the diluted plasma is added zinc glycinate to give a concentration of 25 mM Zn. The mixture is adjusted to pH 6.8. After 2 hours to overnight at 2 to 4C, the PGP is removed by centrifugation at 2 to 4 C. The PGP is dissolved in 0.5 M EDTA (ethylenediaminetetraacetic acid) solution, pH 7.0, a quantity of EDTA equivalent to the amount of added zinc being used. The dissolved PGP is dialyzed with stirring against large volumes of 0.15 M NaCl solution containing 4 mM ascorbic acid adjusted to pH 6.4 at 2 to 4 C overnight.

The dialyzed PGP is diluted to one-half of the plasma volume with cold 0.15 M NaCl and 4 mM ascorbic acid solution adjusted to pH 6.4. Zinc glycinate is added to a 25-mM concentration, and the mixture is adjusted to pH 5.8. After 2 hours to overnight a precipitate is collected by centrifugation at 2 to 4 C. The precipitate is dissolved as before in 0.5 M EDTA, pH 7.0, and is dialyzed overnight against large volumes of 0.15 M NaCl and 4 mM ascorbic acid solution at pH 6.4.

After dialysis, insoluble fibrinogen is removed by centrifugation, and the protein content of the solution is estimated by nitrogen determination or by optical density measurement. Final purification is achieved by chromatographic separation on DEAE cellulose. The milligrams of protein per unit of wet resin volume should not exceed 3. The column is prepared and equilibrated in 0.02 M sodium acetate and 4 mM ascorbic acid, pH 7. Elution is by variable gradient, the column being fed from a mixing chamber which at first contains 0.02 M sodium acetate and 4 mM ascorbic acid, pH 7, with which is gradually mixed 0.2 M acetate buffer, pH 4.5, containing 4 mM ascorbic acid. Protein is precipitated from the eluates at pH 7 by 20 mM Zn. The precipitates are dissolved in EDTA as before and are dialyzed. The preparation is then ready for assay. Solutions of the active fraction may be sterilized by filtration through Millipore filters and stored under hydrogen with little loss of activity. Table III presents data obtained from normal human plasma.

From the inception of this study, plasma from schizophrenic and other psychotic subjects has been fractionated and tested simultaneously with that from normal donors.

Different amounts of an active PGP fraction have been injected into rats and the CTD values for each dose measured. A plot of PGP dose against the CTD yields good logarithmic dose response curves.

TABLE III

Precipitation of Active Globulin from PGP Prepared from Normal Human Plasma at 25 mM Zn^{++}, 1 Plasma Volume, pH 5.8, 0.15 Ionic Strength, 4 mM Ascorbic Acid

Sample	No. Donors	No. Rats Injected	Mean CTD (min-sec)	Relative Purity
Plasma*	8	55	136	1
PGP†	32	155	549	3
SPPS*	9	20	45	-
25 mM precipitate‡	25	145	393	20
25 mM supernatant‡	10	40	58	-
Chromatographed Product§	8	145	1230	500

*Each injection equivalent to amount of fraction in 1 to 2 ml plasma per 100 g body weight.
†Each injection equivalent to amount of fraction in 1 to 5 ml plasma per 100 g body weight.
‡Each injection equivalent to amount of fraction in 3 to 5 ml plasma per 100 g body weight.
§Each injection equivalent to amount of fraction in 5 ml of plasma per 100 g body weight.

It will be seen in Table IV that greater CDT consistently is produced by fractions prepared from the plasma of psychotic than by fractions prepared from normal donors. This differential is maintained at each step of the purification. The CDT differences are significant (P<0.01) except, as earlier mentioned, for those between the nonschizophrenic psychotic and control subjects. These findings are believed to corroborate the existence of an abnormality in the plasma protein of schizophrenic persons, as reported by Heath et al. [1,2]. Although we prefer the zinc preparative procedure reported, because of its speed and simplicity, the procedure currently used by Heath and his associates for the isolation of taraxein produces, in our hands, fractions from both normal and psychotic subjects giving data comparable to those reported here. The present study is most readily interpretable as suggesting an alteration in schizophrenia, either of the quantity or of the quality, of a normal plasma globulin. It does not preclude, however, that the higher climb time delays produced by the globulin prepared from the plasma of psychotic subjects is due to a protein which is not present in normal plasma. Such a new protein would, however, have solu-

TABLE IV

Comparison of Fractions Prepared and Tested Simultaneously
from Normal and Psychotic Donors

Sample	No. Donors	No. Rats Injected	Mean CTD (min-sec)	% CTD of Patients Over Controls
Plasma	8 Nonpsychotic	55	136	
	13 Schizophrenic	92	197	45
PGP	12 Nonpsychotic	40	818	
	13 Schizophrenic	40	1112	36
25 mM Zn^{++} ppt.	13 Nonpsychotic	65	353	
	17 Schizophrenic	85	841	136
25 mM Zn^{++} ppt.	12 Nonpsychotic	60	320	
	14 Nonschizophrenic psychotics	84	372	16

bility characteristics entirely comparable to those of a normal plasma globulin.

Our observations suggest, although they do not yet prove, that there is increased activity and stability of the globulin as purification proceeds. This might suggest the gradual elimination of an inhibitor or of a destructive agent or of both during the isolation.

The studies have led us to various attempts further to identify the active substance. Our protein extraction procedures all involve many hours of dialysis against saline solutions. One would thus expect that all dialyzable molecules would have been removed. However, in the course of a variety of experiments we dialyzed some active PGP fractions from patients against less active PGP fractions from normal controls. The dialysis was through cellophane for eighteen to twenty-four hours. To our surprise, we found invariably that the less active fractions markedly gained activity as measured by our rat tests and the active fractions correspondingly lost it [8]. These experiments have been often repeated by us and are unequivocal. The results suggest that a small molecule was trasferred across the membrane from the active globulin to receptors on the less active globulin. Such transfers did not occur with protein solutions used as controls other than the PGP moities in our experiments. However, we also found that Fraction III as isolated by the techniques of Sanders et al. [9], that contain the same active globulins as our PGP fractions, also showed this exchange of activity between active and inactive fractions. These results could be accounted for either by the transfer of a small active prosthetic group directly from active globulin fractions of psychotic subjects to less active globulins of control subjects, or, on the other hand, they might reflect the transfer of an inhibitor of the active substance from the less active samples of plasma from normal subjects to those of the more active fractions of the psychotic patients. This finding is of special interest since it suggests a possible mechanism for the transfer of activity across the blood brain barrier. This barrier would be expected to be impermeable to large globulin molecules, as is the cellophane membrane. However, a small active molecule bound to protein might be exchanged across the blood brain barrier with a corresponding globulin synthesized in the brain. We do not know what this small molecule may be. It might be an indole or a biogenic amine or something quite different. All attempts to separate and isolate it from the carrier protein have so far been unsuccessful.

We have sought indices of effects of our substance on the central nervous system other than that of confusing and slowing the rat's ability to climb. Koella and Wells[15] have reported studies of effects of injections of the psychotomimetic drug LSD on optically evoked potentials in the nonanesthetized rabbit. Using a similar procedure Koella has studied the effects of injected PGP samples from normal subjects and schizophrenic patients on the cortical potentials evoked by flashes of light to the eyes of unanesthetized rabbits with chronically implanted electrodes [13]. It was found that active fractions from psychotic subjects produce similar effects on the evoked potentials to those of LSD. The relatively inactive PGP fractions from normal control subjects have no effect on the evoked potentials. Both PGP extracts from the patients and injections of LSD markedly decrease the variability of the amplitude and wave pattern of repetitively evoked potentials. The decrease in variability following the injection of LSD lasted for about 15 minutes and that of PGP samples for an average of 8 minutes. These effects on variability for both substances are statistically highly significant. Latency of cortical responses to the light flashes is also significantly reduced after injections of PGP samples from schizophrenic but not by samples from normal control subjects. There is also a reduction of variability of latency, but this is not as marked as is the reduction of variability of amplitude. The similarity of effects of the psychotomimetic drug LSD and the more active PGP samples from patients in these tests, as well as in the rat climb test, indicates similar actions of these substances on the brains of the animals.*

*Marrazzi et al. (in the symposium volume Inhibition of the Nervous System and Gamma Aminobutyric Acids, Pergamon Press, New York, 1960, p. 534; Fed. Proc. 18:419, 1959; and personal communication) have reported that they have demonstrated a cerebral synaptic inhibitor of transcallosal conduction in the cat present in normal human serum. Serum or serum fractions are injected into the ipsilateral artery and produce inhibition similar to that resulting from injection of the LSD, serotonin, and some other biogenic amines. Only aged and not fresh whole serum shows that effect. They have also reported that a taraxein sample sent them by Heath and Leach similarly acts as an inhibitor. They have extracted for testing, albumin and globulin fractions from normal serum and have also tested albumin and globulin fractions sent by the Protein Foundation. They found maximum inhibitory activity in the albumin fractions and less in the globulin fractions. These fractions lost activity with aging. The inhibitory action occurs so promptly (seconds) that they believe a small molecule may be involved in passing the blood brain barrier. As in our own studies, they were unable to separate this possible small molecule from the protein by ultrafiltration. They have not as yet made comparisons of serum or its fractions from schizophrenic and nonpsychotic subjects.

Those findings are both interesting and puzzling, since our active substance and taraxein are composed primarily of globulins and our albumin fractions are not active in our tests. Marrazzi finds that aging enhances the activity of whole serum in inhibiting the transcallosal response, but aging destroys the activity of plasma fractions and of taraxein. We also found this loss of activity in our tests if the samples were unprotected by hydrogen storage or ascorbic acid. Of course different bioassay tests are involved and ours are fractions of plasma rather than serum, but clearly more clarifying work is needed.

Koella has pointed out that sensory deprivation may induce psychotic symptoms such as hallucinations in man by reducing afferent impulses impinging on the central nervous system, thus reducing the irregular afferent bombardment of cortical centers. The decreased variability of cortical potentials induced by light flashes in animals following both LSD and injections of active PGP extracts from psychotic patients is highly suggestive, since presumably sensory deprivation and the actions of these substances may have similar effects on sensory receptive areas.

Ulrich Schaeppi in our laboratory has made pharmacological tests of our active fractions on rabbits and cats [13]. He finds them to have no effects as stimulants or inhibitors of the peripheral autonomic nervous system as judged by a variety of pharmacological tests.

Earlier in this paper we mentioned that Sanders et al.[9] were led to consider that an inhibitor of their active globulin might be contained in normal plasma. The evidence for this came from the finding that with increasing purification and removal of extraneous protein, differences in activity between samples from normal and psychotic subjects were lost, i.e., all purified fractions were equally high in activity. This led them to reexamine certain of their supernatant fractions that had been discarded in the course of processing in hopes of finding a solution that would inhibit their active globulin fractions [16]. In 27 experiments they injected extracts of one of their previously discarded supernatants from normal subjects into their rats 15 minutes before injecting their active fractions. In 19 of the 27 experiments they found the activities of the active fractions to be significantly reduced in the rat tests, i.e., the CTD values were reduced following the injection of the presumed inhibitor.

We also have prepared the inhibitors by the methods of Sanders et al.[16] from normal plasma and injected them into rats 15 minutes before injecting our active PGP fractions. We found (unpublished) in nine experiments a relation indicating that an inhibitor reduced the PGP response in proportion to the logarithm of the CTD activity of the particular PGP sample.* It is clearly desirable to learn more about this possible inhibitory substance because of its implications for therapeutic use in relation to the psychoses.

---

*The "inhibition" decreased the effect of highly active samples, but this inhibition became less marked as the original activity of the samples approached a particular lower value (CTD 550). Below this value, injections of the inhibition potentiated sample activity. Samples of lowest activity showed greatest potentiation.

OTHER STUDIES

We have reviewed studies from Tulane, from the laboratories of Merck Sharp & Dohme, and from the collaborative efforts of the Worcester Foundation with the Protein Foundation. The findings of all three groups point to a globulin that may play a role in the major psychoses. Earlier in the discussion we mentioned a fourth group who have independently produced evidence for a protein factor similar to ours involved in psychotic behavior.

Frohman et al.[17, 18] from the Lafayette Clinic in Detroit have produced evidence for the presence of a globulin in blood of schizophrenic patients very similar in properties to our purified globulin fractions. Their globulin fractions appear to modify carbohydrate metabolism of cells in characteristic ways.

The Detroit workers studied the carbohydrate metabolism of erythrocytes from normal persons and schizophrenic patients by the use of C14-labeled hexose-6-phosphate and hexose-1-phosphate as tracers. They found that when 10 units of insulin were administered as a stressor to schizophrenic patients and to normal control subjects that the production of energy-rich ATP of the cells from normal persons was increased but that of the patients' cells was not. The red blood cells of the schizophrenic subjects thus responded less effectively to this insulin challenge than did those of the controls.

There are two interrelated pathways of glucose metabolism, the Embden-Meyerhof cycle of anaerobic metabolism involving primarily hexose-1-phosphate as substrate and the hexose monophosphate shunt utilizing hexose-6-phosphate as substrate. The former pathway is primarily concerned with energy metabolism via the production and utilization of ATP and the latter with the synthesis of ribose for the production of nucleic acids necessary ultimately for protein formation. The insulin decreases the percent of carbohydrate metabolism through the shunt in erythrocytes from normal persons and favors the Embden-Meyerhof cycle. This effect does not occur in the erythrocytes of schizophrenic patients, as indicated by the C14 tracer studies.

The Detroit group found, however, that if erythrocytes of normal persons were incubated in the plasma of schizophrenic patients these cells then behaved metabolically like those from schizophrenic patients. This led them to the conclusion that there was a factor in plasma from schizophrenic patients that was responsible for this shift in metabolism. Frohman et al.[18] accordingly used chicken erythrocytes as test preparations and studied their carbohydrate metabolism after incubation in plasma from normal persons or from schizophrenic patients. They used the ratio of the cells' lactic acid to pyruvic acid production as a measure of hydrogen transport since Stoltz et al. in 1948 had shown this to be a measure of the oxidizing activity of tissues. Incubation in plasma from schizophrenic subjects significantly increased this ratio. Thus, a factor in the plasma of schizophrenic patients accentuates the anaerobic metabolism of the bird erythrocytes.

The Detroit group has presented evidence that the factor in plasma from schizophrenic subjects altering cell metabolism is probably an alpha globulin. This appears to have properties similar to those of taraxein and to our active globulin and of the concentrated globulin fraction of the Merck Sharp & Dohme group. Frohman et al. [18] used quite different isolation procedures from those of the other three groups.

None of the factors so far discussed may be regarded as one pure protein—all are clearly mixtures despite the concentration and refinement procedures used. The active protein appears to be either an alpha or beta globulin. Frohman and co-workers also have presented evidence that a small molecule may be combined with the globulin. They regard it as probable that their globulin factor may also be present in the plasma of normal persons but with more of it in the plasma from schizophrenic patients.*

Recently two groups in the Soviet Union [19, 20] have used the procedure of Heath et al. and have obtained globulin fractions from the plasma of schizophrenic patients that modify learned behavior patterns in mice. Space limitations preclude a critical discussion of these findings, but they further substantiate the findings from the American laboratories.

DISCUSSION AND SUMMARY

We have reviewed work from four groups indicating the existence of a globulin in human blood probably associated with a tightly bound small molecule. This active complex displays, on the average, considerably greater activity by several test procedures if it is extracted from the plasma of schizophrenic patients in contrast to that from normal controls.

*Personal communication.

Is this factor causally related to psychosis in man or is it an incidental by-product of the psychosis? The only direct evidence to date for its playing a causal role is that of the Tulane group, which reports that injected taraxein produces transient psychoses in man. This is the only one of the four groups whose work is here reviewed that has administered it to man. We have wished to obtain more information about the substance before testing its possible psychotogenic effects on man.

We think it especially interesting that evidence both from the Merck Sharp & Dohme group and from our group suggests the presence of an inhibitor or regulator of the activity of these globulin fractions in normal plasma that may block the actions of the possible psychotogenic factor as indicated by our rat tests. Further investigations of this inhibitor are under way.

REFERENCES

1. Heath, R. G., Martens, S., Leach, B. E., Cohen, M., and Angel, C.: Effect on behavior in humans with the administration of taraxein, Am. J. Psychiat. 114:14, 1957.

2. Heath, R. G.: Transactions of the Josiah Macy, Jr. Foundation 4th Conference on Neuropharmacology, 1957.

3. Robins, E.: Transactions of the Josiah Macy, Jr. Foundation 4th Conference on Neuropharmacology, 1957.

4. Siegel, M., Niswander, G. E., Sachs, E., and Stavros, D.: Taraxein, fact or artifact? Am. J. Psychiat. 115:819, 1959.

5. Melander, B., and Martens, S.: The mode of action of taraxein and LSD, Dis. Nerv. Syst. 19:478, 1958.

6. Winter, C. A., and Flataker, L.: Efect of blood plasma from psychotic patients upon performance of trained rats, A.M.A. Arch. Neurol. Psychiat. 80:441, 1958.

7. Ghent, L., and Freedman, A. M.: Comparison of normal and schizophrenic serum on motor performance in rats, Am. J. Psychiat. 115:465, 1958.

8. Bergen, J., Pennell, R. B., Freeman, H., and Hoagland, H.: Rat behavior changes in response to a blood factor from normal and psychotic persons, A.M.A. Arch. Neurol. 2:146, 1960.

9. Sanders, B. E., Flataker, L., Boger, W. P., Smith, E. V. C., and Winter, C. A.: Effect of protein fractions of normal and schizophrenic serum on rat performance. Vox Sanguinis 4:68, 1959.

10. Cohn, E. J., Strong, L. E., Hughes, Jr., W. L., Mulford, D. J., Ashworth, J. N., Melin, M., and Taylor, H. L.: Preparation and properties of serum and plasma proteins. IV. A system for the separation into fractions of the protein and lipoprotein components of biological tissues and fluids, J. Am. Chem. Soc. 68:459, 1956.

11. Lever, W. F., Gurd, F. R. N., Uroma, E., Brown, R. K., Barnes, B. A., Schmid, K., and Schultz, E. L.: Chemical, clinical and immunological studies on the products of human plasma fractionation. XL. Quantitative separation and determi-

nation of the protein components in small amounts of normal human plasma, J. Clin. Invest. 30:99, 1951.

12. Surgenor, D. M., Pennell, R. B., Alemeri, E., Batchelor, W. H., Brown, R. K., Hunter, M. J., and Mannick, V. L.: Preparation and properties of serum and plasma proteins. XXXV. A system of protein fraction using the zinc complexes, Vox Sanguinis 5:272, 1960.

13. Bergen, J. R., Koella, W. P., Freeman, H., and Hoagland, H.: A human plasma factor inducing behavioral and electrophysiological changes in animals in Symposium on some biological aspects of schizophrenic behavior, Ann. N.Y. Acad. Sci. 96: 469, 1962.

14. Bergen, J. R., Saravis, C., Pennell, R. B., and Hoagland, H.: Stabilization of a human blood factor causing behavior changes in rats, J. Neuropsychiat. 2:201, 1961.

15. Koella, W. P., and Wells, C. H.: Influence of LSD-25 on optically evoked potentials in the nonanesthetized rabbit, Am. J. Physiol. 1181:196, 1959.

16. Sanders, B. E., Smith, E. V. C., Flataker, L., and Winter, C. A.: Symposium on some biological aspects of schizophrenic behavior, Ann. N.Y. Acad. Sci. 96:448, 1962.

17. Frohman, C. E., Czajkowski, N. P., Luby, E. D., Gottlieb, J. S., and Senf, R.: Further evidence of a plasma factor in schizophrenia, A.M.A. Arch. Gen. Psychiat. 2:263, 1960.

18. Frohman, C. E., Luby, E. D., Tourney, G., Beckett, P. G. S., and Gottlieb, J. S.: Steps towards isolation of a serum factor in schizophrenia, Am. J. Psychiat. 117:401, 1960.

19. Mekler, L. B., Lepteva, N. N., Lozovsky, D. V., and Balesina, T. I.: J. Neuropath. Psychiat. (U.S.S.R.) 58:703, 1958.

20. Braynes, S. N., Kaversnevak, E. D., Korshov, B. A., and Kuchina, E. B.: Probl. Exp. Path. (U.S.S.R.), Mar. 1960.

CHAPTER 30

Behavioral Adaptations After Parietal Cortex Ablation in the Neonate Macaque

By L. AARONS, PH.D., J. SCHULMAN, M.D.,
J. H. MASSERMAN, M.D., AND G. P. ZIMMAR, M.A.

A considerable body of evidence supports the view that the restriction or deprivation of early sensory experiences has a detrimental effect upon the development of social relations in a variety of mammals. The recent studies of Harlow and Zimmermann [1] indicate that in the infant monkey somesthetic sensations are essential for the perception of "mothering" and underlie the growth of affectional responses. Most of the interest in disturbed mother-child relations in humans has centered around the mother's role; however, some authors have considered the possibility of receptive deficiencies in the child itself. Owen [2], for example, stated, " . . . many of the emotional disorders of childhood might be predicated upon faulty ego formations based not entirely upon unfortunate integrations with people important to the child, but upon faulty or irregular maturation of the nervous system, rendering perception of reality for these children different from that of other children, and thus making integrations with other people difficult." Escalona [3] suggested " . . . a schizophrenic process may be set in motion if a child in early infancy has organismic characteristics which make it impossible for him to interact with the mother in the normal way. . . ." Mahler et al. [4] reported " . . . we found that from a very early age there was an intrinsic inability to form affective contact with people . . ."

The present study is an initial attempt to explore experimentally the functions of the parietal lobe in the sensory integrations under-

This investigation was supported in part by Grant 1719 from the Mental Health Fund of the Illinois Department of Public Welfare and Research Grant M-2312 from the National Institutes of Health, Public Health Service.

lying the development of adaptive social-emotional patterns of behavior in the neonate macaque.

EXPERIMENTAL METHODS

Subjects

Four male and one female infant monkeys (*Macaca mulatta*) were separated from their mothers at birth and given optimal human care from two to eleven months in the homes of the investigators. The animals are designated as follows*:

M_8; normal male infant reared at home for 8 weeks.

M_{44}; normal male infant reared at home for 44 weeks.

M_{16p}; normal male infant reared at home for 16 weeks with OM_{20p} and then paired and caged with OM_{20p} in the laboratory.

OF_{10i}; parietal decorticated female reared at home for 10 weeks and then isolated in the laboratory.

OM_{20p}; parietal decorticated male reared at home for 20 weeks and then caged with M_{16p} in the laboratory.

Developmental Records

All animals were observed for the development of feeding habits, body weight, locomotor and manipulatory skills, reflex responses, play and exploration patterns, motor stereotypies, intra- and interspecies sociability, emotional reactions to novel objects or situations, illness, and idiosyncratic responses to specific events outside formal testing situations. Representative samples of the various developmental and test behavior were recorded on motion picture film [6].†

Surgery ‡

Following a neonate observation period of twenty-four hours to confirm normality, the parietal cortices were removed bilaterally six days apart on two monkeys (OF_{10i} and OM_{20p}). Open-field operations were performed under aseptic conditions with procaine anesthesia while the animal was restrained in a specially con-

---

*Male is indicated by the letter M, female by F, operated by O; the subscript indicates weeks of rearing at the experimenter's home, after which the animal was either isolated (i) or paired (p) in the laboratory.

†Copies are available from the Psychological Cinema Register, State College, Pennsylvania.

‡The authors are indebted to Drs. James E. Keplinger and Edir Siqueira for the surgery.

structed head-holder. The ablations carried out by aspiration (OF_{10i}) and resection (OM_{20p}) encompassed the postcentral, superior and inferior parietal gyri. Cortical hemorrhage was controlled by saline-soaked pledgets and by minimal cautery. The histologic verification of the lesions is being postponed until longitudinal behavior studies are completed.

Discrimination Training

Preliminary observations of sensory discrimination in an apparatus adapted from Josephine Blum [5] were begun when the monkeys were five months of age. This consisted of plywood boards fastened at right angles (vertical 24 by $6\frac{1}{2}$ by $\frac{1}{2}$ in. and horizontal 20 by 16 by $\frac{1}{2}$ in.) and mounted on tracks for presentation of choice trials (Fig. 1). To obtain a grape food reward, the monkey reached through an adjustable aperture ($\frac{1}{2}$ to 8 in.) to grasp and remove stimuli objects that served as handles for cups (2 in. diameter, $\frac{1}{2}$ in. height) fitted into recessed food wells.

The initial problem presented a $\frac{1}{2}$ in. diameter metal ring as

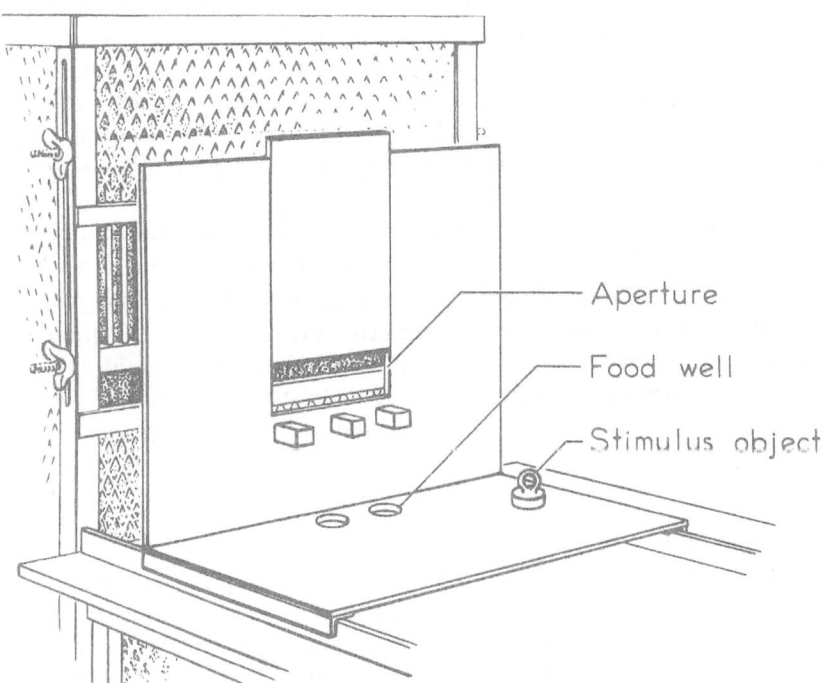

Aperture

Food well

Stimulus object

FIG. 1. Schematic diagram of somatosensory discrimination apparatus.

the positive stimulus and a $1\frac{1}{2}$ by $\frac{1}{2}$ in. wooden cylinder as the negative one. Twenty choices in irregular sequence were administered from three to six days each week. A modified procedure provided a maximum of three separate presentations, the last remaining until a correct choice was made; however, only the first responses were counted in learning scores, the arbitrary criterion for which was set at 20 successive correct choices in two consecutive sessions.

Although preliminary training allowed sequential viewing and manipulation of the stimuli, visual inspection was eliminated by gradually reducing the aperture so that only tactile cues remained. Subsequent discrimination problems employed form (a positive 1 by 1 by $\frac{1}{2}$ in. diamond vs. a negative 1 by $\frac{5}{8}$ in. square-ended prism) and hardness (a $1\frac{1}{8}$ by 1 by $\frac{1}{2}$ in. rectangular block of sponge rubber, positive, vs. an equal weight of balsa wood, negative, both sewed up in cloth covers).

Social Interaction Testing

After from three to five months of laboratory experience, normal and operated animals were paired according to a counterbalanced latin-square sequence of seven sessions for each combination in an unfamiliar test chamber (30 by 24 by 24 in.), opaque except for vertical bars in the front. Sessions lasted for 15 minutes, during which time the quality and frequency of social responses were recorded for each 5-minute interval.

Records included initiatory and reciprocatory behavior categorized as follows: (1) oral contacts: nipping, biting, mouthing, (2) manual contacts: tugging, grasping, pulling, nongrooming handling, (3) grooming: systematic fur picking, (4) mounting: grasping and straddling dorsal surface of partner, and (5) vocalization: high-pitched "coo," barks, or whines. Each monkey was then observed separately after the first and second pairings.

RESULTS

Developmental Characteristics

Content analysis of the written and photographic records showed, somewhat surprisingly, that the physical development, locomotor and manipulatory abilities, feeding habits, and patterns of spontaneous play and exploration were not significantly different in the parietal decorticate and normal infants. Equivalent gains in body weight over the first forty weeks are shown in Fig. 2.

As Kennard [7, 8] had observed in adult and infant monkeys, minor variations among animals in sitting, creeping, walking, running, jumping, and climbing behavior were not significantly related to the parietal lesions. Patellar deep-tendon reflexes and visual placing responses were also intact for the upper and lower limbs of all animals; however, tactual placing responses were completely absent for all limbs in the operated female (OF_{10i}) and absent in the upper limbs but present and slow in the lower limbs of the operated male (OM_{20p}). A consistent difference between the parietal and normal infants appeared also in oral activities, in that the former exhibited more non-food-rewarded sucking behavior during bottle feeding and also tended to employ the mouth rather than normal hand contacts in the exploration of both edible and nonedible objects.

Motor Patterns

All infants reared at home exhibited thumb sucking instead of the great-toe sucking pattern observed in laboratory animals. Motor stereotypies, such as rocking or swaying of the torso and

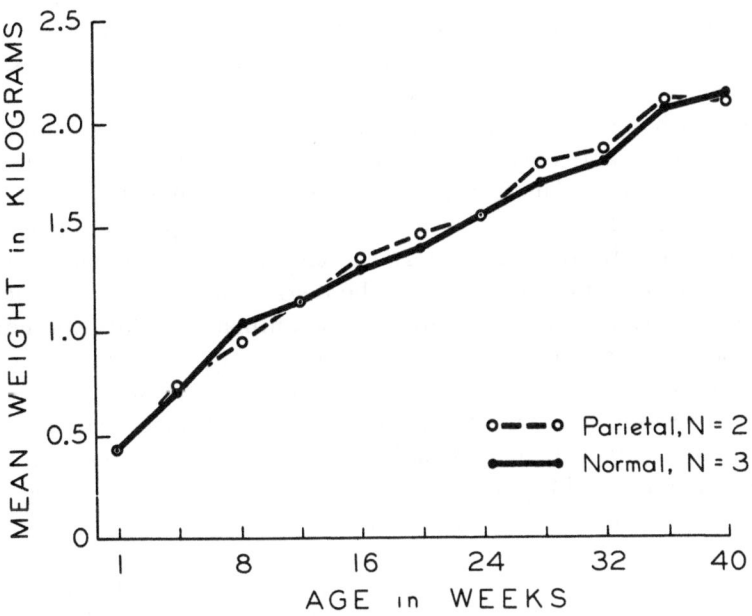

FIG. 2. Equivalent increments of body weight for parietal and normal infants for the first forty weeks of age.

rubbing or stroking of the body or parts of the cage, commonly seen in laboratory-raised animals did not appear in those reared at home. However, OM_{20p} frequently engaged in well-coordinated back flips and OF_{10i} in continual circling activity on a cage ledge. The home-reared infants may thus be regarded as intermediate between macaques born and raised in the wild and laboratory animals raised in isolation.

Exploratory Behavior

When confronted with new situations, e.g., a tree, a field, strange animals, or older monkeys (including their own mothers), all of our home-reared infants would seek refuge with their human parent surrogates and use them as a base for exploration. The range, intensity, and frequency of contact responses directed at humans both in the caged and free situation was highly related to the duration of human domiciliary care prior to removal to the laboratory. For example, OF_{10i} sought contact with various familiar people while in its cage, but would cling only to the experimenter if picked up in the open room. M_{16p} would retreat from or barely tolerate contact with unfamiliar humans while caged, but sought refuge with the experimenter when losing in play fights with OM_{20p} in the open room. OM_{20p} more readily accepted and sought contact with unfamiliar people when caged, and played hide-and-seek with or clung to people when loose in the laboratory. M_{44}, after eight months of home care, freely approached strange humans, both adult and children, and engaged in numerous play activities. Both M_{16p} and OM_{20p} were sexually responsive to the experimenter, exhibiting erections on the average of once a week during play and handling.

Consistently also, an inverse relationship was found between the extent of home rearing and the degree of disturbance elicited by presentation of novel inanimate and animate stimuli whether or not the experimenter was present. Thus, M_{44} after eight months showed a prompt, confident, and integrated investigatory pattern of visual examination, smell, touch, and taste of novel stimuli: e.g., he readily approached and handled a live snake and mouse on their first exposure. OM_{20p} likewise aggressively explored strange objects; in contrast, M_{16p} showed an initial reluctance followed by gradually increased investigatory approaches, whereas OF_{10i} when alone exhibited grimaces and prolonged delays in exploratory contacts. Consistently, M_8 was the most inhibited animal in all unfamiliar situations.

Discrimination Performance

Here the operated animals showed the most marked defects. M_{16p} mastered preliminary training for prompt and successful tactual manipulation of stimuli and food rewards in three days, whereas both OM_{20p} and OF_{10i} showed impaired motor dexterity and required thirty days to achieve a satisfactory level of performance. However, the absence of other manipulating deficits may be inferred from the equivalent performances of M_{10p}, OM_{20p}, and OF_{10i} on the visual-tactual problem (Table I). The slightly better scores of OM_{20p} and OF_{10i} are not necessarily indicative of an increased speed of learning, since the operated animals had greater opportunity to acquire facility in differentiation during their prolonged initial training.

M_{16p} learned to discriminate both form and hardness cues, whereas OM_{20p} failed to discriminate form with more than twice as many trials and hardness with 50% more trials to date. M_{16p}'s performance on the form discrimination is within the range of the preoperative scores (trials 311 to 617, errors 93 to 295) on a problem identical with that presented to the four monkeys studied by Blum [5]; OM_{20p}'s failure to discriminate form cues also confirms the tactile disturbance noted in the parietal monkey studied by Orbach and Chow [9].

TABLE I

Scores on Discrimination Problems*

Animal	Visual to Tactual— Multiple Cues		Tactual—Single Cue			
			Form		Hardness	
	Trials	Errors	Trials	Errors	Trials	Errors
M_{16p}	200	48	566	193	220	44
OM_{20p}	175	60	(1177)	(593)	(305)	(150)
OF_{10i}	150	30	not tested			

*Trials and errors required to reach a criterion of 20 successive correct choices on each of the problems. Scores in parenthesis indicate criteria not met. Visual, multiple cue: wooden cylinder vs. metal ring. Tactual form: diamond vs. square-ended prism; Hardness: sponge rubber block vs. wooden block.

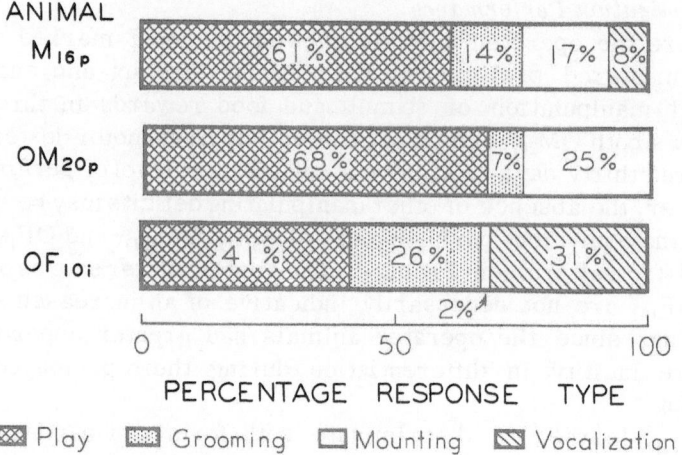

FIG. 3. A comparison of the similarities and differences in the over-all relative incidence of social responses by individual animals.

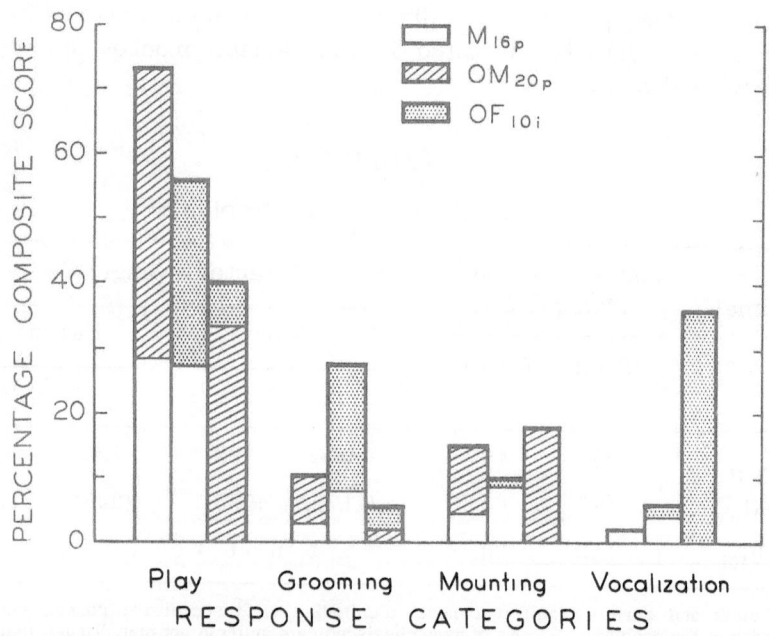

FIG. 4. The proportionate representation of response frequencies within and between pairs of monkey combinations depicting interaction effects of the extent of prior home-rearing experience in the distribution of social response types.

Social Interactions*

Predominating oral and secondary manual contacts in play behavior (tumbling, mauling, and wrestling) accompanied by "non-fearful" vocalizations were observed in all pairs, with the general tenor of a session being determined by the dominant animal in the specific pairing. Thus, OM_{20p}'s mounting and grooming were reciprocated by M_{16p}; M_{16p} mounted OF_{10i} on her sexual presentation and was groomed by her, and she responded similarly to OM_{20p}. The intensification of grooming activities by the parietal infants as compared to the normal may be interpreted as a compensation for decreased tactile sensitivity. On the other hand, the fact that the parietal animal with restricted home care (OF_{10i}) exhibited more than double the amount of grooming than the parietal with extensive experience is taken as indicating a summative interaction effect of extent of prior home rearing and intraspecies transactions. These relationships were marked in the first session for each pair and were maintained at a slightly lower level subsequently; in contrast, the frequency of playful interactions was much greater initially and then showed a steady decline (Fig. 5).

*Individualized raw totals of interanimal responses for the three combinations of monkeys in an unfamiliar cage are given in Table II, composite relative proportions for each monkey are depicted in Fig. 3, and the percentage of each animal's responses in pairs by scored categories in Fig. 4. Although the small sample size precludes statistical treatment of the data, valid and reliable analysis, free from the hazards of an intermediate parental anamnesis [10], is afforded by the intensive single-case approach employed in this study.

TABLE II

Composition of Social Responses (total frequencies)

| | Animals Interacting | | | | | |
Item	M_{16p}	OM_{20p}	M_{16p}	OF_{10i}	OM_{20p}	OF_{10i}
Oral play	55	80	93	109	59	17
Manual play	19	36	31	29	41	5
Grooming	9	18	37	90	5	13
Mounting	12	26	41	7	55	0
Vocalization	6	0	21	9	0	111

The vocalizations of M_{16p} were mainly play squeaks; those of OF_{10i} were correlated with a general excitement during play, whereas OM_{20p} never vocalized except in protest when M_{16p} was removed for pairing with OF_{10i}. Grooming for all animals was mainly limited to the partner's back and forearm and no self-grooming occurred. Both parietal animals showed impairment of the fine-finger movements requisite to normal grooming, OF_{10i} being slightly better skilled than OM_{20p}.

Sexual Behavior

Mountings by OM_{20p} on OF_{10i} were usually carried out with an erection, pelvic thrusting, no foot clasping, and irregular hip

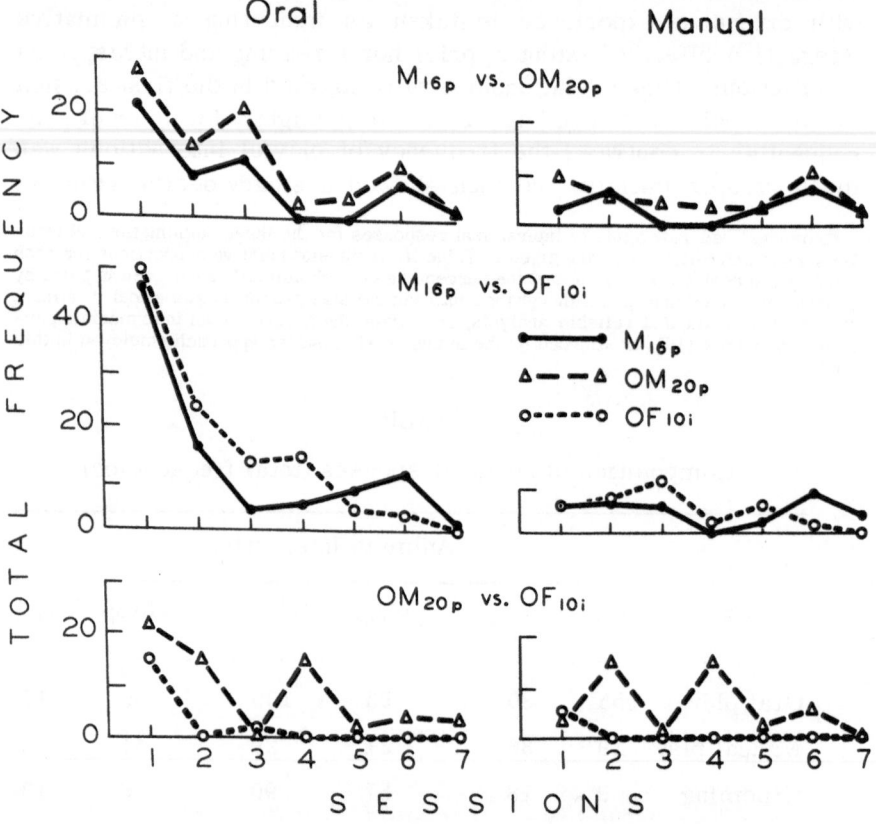

FIG. 5. Initial predominance and subsequent decline of oral contacts in the play behavior of parietal and normal monkeys during social interactions in an unfamiliar cage.

clasping about 50% of the time; and, despite rare insertions, ejaculation occurred on an average of once per session. Mountings by OF_{10i} were minimal and with few thrusts; these were confined to M_{16p} who, however, did not assume a female sexual posture (elevation and turning of hindquarters toward the partner) but remained standing or sitting.

Despite the adequate and frequent sexual presentation of OF_{10i}, the mounting responses of M_{16p} and OM_{20p} were poorly integrated and resembled those reported by Mason [11] for a group of adolescent monkeys reared in the laboratory with intraspecies social contacts restricted to a few brief periods during the first year of life. However, these inadequacies of sexual technique are not significantly different from those seen in normal pairs during the first year of life and probably precede the establishment of effective sexual behavior.

DISCUSSION

Harlow and Zimmermann [1] initially proposed that bodily contact was the primary variable in affective socialization, whereas Bowlby added that deprivations of maternal clinging also produced adverse effects. With respect to these tenets, the finding of greatest import in this study was the development of strong positive attachments to human mother surrogates by infant monkeys whose tactual sensitivity and motor dexterity were impaired by neonate lesions of the parietal cortex. Moreover, these infants failed to exhibit the crouching, rocking, body clutching, convulsive jerking, or other patterns of reaction to stress regarded by Harlow and Zimmermann as analogous to the autisms observed in deprived and institutionalized children. Instead, the relative equanimity in exploring novel objects and the degree of affiliation with humans and later with monkey peers of either sex varied directly in both normal and parietal infants with the length of home rearing and human mothering.

This interpretation is strengthened by the relative lack of affective disturbances in these monkeys, a result particularly striking in view of Hebb's dictum that "sensory and motor capacities after damage to the infant brain tend to reach a higher level than that attained after destruction of the same regions at maturity" [12, p. 292] and our own evidence [13, 14] that cerebral lesions in young monkeys produce a lesser amelioration of neurotic behavior and a greater impairment of postoperative readaptations than did corresponding lesions in adult animals. On the other hand, the adequate social interactions of our parietal decorticate animals exemplify the compensatory effects of favorable postoperative experience [15].

SUMMARY

Five infant macaques separated from their mothers at birth were given varying amounts of optimal human mothering experiences in home environments. Two of the infants were operated on during the first week of life for bilateral ablation of the parietal cortex.

Analysis of data contained in daily written and photographic records, physical measurements, and standardized tests of the infants for from three to sixteen months of age revealed the following:

1. Body weight, physical stature, locomotor and manipulatory abilities, play behavior, and simple visual-tactual discrimination learning were statistically equivalent in the parietal and normal infants.

2. The only consistent differences were deficits in tactile sensitivity and motor dexterity and an increased tendency to oral exploration in the adaptive behavior of infants with parietal lesions.

3. The parietal infants developed normal affective behavior to human mother surrogates and to monkey peers.

4. Affiliative patterns with humans, equanimity in the exploration of unfamiliar situations and novel objects, and sociability with age peers during the first year of life were positively related both in our normal and parietal decorticate monkeys to the duration of human domiciliary care.

REFERENCES

1. Harlow, H. F., and Zimmermann, R. R.: Affectional responses in the infant monkey, Science 130:421, 1959.

2. Owen, M.: Perception of three simultaneous tactile stimuli in emotionally disturbed children and its relation to their body image concept, J. Nerv. Ment. Dis. 121:397, 1955.

3. Escalona, Sibyll: Emotion development in the first year of life, in Senn, M. J. E., Ed.: Problems of Infancy and Childhood, Josiah Macy, Jr. Foundation, Trans. Sixth Conf., 1953, pp. 11−92.

4. Mahler, M. S., Ross, J. R., Jr., and DeFries, Z.: Clinical studies in benign and malignant cases of childhood psychosis (schizophrenia-like), Am. J. Ortho-Psychiat. 19:295, 1949.

5. Blum, Josephine, S.: Cortical organization in somesthesis: Effects of lesions in posterior associative cortex on somatosensory function in *Macaca mulatta*, Comp. Psychol. Mongr. 19:219, 1945.

6. Aarons, L., Bernstein, I. S., and Masserman, J. H.: Early Behavior of a Home-Reared Macaque, Motion Picture, 400 feet, Psychological Cinema Register, State College, Pa., 1961.

7. Kennard, M. A., Spencer, S. S., and Fountain, G.: Hyperactivity in monkeys following lesions of the frontal lobes, J. Neurophysiol. 7:512, 1941.

8. Kennard, M. A.: Reactions of monkeys of various ages to partial and complete decortication. J. Neuropath. Exp. Neurol. 3:289, 1944.

9. Orbach, J., and Chow, K. L.: Differential effects of resections of somatic areas I and II in monkeys, J. Neurophysiol. 22:195, 1959.

10. McGraw, M. B., and Molloy, L. B.: The pediatric anamnesis inaccuracies in eliciting developmental data, Child. Develop. 12:255, 1941.

11. Mason, W. A.: The effects of social restriction on the behavior of rhesus monkeys: I Free social behavior, J. Comp. Physiol. Psychol. 53:582, 1960.

12. Hebb, D. O.: Organization of Behavior, John Wiley & Sons, Inc., New York, 1949, p. 335.

13. Masserman, J. H., Levitt, M., McAvoy, T., Kling, A., and Pechtel, C.: The amygdalae and behavior, Am. J. Psychiat. 115:14, 1958.

14. Pechtel, C., Masserman, J. H., and Aarons, L.: Differential responses in young vs. old animals to training, conflict, drugs and brain lesions, ibid. 116:1018, 1960.

15. Pechtel, C., and Masserman, J. H.: Cerebral localizations: not where but in whom, Am. J. Psychiat. 116:51, 1959.

Discussion by Eugene Ziskind, M.D.

The authors have conducted painstaking experiments in that interesting area of behavior research on infant animals subjected to sustained specific sensory deprivations. Their conclusions are at variance with those of Harlow and Zimmerman. I will discuss the experimental results and add some comments about acute sensory deprivation experiments in man.

Three questions about the new experimental data have a bearing on the conclusions:

1. Was the somesthetic sensation necessary for the preferential distinction shown by Harlow's infant monkeys between cloth-covered wooden and "naked" wire dolls eliminated? Removal of the entire parietal lobe does not deprive the animal of all somesthetic sensation [5, pp. 219, 245]. Furthermore, the partially intact tactual placing responses indicate that at least in this one animal all the parietal cortex was not removed.

2. Is it possible that the operative side-effects of increased oral behavior and hyperactivity masked an induced deficiency in "socialization and affection"? The latter behavior is interpreted in these experiments chiefly through motor activities.

3. Could the increased and prolonged human mothering in Aarons' experiment compensate through other channels for a deficiency related originally to somesthetic sensory deprivation?

Should the possibilities raised prove to be verities, the conclusions would be invalidated. Comparisons between the two sets of experiments would have been simpler if the authors had merely substituted parietal ablated animals in Harlow and Zimmermann's studies, with as few additional changes as necessary. This is particularly so since the variables within the five animals of our authors include differences in duration of human mothering, in cage rearing with peers, in degree of intact parietal brain tissue, in amounts of oral behavior, and in sex.

When one comes to interpretations of the data, there are still more questions. Measurements in the emotional sphere, even in man, are notoriously difficult, and often lacking in reliability. How much more is this true in animal experiments where "operational definitions" involve substitutions which are often very different from the real thing? To be more specific, the "approach" or "avoidance" response to strange and novel stimuli utilized in both sets of experiments are not synonymous with affection and fear and may have other explanations. Hence, even though the experiments of Aarons and co-workers are a closer approximation than those of Harlow to natural human mothering and the development of affection, the behavioral responses assumed to reflect the latter may be in error.

These questions are raised merely to indicate that the variables involved are great. Perhaps reference to the complexities in the simpler related field of acute "sensory deprivation" experiments in man may serve to further emphasize the cautions necessary in reaching valid conclusions. Although my experience has been with patients binocularly patched on an eye ward, the following remarks apply extensively to other sensory deprivation experiments. Hebb and his co-workers excited the scientific world eight years ago when they reported that all subjects who remained in their experimental isolation chamber for more than three days developed hallucinations. It has formerly been known that some individuals developed mental symptoms due to special types of isolation, the so-called paranoias of solitary confinement in prisons, of the hard-of-hearing, and of language-deprived refugees. Hebb's experiments, however, pointed to a universal response with symptoms formerly thought to occur only in specially predisposed individuals. To date there is no general understanding on how these symptoms are formed. In fact, there is little agreement as to exact delineation of the symptoms.

These failures to progress, despite numerous researches throughout the world, may be due to lack of control of the large number of variables in individual experiments and from experiment to experiment. Some of these related to causative factors are shown in Table 1.

In addition, the responses vary widely and their descriptions are not sufficiently refined. Until some invariable behavioral responses are set up, comparisons between different experimental approaches may be difficult or impossible. Take, for instance, the effect on perceptual processes. True hallucinations, hypnagogic hallucinations, other pseudohallucinations, eidetic imagery, dreams, daytime reveries, and accentuated mental imagery are all reported as hallucinations.

There are therefore complexities in sensory deprivation experiments both as to causative factors (factors of input) and as to response (factors of output). In the sensory deprivation experiments in animals, complicated as they are by factors of phylogeny, ontogeny, and enduring (chronic) operative neurophysiologic differences, many of the confusing variables still apply and are, indeed, compounded. Analysis of some of these variables has already pointed up new orientations in this field of research.

Our own experience, reported elsewhere, reveals that the majority of symptoms occur in periods of half sleep and half wakefulness and that they are part of a syndrome of impaired mental functions related to reduced conscious awareness, attention, and logic. Our data raise the question whether sensory deprivation is even one of the necessary conditions. The picture of acute sensory deprivation is, however, quite different from the chronic, persistent sensory deprivation during maturation.

I would prefer that these evaluative remarks not be taken as nihilistic. The approach of our authors and their related colleagues is a most important one.

TABLE 1

Variables in Sensory Deprivation Experiments

I. Alterations in Sensory Stimulation

1. Quantitative:	deprivation, excess
2. Variation:	invariance
3. Parameters:	vividness, pitch, frequency, constancy, etc.
4. Modalities: (number)	one or combination of visual, auditory, tactile, and proprioceptive
5. Duration:	acute, subacute, chronic

II. Concordant Persistent Factors

1. Sensory deprivation *per se*
2. Immobilization
3. Confinement
4. Interpersonal isolation

III. Concordant Intermittent Factors

1. Hypnagogic and other periods of reduced awareness
2. Subconscious urges, irritations, and motivations

There is a need for a tremendous amount of data, which also means refinements of techniques and much more experimentation, as indeed has been stated by our essayists. Until such time, conclusions regarding human behavior should be chary. Dr. Aarons has already had a notable tutelage with Dr. Reisen in this area of research and now with Dr. Masserman, and he and his colleagues should have further interesting material in years to come.

CHAPTER 31

Disordered Perception of Simultaneous Stimulation of Face and Hand: A Review and Theory

By MAX POLLACK, PH.D., AND MAX FINK, M.D.

Since its reintroduction by Morris B. Bender during World War II, the method of double simultaneous stimulation has attracted wide attention in neurology and psychiatry. This paper is concerned with one facet of the many studies in this area, namely, the perception of simultaneous tactile stimulation of the face and hand—the face-hand test. In a series of studies, Bender and his associates Fink, Green, and Jaffe [1-11] have shown this task to have clinical value as a measure of cerebral function, with applications in studies of brain damage, mental age, and altered states of consciousness.

THE TEST

The face-hand test consists of repeated trials of simultaneously touching the subject, whose eyes are closed, on the cheek and the dorsum of the hand. The usual order of stimulation is shown in Table I. Normal adults make errors only on the initial trials, correctly reporting both stimuli within ten trials. Brain-damaged patients with severe mental changes ("organic mental syndrome"), however, make persistent errors beyond ten trials. When errors are made, they occur in the recognition of the hand stimulus, whereas the cheek stimulus is correctly reported.

The errors in the recognition of the hand stimulus are of two types: (1) extinction, i.e., failure to report the stimulus and (2) displacement or mislocalization of the hand stimulus to another part of the body, usually the other cheek. In patients with severe alterations of brain function the hand stimulus is sometimes displaced

Aided in part by Grant MY-2092 of the National Institute of Mental Health, National Institutes of Health, U. S. Public Health Service.

into extrapersonal space (exosomesthesia) [12]. This pattern of persistent errors in the hand stimulus and correct face localization has been called "face dominance," and is part of a general body order of dominance determined by simultaneous tactile testing [4].

Bender and Fink [2] have found the face-hand test useful in differentiating adult hospitalized psychiatric patients from those with behavioral changes due to massive brain lesions. In contrast to patients with "organic psychoses," adult schizophrenic patients do not make persistent errors. Their perceptual pattern is similar to that of normal adults.

Fink and Bender [5] have also shown that young children make the same kind of errors in cutaneous perception as do adults with altered brain function. Below the age of six years almost all normal children have a positive face-hand test result; i.e., they fail to identify both stimuli correctly within ten trials. The children are face dominant in that they report the face stimulus but not the hand stimulus. Younger children fail to perceive the hand stimulus even when tested with the eyes open. However, by the age of four years simultaneous stimulations of symmetric body areas, e.g., both cheeks and both hands, are correctly identified [5, 13].

The face-hand test is related to mental age in normal children

TABLE I

Presentation of Face-Hand Stimuli

1.	right cheek-left hand
2.	left cheek-right hand
3.	right cheek-right hand
4.	left cheek-left hand
5.	right cheek-left cheek
6.	right hand-left hand
7.	right cheek-left hand
8.	left cheek-right hand
9.	right cheek-right hand
10.	left cheek-left hand

[5,14], mentally retarded adults [7,15] and in mentally retarded children [7,13,16]. Children or adults whose mental ages are above seven years, as defined by psychometric examinations, have a negative result. The test has found increased usefulness with problems where the standard neurological examination is frequently noncontributory, as in children with learning disorders [17-22] in psychiatric populations, particularly children with behavior disorders [13,14,21,23], and in aged persons [8,24-26].

THEORETIC VIEWS

In 1954, Bender, Green, and Fink [4] reviewed the then existing theories that attempted to account for the order of dominance of body parts when examined by this method. They concluded that the psychophysical "body image," attention, and learning theories were unacceptable explanations, stating: "No one theory adequately explains the organization of this pattern. Learning and maturation are probable factors, but it appears to be most inherent. The pattern is found in the normal subject but is accentuated in the presence of disease of the brain."

Considerable confusion still exists concerning the status of these theories. The initial reports of Bender and his associates [1] concerned the demonstration of minimal hemisensory defects through the simultaneous stimulation of the intact and homologous defective body parts. In such patients, sensory extinction was unrelated to their mental state. Subjects with focal sensory defects do not make persistent errors on the face-hand test unless they have associated mental changes, but do show consistent asymmetry when stimulated bilaterally. Previous reviews by Denny-Brown, Meyer, and Horenstein [27] and Critchley [28] have emphasized this phenomenon and have attributed the defects to an impairment of the parietal lobe. Critchley indicated that the failure to report one stimulus in a defective part was due to inattention, but he failed to distinguish between patients with a hemisensory defect with mental impairment and those without mental impairment. This confusion has led other investigators to regard defects in the face-hand test as a manifestation of parietal lobe dysfunction [20].

Another view ascribes the inability of young children and adults with brain disease to perceive the hand stimulus to a defect in body image concept. Both Cohn [18] and Linn [29] have ascribed the pattern of face dominance to an undeveloped body image in children and as a regressed body image in adults with brain disease. Linn claims that the face and hand are "fused" in development, and are not "defused" until maturity. Such reasoning appears circular, for hand dominance could be just as easily explained.

Linn's hypothesis of an early syncretic state appears to be contradicted by Hooker's study [30] of responses to tactile stimulation in three and four-month-old fetuses. On simultaneous stimulation of facial and palmar tactile areas, the typical palmar reflex is extinguished.

A body image explanation is also based on observations that the face-hand test performance is correlated with the development of children's human figure drawings from a stage where only the head is drawn to a more complete representation of the body [18, 29]. Similar types of drawings are seen in patients with an organic mental syndrome. Thus, Cohn [31] has assumed a literal relation between the drawings of a large head and face dominance. Owen [32] has tested this hypothesis in school children and concluded that body image data, as constructed from drawings, stories, interviews, and simultaneous tactile tests, were not intrinsically related but were parallel facets of general psychological development. A more stringent control was employed by Pollack and Gordon [33] in a study in which figure drawings, copying of simple geometric figures, and face-hand test performance were obtained. While the mental age of the figure drawings correlated with face-hand test performance, the correlation between the copying of a diamond-shaped figure and face-hand test performance was also significant. These data could be interpreted more parsimoniously as a lack of perceptual-cognitive integration rather than a "body-image" defect.

Another aspect of the body image hypothesis is reflected in studies of subjects with supposed alterations in body image. Studies of subjects with sensory handicaps, blindness, and deafness have shown that the pattern of double simultaneous tactile perception is identical with that in normal subjects [4]. A study of subjects with their hands in different positions during testing showed that this modification made little difference in performance [34]. Pollack and Goldfarb [14] tested children and had them place one hand on a cheek. When the hand and the uncovered cheek were touched, the children withdrew the hand and pointed to the cheek beneath it.

It would appear that the data for a body image concept fails to explain the patterns of perceptual errors observed.

AN EXPLANATION

We believe that errors in face-hand perception are best explained in the matrix of a sensory threshold-mental set hypothesis. The theory rests on the assumption that there is a fundamental difference in cutaneous threshold between hand and cheek that accounts for face dominance and that face dominance is maintained in young children and patients with brain disease because of a generalized learning defect—an inability to alter a mental set induced by the test procedure. This hypothesis was previously advanced by Korin and Fink [35].

In their study using fixed electrodes Korin and Fink [36] indicated that the threshold for the perception of an electric pulse is approximately four times higher in the hand as compared to the cheek (Table II). Under these conditions the order of body part

TABLE II

Threshold for Electric Stimuli and Body Part Dominance *

	Right Cheek	Left Cheek	Right Hand	Left Hand	Right Leg	Left Leg
Mean Threshold (volts)	6.7	7.8	29.2	22.2	24.5	19.5

Stimuli Combinations	Mean Extinctions of Cheek	Mean Extinctions of Hand	Difference	P
Hand and cheek at threshold	1.5	1.5	0.0	NS
Hand at suprathreshold and cheek at threshold	2.3	0.2	2.1	0.01
Cheek at suprathreshold and hand at threshold	0.3	1.3	1.0	0.01

*After Korin and Fink [32].

dominance could be manipulated by altering the ratio of current intensity applied to different body parts (Table II). When the current was adjusted so that the hand stimulus was at suprathreshold and the cheek at threshold, the hand was dominant. Body part dominance could be achieved by a 10% rise in threshold in one body part. One aspect of the hypothesis encompasses these psychophysical relationships.

But, this difference in threshold does not explain the failure of preschool children and confused adults to learn this simple task. The second aspect can best be understood by going over the test procedure in detail. The instruction to the subject is that he will be touched and to report what he felt. The initial implicit expectancy is for a single stimulus, and the face area, having a lower sensory threshold, is consequently more readily perceived. Thus, many normal subjects report only the cheek stimulus on the initial trial, although some believe that they were touched in more than one area and request another trial. After the second trial the subject, if he has not already identified both stimuli, is given a verbal clue by being asked if he had been touched "anywhere else." In the usual face-hand procedure, symmetrical stimuli are presented at the fifth and sixth trials. These face-face and hand-hand stimulations are almost always perceived correctly, probably because there is little difference in threshold. These trials serve as nonverbal learning cues for the concept of twoness as well as hand localization.

After these two trials many normal dull subjects firmly grasp the meaning of the test. Brain-damaged patients with positive face-hand test performance frequently retain the set for twoness and perceive the face and hand correctly on the trial following the symmetric trials. However, those with severe mental changes cannot retain this set and return to the previous mode of face dominance. This is equally true under conditions of testing with the subject's eyes open. These differences may account for the marked individual differences in performance in patients with severe brain disease.

CONCLUSION

We believe that the failure to localize the hand stimulus (face-dominance) on repeated simultaneous tactile tests in children, in mentally defective and brain-damaged adults, and in various states of altered consciousness, may best be understood within the framework of a psychophysical (relative sensory threshold)-mental set (failure to learn the set for "twoness") hypothesis. The method of double simultaneous stimulation is an excellent tool for the study of cerebral processes. The face-hand test is particularly intriguing because of its simplicity and applicability; it comes close to a culture-free test. Because of its importance, it will continue to attract students and through their investigations increase our knowledge of the cerebral mechanisms underlying learning.

REFERENCES

1. Bender, M. B.: Disorders in Perception. Springfield, Charles C. Thomas, 1952.

2. Bender, M. B., and Fink, M.: Tactile perceptual tests in the differential diagnosis of psychiatric disorders, J. Hillside Hosp. 1:21, 1952.

3. Bender, M. B., Fink, M., and Green, M.: Patterns in perception on simultaneous tests of face and hand, A.M.A. Arch. Neurol. Psychiat. 66:355, 1951.

4. Bender, M. B., Green, M. A., and Fink, M.: Patterns of perceptual organization with simultaneous stimuli, ibid. 72:223, 1954.

5. Fink, M., and Bender, M. B.: Perception of simultaneous tactile stimuli in normal children, Neurology 3:27, 1952.

6. Fink, M., Green, M. A., and Bender, M. B.: The face-hand test as a diagnostic sign of organic mental syndrome, ibid. 2:48, 1952.

7. Fink, M., Green, M. A., and Bender, M. B.: Perception of simultaneous tactile stimuli by mentally defective subjects, J. Nerv. Ment. Dis. 117:43, 1953.

8. Green, M. A., and Bender, M. B.: Cutaneous perception in the aged, A.M.A. Arch. Neurol. Psychiat. 69:577, 1953.

9. Green, M. A., and Fink, M.: Standardization of the face-hand test, Neurology, 4:211, 1954.

10. Jaffe, J., and Bender, M. B.: Perceptual patterns during recovery from general anesthesia, J. Neurol. Neurosurg. Psychiat. 14:316, 1951.

11. Jaffe, J. and Bender, M. B.: The factor of symmetry in the perception of two simultaneous cutaneous stimuli, Brain 75:167, 1952.

12. Shapiro, M. F., Fink, M., and Bender, M. B.: Exosomesthesia or the phenomenon of displacement of sensation into extra-personal space, A.M.A. Arch Neurol. Psychiat. 68:481, 1952.

13. Pollack, M., and Gordon, E. W.: The face-hand test in retarded and nonretarded emotionally disturbed children, Am. J. Ment. Defic. 64:758, 1959.

14. Pollack, M., and Goldfarb, W.: The face-hand test in schizophrenic children, A. M. A. Arch. Neurol. Psychiat. 77:635, 1957.

15. White, R. P.: Face-hand test responses of psychotic and mentally defective patients, ibid. 77:120, 1957.

16. Swanson, R.: Perception of simultaneous tactual stimulation in defective and normal children, Am. J. Ment. Defic. 61:743, 1957.

17. Cohn, R.: On certain aspects of the sensory organization of the human brain. II. A study of rostral dominance in children, Neurology 1:119, 1951.

18. Cohn, R.: Role of "body image concept" in pattern of ipsilateral clinical extinction, A.M.A. Arch. Neurol. Psychiat. 70:503, 1953.

19. Cohn, R.: Delayed acquisition of reading and writing abilities in children, Arch. Neurol. 4:153, 1961.

20. Drew, A.: A neurological appraisal of familial congenital word-blindness, Brain 79:440, 1956.

21. Kehne, C. W.: The role of the school and its psychiatric implications in the personality development of hyperactive brain damaged and non-brain damaged children, Presented at the 117th Annual Meeting, American Psychiatric Association, May, 1961, Chicago.

22. Rabinovitch, R. D., Drew, A. I., De Jong, R. N., Ingram, W., and Withey, L.: A research approach to reading retardation, Proc. Assoc. Res. Neur. Ment. Dis. 34:363, 1954.

23. Pollack, M.: Brain damage, mental retardation, and childhood schizophrenia, Am. J. Psychiat. 115:422, 1958.

24. Kahn, R. L., Goldfarb, A. I., Pollack, M., and Gerber, I. E.: The relationship of mental and physical status in institutionalized aged persons, ibid. 117:124, 1960.

25. Kahn, R. L., Goldfarb, A. I., Pollack, M., and Peck, A.: Brief objective measures for the determination of mental status in the aged, ibid. 117:326, 1960.

26. Pollack, M., Kahn, R. L., and Goldfarb, A. I.: Factors related to individual differences in perception in institutionalized aged subjects, J. Gerontol. 13:192, 1958.

27. Denny-Brown, D., Meyer, J. S., and Horenstein, S.: The significance of perceptual rivalry resulting from parietal lesions, Brain 75:433, 1952.

28. Critchley, McD.: Phenomenon of tactile inattention with special reference to parietal lesions, ibid. 72:538, 1949.

29. Linn, L.: Some developmental aspects of the body image, Internat. J. Psychoanal. 36:1, 1955.

30. Hooker, D.: Early human fetal behavior, with a preliminary note on double simultaneous fetal stimulation. Proc. Assoc. Res. Nerv. Ment. Dis. 33:99, 1954.

31. Cohn, R.: On certain aspects of the sensory organization of the human brain: A study in rostral dominance as determined by ipsilateral simultaneous stimulation, J. Nerv. Ment. Dis. 113:471, 1951.

32. Owen, M.: Perception of simultaneous tactile stimuli in emotionally disturbed children and its relation to their body image concept, ibid. 121:397, 1955.

33. Pollack, M., and Gordon, E. W.: Cutaneous perception and the body-image concept in abnormal children, in preparation.

34. Pasik, T., and Pasik, P.: Face-hand test and background activity, Neurology 7:466, 1957.

35. Korin, H., and Fink, M.: The role of set in perception of simultaneous tactile stimuli, Am. J. Psychol. 72:384, 1959.

36. Korin, H., and Fink, M.: Role of stimulus intensity in perception of simultaneous cutaneous electrical stimuli, J. Hillside Hosp. 6:241, 1957.

Membership Roster
Society of Biological Psychiatry

(Membership to date: Active – 192, Honorary – 3, Senior – 25,
TOTAL 220) (S – denotes Senior; H – Honorary)

SPAFFORD ACKERLY, M. D. (1947) (S)
206 East Chestnut Street
Louisville 2, Kentucky

FRANZ ALEXANDER, M.D. (1955)
Mount Sinai Hospital
8720 Beverly Boulevard
Los Angeles 48, California

LEO ALEXANDER, M.D. (1956)
433 Marlborough Street
Boston 15, Massachusetts

WALTER C. ALVAREZ, M. D. (1958)
700 North Michigan Avenue
Chicago 11, Illinois

HENRY E. ANDREN, M.D. (1955)
7600 Carroll Avenue
Takoma Park, Maryland

MORRIS HERMAN APRISON, Ph.D. (1960)
Indiana University Medical Center
Dept. of Psychiatry & Biochemistry
Indianapolis, Indiana

WINIFRED ASHBY, Ph.D. (1949) (S)
Route 2, Box 67
Lorton, Virginia

ALBERT FRANCIS AX, Ph.D. (1060)
Lafayette Clinic
951 East Lafayette
Detroit 7, Michigan

FRANK J. AYD, JR., M.D. (1955)
6231 York Road
Baltimore 12, Maryland

HASSAN AZIMA, M.D. (1956)
1025 Pine Avenue
Montreal 2, Canada

*PERCIVAL BAILEY, M.D. (1946) (H)
912 South Wood Street
Chicago, Illinois

WALTER W. BAKER, M.S. (1961)
Assoc. Prof. Pharmacology & Psychiatry
Jefferson Medical College
Philadelphia, Pennsylvania

H. THOMAS BALLANTINE, M.D. (1956)
Massachusetts General Hospital
Boston 14, Massachusetts

†LAURETTA BENDER, M.D. (1955)
Department of Mental Hygiene
Creedmoor State Hospital
Queens Village, New York

MORRIS B. BENDER, M.D. (1947) (S)
1150 Park Avenue
New York 28, New York

‡ABRAM E. BENNETT, M.D. (1947) (H)
2000 Dwight Way
Berkeley 4, California

IVAN F. BENNETT, M.D. (1957)
R.R. 18, Box 285
Indianapolis 24, Indiana

FRANK MILLAN BERGER, M.D. (1960)
227 Prospect Avenue
Princeton, New Jersey

LOUIS BERLIN, M.D. (1050)
99 Pennsylvania
Mount Vernon, New York

NEWTON BIGELOW, M.D. (1960)
Marcy
New York

EDWARD G. BILLINGS, M.D. (1959)
1820 High Street
Denver 18, Colorado

*President – 1948
†President – 1961
‡President – 1952

BENJAMIN BOSHES, M.D. (1960)
Northwestern University Medical School
303 East Chicago Avenue
Chicago 11, Illinois

KARL M. BOWMAN, M.D. (1946) (S)
Langley Porter Clinic
Second and Parnassus Avenues
San Francisco 22, California

JOHN PAUL BRADY, M.D. (1960)
Indiana University Medical School
Indianapolis 7, Indiana

WAGNER H. BRIDGER, M.D. (1960)
Albert Einstein College of Medicine
Bronx, New York

HENRY W. BROSIN, M.D. (1947)
University of Pittsburgh
School of Medicine
Western Psychiatric Institute & Clinic
3811 O'Hara Street
Pittsburgh 13, Pennsylvania

BARBARA B. BROWN, Ph.D. (1960)
3477 Beverly Glen Boulevard
Sherman Oaks, California

MARTHA BRUNNER-ORNE, M.D. (1958)
88 Marlborough Street
Boston 16, Massachusetts

ENOCH CALLAWAY, M.D. (1959)
The Langley Porter Neuropsychiatric Institute
Parnassus & First Avenues
San Francisco 22, California

D. EWEN CAMERON, M.D. (1955)
Allan Memorial Institute
1025 Pine Avenue West
Montreal 21, Quebec, Canada

JOHN D. CAMPBELL, M.D. (1951)
400 Peachtree Street, N.E.
Atlanta 3, Georgia

JOSEPH CHUSID, M.D. (1950)
3390 Emeric Avenue
Wan Tagh, New York

HERVEY M. CLECKLEY, M.D. (1956)
1423 Harper Street
Augusta, Georgia

R.A. CLEGHORN, M.D. (1959)
1025 Pine Avenue West
Montreal, Quebec, Canada

STANLEY COBB, M.D. (1946) (S)
Massachusetts General Hospital
Boston, Massachusetts

IRVIN M. COHEN, M.D. (1958)
641 Hermann Professional Building
Houston 25, Texas

MANDEL COHEN, M.D. (1947)
Massachusetts General Hospital
Boston, Massachusetts

SANFORD IRWIN COHEN, M.D. (1960)
Department of Psychiatry
Duke University Medical Center
Durham, North Carolina

SIDNEY COHEN, M.D. (1960)
13020 Sky Valley Road
Los Angeles 49, California

JONATHAN COLE, M.D. (1959)
National Institute of Mental Health
Bethesda, Maryland

ERMINIO COSTA, M.D. (1958)
N.I.H. National Heart Institute
Laboratory of Chemical Pharmacology
Bethesda 14, Maryland

RUSSELL T. COSTELLO, M.D. (1955)
630 Fisher Building
3001 West Grand Boulevard
Detroit, Michigan

CHESTER W. DARROW, Ph.D. (1954)
5802 South Blackstone
Chicago 37, Illinois

CHARLES DAVISON, M.D. (1950) (S)
1155 Park Avenue
New York, New York

HERMAN C. B. DENBER, M.D. (1955)
600 East 125th Street
New York 35, New York

JAMES M. DILLE, M.D. (1959)
Dept. of Pharmacology
School of Medicine
University of Washington
Seattle 5, Washington

ALBERTO DI MASCIO, M. A. (1959)
74 Fenwood Road
Boston, Massachusetts

HENRY W. DODGE, JR., M.D. (1961)
2010 Wilshire Blvd.
Los Angeles 57, California

PHILIP ROGERS DODGE, M.D. (1960)
117 Revere Street
Boston 14, Massachusetts

ARTHUR L. DREW, M.D. (1960)
Indiana University Medical Center
1100 West Michigan Street
Indianapolis, Indiana

EDWIN M. DUNLOP, M.D. (1961)
9 School Street
Attleboro, Massachusetts

JOEL J. ELKES, M.D. (1960)
9902 Cedar Lane
Bethesda, Maryland

R. J. ELLINGSON, Ph.D. (1959)
403 South 49th Street
Omaha, Nebraska

FRED ELMADJIAN, Ph.D. (1961)
Worcester Foundation for Experimental Biology
Shrewsbury, Massachusetts

GUY M. EVERETT, Ph.D. (1956)
Department of Pharmacology
Abbott Laboratories
North Chicago, Illinois

*HOWARD D. FABING, M.D. (1950)
2314 Auburn Avenue
Cincinnati, Ohio

JOSEPH F. FAZEKAS, M.D. (1955)
171 Harrison Avenue
Boston 11, Massachusetts

MYRON FELD, M.D. (1959)
5459 Oleta
Long Beach, California

CHARLES D. FERSTER, Ph.D. (1960)
5680 Winthrop Avenue
Indianapolis, Indiana

MAX FINK, M.D. (1959)
Dept. of Experimental Psychiatry
Hillside Hospital
Glen Oaks, L.I., New York

KNOX H. FINLEY, M.D. (1952)
450 Sutter Street
San Francisco, California

ROLAND FISCHER, Ph.D. (1956)
Research Division, C.P.I.H.
473 West 12th Avenue
Columbus, Ohio

HAMILTON FORD, M.D. (1953)
112 North Boulevard
Galveston, Texas

JOEL FORT, M.D. (1959)
2712 Shasta Road
Berkeley 8, California

ALFRED M. FREEDMAN, M.D. (1955)
161 West 86th Street
New York 24, New York

HARRY FREEMAN, M.D. (1961)
8 Course Brook Road
Sherborn, Massachusetts

WALTER FREEMAN, M.D. (1948) (S)
877 Fremont
Sunnyvale, California

WALTER J. FREEMAN, III M.D. (1961)
30 Menlo Place
Berkeley 7, California

FRITZ FREYHAN, M.D. (1959)
503 Medical Arts Building
Wilmington, Delaware

ARNOLD P. FRIEDMAN, M.D. (1959)
71 East 77th Street
New York, New York

SABIT GABAY, Ph.D. (1961)
Res. Facility
Rockland State Hospital
Orangeburg, New York

The Beverly Hills Medical Clinic
133 South Lasky Drive
Beverly Hills, California

WILLIAM J. GALLAGHER, M.D. (1959)
100 Barnard Rd.
Manteno, Illinois

†WILLIAM HORSLEY GANTT, M.D. (1952)
Phipps Clinic, Johns Hopkins Hospital
Baltimore 5, Maryland

RALPH W. GERARD, M.D. (1947)
Mental Health Research Institute
University of Michigan
Ann Arbor, Michigan

FRANCIS J. GERTY, M.D. (1947) (S)
912 South Wood Street
Chicago 12, Illinois

WILLIAM C. GIBSON, M.D. (1953)
UBC—Crease Clinic Research Unit
The University of British Columbia
Vancouver, British Columbia

EDWIN F. GILDEA, M.D. (1959)
4940 Audubon
St. Louis, Missouri

MARGARET CRANE LILLIE GILDEA, M.D. (1959)
4500 West Pine Blvd.
St. Louis 8, Missouri

DOUGLAS GOLDMAN, M.D. (1957)
320 Provident Bank Building
Cincinnati 2, Ohio

JACQUES S. GOTTLIEB, M.D. (1959)
951 East Lafayette
Detroit 7, Michigan

MILTON GREENBLATT, M.D. (1956)
74 Fenwood Rd.
Boston 15, Massachusetts

*President – 1955
†President –|1960

ROBERT C. GRENELL, Ph.D. (1958)
Psychiatric Institute
University of Maryland Hospital
Baltimore 1, Maryland

MARTIN GROSS, M.D. (1950)
334 East Main Street
Westminster, Maryland

WARD C. HALSTEAD, Ph.D. (1947)
The University of Chicago
Department of Medicine
950 E. 59th Street
Chicago 37, Illinois

TITUS H. HARRIS, M.D. (1948) (S)
112 North Boulevard
Galveston, Texas

ABE HAUSER, M.D. (1959)
1119 Lovett Boulevard
Houston, Texas

LOUIS HAUSMAN, M.D. (1947) (S)
140 East 54th Street
New York, New York

ROBERT G. HEATH, M.D. (1956)
Tulane University, School of Medicine
1430 Tulane Avenue
New Orleans 12, Louisiana

CHARLES D. HENDLEY, Ph.D. (1960)
Schering Corporation
Bloomfield, New Jersey

*HAROLD E. HIMWICH, M.D. (1947) (S)
Research Director
Galesburg State Research Hospital
Galesburg, Illinois

WILLIAMINA A. HIMWICH, Ph.D. (1956)
Galesburg State Research Hospital
Galesburg, Illinois

HUDSON HOAGLAND, Ph.D. (1959)
Worcester Foundation for Experimental Biology
Shrewsbury, Massachusetts

GEORGE EDGAR HOBBS, M.D. (1961)
117 Bloomfield Drive
Orchard Park
London, Ontario, Canada

†PAUL H. HOCH, M.D. (1949)
722 West 168th Street
New York, New York

ABRAM HOFFER, M.D. (1959)
University of Saskatoon
University Hospital
Saskatoon, Saskatchewan

LESLIE B. HOHMAN, M.D. (1952)
School of Medicine
Duke University
Durham, North Carolina

WILLIAM L. HOLT, JR., M.D. (1953)
47 Douglas Road
Delmar, New York

MAX K. HORWITT, Ph.D. (1960)
L. B. Mendel Research Laboratory
Elgin State Hospital
Elgin, Illinois

DAVID J. IMPASTATO, M.D. (1959)
40—Fifth Avenue
New York 11, New York

SAMUEL D. INGHAM, M.D. (1946) (S)
876 Victoria Avenue
Los Angeles 5, California

NADOR DORIN ISCHLONDSKY, M.D. (1953)
225 Central Park West
New York 24, New York

ELINOR R. IVES, M.D. (1953)
5636 Berkshire Drive
Los Angeles 32, California

ROBERT F. JEANS, M.D. (1960)
1209 East Madison Park
Chicago 15, Illinois

GEORGE A. JERVIS, M.D. (1960)
Thiells
New York

CHARLES H. JONES, M.D. (1960)
Butler Health Center
333 Grotto Avenue
Providence 6, Rhode Island

LOTHAR B. KALINOWSKY, M.D. (1947)
115 East 82nd Street
New York 28, New York

FRANZ J. KALLMANN, M.D. (1961)
722 West 168th Street
New York 32, New York

GORDON R. KAMMAN, M.D. (1951)
1044 Lawry Medical Arts Building
St. Paul 2, Minnesota

LOUIS J. KARNOSH, M.D. (1947) (S)
22299 Parnell Rd.
Cleveland 22, Ohio

‡MARGARET A. KENNARD, M.D. (1947)
144 Tarrytown Road
Manchester, New Hampshire

SEYMOUR S. KETY, M.D. (1958)
National Institute of Health
Bethesda 14, Maryland

VERNON J. KINROSS-WRIGHT, M.D. (1957)
1200 M.D. Anderson Blvd.
Houston 25, Texas

*President – 1954
†President – 1959
‡President – 1956

NATHAN S. KLINE, M.D. (1955)
Director of Research
Research Facility
Rockland State Hospital
Orangeburg, New York

WALTER O. KLINGMAN, M.D. (1956)
112 North Boulevard
Galveston, Texas

HEINRICH KLÜVER, PH.D. (1947)
Culver Hall
University of Chicago
Chicago, Illinois

WERNER P. KOELLA, M.D. (1961)
Worcester Foundation for Experimental Biology
Shrewsbury, Massachusetts

GEORGE B. KOELLE, M.D. (1956)
Department of Pharmacology
Graduate School of Medicine
University of Pennsylvania
Philadelphia 4, Pennsylvania

YALE DAVID KOSKOFF, M.D. (1961)
5500 Hobart Street
Pittsburgh 17, Pennsylvania

ELSE B. KRIS, M.D. (1958)
94 Ocean Avenue
Bay Shore, L.I., New York

ORTHELLO LANGWORTHY, M.D. (1947)
800 Malvern Avenue
Ruxton 4, Maryland

BYRON E. LEACH, Ph.D. (1960)
1430 Tulane Avenue
New Orleans, Louisiana

STANLEY LESSE, M.D. (1959)
15 West 81st Street
New York, New York

SOL LEVY, M.D. (1951)
363 Paulsen Medical & Dental Building
Spokane 1, Washington

NOLAN D. C. LEWIS, M.D. (1947) (S)
5 Rivercrest Road
New York 71, New York

WLADIMIR T. LIBERSON, M.D. (1960)
Veterans Administration Hospital
P. O. Box 28
Hines, Illinois

HARRY R. LIPTON, M.D. (1956)
400 Peachtree Street, N.E.
Suite 243
Atlanta, Georgia

* ROLAND P. MACKAY, M.D. (1946)
8 South Michigan Avenue
Chicago, Illinois

SIDNEY MALITZ, M.D. (1960)
New York State Psychiatric Institute
722 West 168th Street
New York, New York

LESTER H. MARGOLIS, M.D. (1952)
1 Baywood Avenue
San Mateo, California

AMEDEO S. MARRAZZI, M.D. (1956)
Veterans Administration Hospital
Leech Farm Road
Pittsburgh 6, Pennsylvania

†JULES MASSERMAN, M.D. (1947)
8 South Michigan Avenue
Chicago 11, Illinois

MABEL G. MASTEN, M.D. (1951)
212 N.W. 93rd Street
Miami Shores, Florida

WARREN S. MC CULLOCH, M.D. (1947)
Research Laboratory of Electronics
Massachusetts Institute of Technology
Cambridge, Massachusetts

‡LADISLAS J. MEDUNA, M.D. (1947) (S)
8 South Michigan Avenue
Chicago 11, Illinois

HUGO MELLA, M.D. (1953)
Apartment 525
333 South Glebe Road
Arlington, Virginia

SIDNEY MERLIS, M.D. (1959)
437 North Windsor
Brightwaters, New York

STANLEY T. MICHAEL, M.D. (1958)
39 East 75th Street
New York 21, New York

JOHN D. MORIARTY, M.D. (1959)
6753 Hollywood Boulevard
Los Angeles 28, California

WILLIAM H. MOSBERG, JR., M.D. (1954)
803 Cathedral Street
Baltimore 1, Maryland

§ J.M. NIELSEN, M.D. (1946) (H)
727 West Seventh Street
Los Angeles 17, California

JOHN I. NURNBERGER, M.D. (1959)
1100 West Michigan
Indianapolis, Indiana

*President—1951
†President—1957
‡President—1953
§President—1947

WALTER OBRIST, Ph.D. (1958)
Department of Psychiatry
Duke University
School of Medicine
Durham, North Carolina

CLARENCE W. OLSEN, M.D. (1952)
1700 Brooklyn Avenue
Los Angeles 33, California

JOHN L. OTTO, M.D. (1953)
112 North Boulevard
Galveston, Texas

BERNARD L. PACELLA, M.D. (1951)
115 East 61st Street
New York 21, New York

JOSEPH B. PARKER, JR., M.D. (1960)
University of Kentucky Medical Center
Lexington, Kentucky

ERNEST H. PARSONS, M.D. (1958)
457 North Kings Highway
St. Louis 8, Missouri

BENJAMIN PASAMANICK, M.D. (1953)
Director of Research
Columbus Receiving Hospital
University Health Center
Columbus, Ohio

FREDERICK L. PATRY, M.D. (1960)
1917 14th Street West
Bradenton, Florida

CURTIS PECHTEL, Ph.D. (1958)
3926 North 12th Street
Milwaukee 6, Wisconsin

HARRY H. PENNES, M.D. (1958)
611 W. 239th Street
Bronx 63, New York

HAROLD PERSKY, Ph.D. (1960)
Inst. Psychiatric Research
Indiana University Medical Center
Indianapolis 7, Indiana

MAGNUS C. PETERSEN, M.D. (1958)
1745 Sixth Street Southwest
Rochester, Minnesota

CARL C. PFEIFFER, M.D. (1956)
New Jersey Neurology & Psychiatric Institute
P. O. Box 1000
Princeton, New Jersey

GEORGE H. POLLOCK, M.D. (1954)
5759 Dorchester Avenue
Chicago 37, Illinois

LORNE DOUGLAS PROCTOR, M.D. (1954)
Division of Neurology & Psychiatry
Henry Ford Hospital
2799 West Grand Boulevard
Detroit 2, Michigan

A. M. RABINER, M.D. (1950) (S)
78 Eighth Avenue
Brooklyn 15, New York

MARGARET READ, M.D. (1959)
400 Division Street
Vermilion, Ohio

HANS H. REESE, M.D. (1947) (S)
1300 University Avenue
Madison, Wisconsin

JOHN DAVIS REICHARD, M.D. (1949) (S)
1541 Palancia Avenue
Coral Gables 34, Florida

CURT P. RICHTER, PH.D. (1947) (S)
Johns Hopkins Hospital
601 North Broadway
Baltimore, Maryland

HELENA RIGGS, M.D. (1951)
150 Hewitt Road
Wyncote, Pennsylvania

FRANCO RINALDI, M.D. (1957)
Abbott Laboratories
North Chicago, Illinois

MAX RINKEL, M.D. (1952)
479 Commonwealth Avenue
Boston, Massachusetts

THEODORE R. ROBIE, M.D. (1955)
676 Park Avenue
East Orange, New Jersey

ELI ROBINS, M.D. (1958)
Washington University
School of Medicine, Dept. of Psychiatry
4580 Scott Avenue
St. Louis 10, Missouri

AUGUSTUS S. ROSE, M.D. (1952)
Medical Center
University of California at Los Angeles
Los Angeles 24, California

LESTER H. RUDY, M.D. (1955)
Illinois State Psychiatric Institute
1601 West Taylor Street
Chicago 12, Illinois

CHARLES RUPP, M.D. (1948)
133 South 36th Street
Philadelphia, Pennsylvania

MELVIN SABSHIN, M.D. (1960)
Psychosomatic & Psychiatric Institute
Reese Hospital
Chicago 16, Illinois

D. V. SIVA SANKAR, Ph.D. (1960)
Children's Unit
Creedmoor State Hospital
Queens Village, New York

GERALD J. SARWER-FONER, M.D. (1959)
4565 Queen Mary Road
Montreal, Quebec, Canada

ARNOLD B. SCHEIBEL, M.D. (1960)
Dept. of Psychiatry & Anatomy
U.C.L.A. Medical Center
Los Angeles 24, California

VICTOR J. SCHENKER, Ph.D. (1960)
141-32 73rd Avenue
Kew Gardens Hills
Flushing 67, New York

JORDAN M. SCHER, M.D. (1961)
679 N. Michigan Avenue
Chicago 11, Illinois

WILLIAM B. SCOVILLE, M.D. (1953)
85 Jefferson Street
Hartford, Connecticut

CHARLES SHAGASS, M.D. (1959)
500 Newton Road
Iowa City, Iowa

BARRY M. SHMAVONIAN, Ph.D. (1960)
Department of Psychiatry
Duke University
Durham, North Carolina

MAXIMILIAN SILBERMANN, M.D. (1954)
893 Park Avenue
New York 21, New York

ALBERT J. SILVERMANN, M.D. (1959)
Medical Center
Duke University
Durham, North Carolina

ALEXANDER SIMON, M.D. (1949)
Langley Porter Clinic
Second and Parnassus Avenues
San Francisco 22, California

JACKSON A. SMITH, M.D. (1953)
Tinley Park State Hospital
Tinley Park, Illinois

*HARRY C. SOLOMON, M.D. (1946) (S)
Boston Psychopathic Hospital
74 Fenwood Rd.
Boston 15, Massachusetts

MEYER SOLOMON, M.D. (1958)
5426 East View Park
Chicago 15, Illinois

MESROP A. TARUMIANZ, M.D. (1954)
Delaware State Hospital
Farnhurst, Delaware

REGINALD M. TAYLOR, M.D. (1952)
722 West 168th Street
New York 32, New York

CORBETT H. THIGPEN, M.D. (1956)
815 Dogwood Lane
Augusta, Georgia

GEORGE N. THOMPSON, M.D. (1946)
2010 Wilshire Boulevard
Los Angeles 57, California

JOSEPH M. TOBIN, M.D. (1960)
261 Jefferson Road
Princeton, New Jersey

THOMAS T. TOURLENTES, M.D. (1958)
Galesburg State Research Hospital
Galesburg, Illinois

MARTIN LEE TOWLER, M.D. (1953)
112 North Boulevard
Galveston, Texas

LOUIS TUREEN, M.D. (1957)
Neuropsychiatric Clinic of St. Louis
457 North Kings Highway
St. Louis 8, Missouri

WERNER TUTEUR, M.D. (1957)
750 South State Street
Elgin, Illinois

GEORGE A. ULETT, M.D. (1956)
54 Picardy Lane
St. Louis 24, Missouri

MONTAGUE ULLMAN, M.D. (1959)
46 East 73rd Street
New York 21, New York

MAURICE VICTOR, M.D. (1959)
Massachusetts General Hospital
Boston, Massachusetts

GERHARD VON BONIN, M.D. (1947) (S)
1853 West Polk Street
Chicago 12, Illinois

ALPHONSE R. VONDERAHE, M.D. (1950) (S)
Associate Professor of Neurology
University of Cincinnati
Cincinnati, Ohio

KARL O. VON HAGEN, M.D. (1953)
2010 Wilshire Boulevard
Los Angeles 57, California

THEODORE J.C. VON STORCH, M.D. (1960)
1333 S. Miami Avenue
Miami 32, Florida

RAYMOND W. WAGGONER, M.D. (1955)
3333 Geddes Road
Ann Arbor, Michigan

*President – 1950

A. EARL WALKER, M.D. (1947)
601 North Broadway
Baltimore 5, Maryland

ARTHUR A. WARD, M.D. (1952)
School of Medicine
University of Washington
Seattle, Washington

ANNETTE C. WASHBURNE, M.D. (1952)
110 East Main Street
Madison, Wisconsin

CHARLES WATKINS, M.D. (1959)
Dept. of Neurology & Psychiatry
Louisiana State University
New Orleans, Louisiana

ISRAEL S. WECHSLER, M.D. (1948) (S)
70 East 83rd Street
New York 28, New York

ARTHUR WEIL, M.D. (1950) (S)
115-06 Park Lane South
Kew Gardens, New York

LOUIS J. WEST, M.D. (1959)
University of Oklahoma Medical Center
800 N.E. 13th Street
Oklahoma City, Oklahoma

ABRAHAM WIKLER, M.D. (1953)
Research Division
U.S. Public Health Service Hospital
Lexington, Kentucky

PAUL H. WILCOX, M.D. (1959)
333 Sixth Street
Traverse City, Michigan

WILLIAM P. WILSON, M.D. (1960)
Dept. of Psychiatry
Duke Medical Center
Durham, North Carolina

GEORGE WINOKUR, M.D. (1959)
4940 Audubon
St. Louis, Missouri

HAROLD WOLFF, M.D. (1947)
New York Hospital
525 East 68th Street
New York 21, New York

*JOSEPH WORTIS, M.D. (1950)
152 Hicks Street
Brooklyn, New York

†S. BERNARD WORTIS, M.D. (1946)
Director, Psychiatric Division
Bellevue General Hospital
New York, New York

PAUL I. YAKOVLEV, M.D. (1947) (S)
21 Addington Road
Brookline 46, Massachusetts

DEWEY K. ZIEGLER, M.D. (1952)
425 East 63rd Street
Kansas City 10, Missouri

EUGENE ZISKIND, M.D. (1949)
2007 Wilshire Boulevard
Los Angeles 57, California

JOSEPH ZUBIN, Ph.D. (1959)
Biometrics Research Unit
722 West 168th Street
New York 32, New York

*President – 1958
†President – 1949

Author Index

All references in **bold type** are to chapters or discussions.

Subject Index

References to topical discussions are in **bold type.**